The Immune System:
Comparative Histophysiology

The Immune System:
Comparative Histophysiology

Agustin G. Zapata
Universidad Complutense de Madrid,
Departamento de Biologia Celular,
Madrid, Spain

and

Edwin L. Cooper
Department of Anatomy and Cell Biology,
UCLA Medical Center, Los Angeles, USA

A Wiley — Interscience Publication

JOHN WILEY & SONS
Chichester · New York · Brisbane · Toronto · Singapore

Other Wiley Editorial Offices

John Wiley & Sons, Inc., 605 Third Avenue,
New York, NY 10158-0012, USA

Jacaranda Wiley Ltd, G.P.O. Box 859, Brisbane,
Queensland 4001, Australia

John Wiley & Sons (Canada) Ltd, 22 Worcester Road,
Rexdale, Ontario M9W 1L1, Canada

John Wiley & Sons (SEA) Pte Ltd, 37 Jalan Pemimpin 05-04,
Block B, Union Industrial Building, Singapore 2057

Library of Congress Cataloging-in-Publication Data:

Zapata, Agustin G.
    The immune system : comparative histophysiology / Agustin G. Zapata
and Edwin L. Cooper.
        p. cm.
    "A Wiley—Interscience publication."
    Includes bibliographical references.
    ISBN 0 471 92361 3
    1. Immune system—Physiology.   2. Immune system—Histology.
3. Immunology, Comparative. I. Cooper, Edwin L.   II. Title.
    [DNLM: 1. Immune System—anatomy & histology. 2. Immune System—
physioloy.   QW 504 C776i]
QR182.C66 1989
616.079—dc20
DNLM/DLC
for Library of Congress   89-21498
                                                               CIP

British Library Cataloguing in Publication Data:

Zapata, Agustin G.
    The immune system : comparative histophysiology.
    1. Vertebrates. Immunology
    I. Title II. Cooper, Edwin L.
    596.029

    ISBN 0 471 92361 3

Printed in Great Britain by Butler and Tanner Ltd, Frome, Somerset

Contents

CONTENTS

8 Lymphoid Aggregations Associated with the Gut, Lungs and Urogenital System   232

Preface

Why did we write this book? We hope you are persuaded, as you read the book, that it is timely, necessary, and unique. There has never been a text which covers aspects of cell biology, histology and current experimental immunology in the broadest context, and at the same time delves into these phenomena in ectothermic vertebrates, birds and a few unique mammals such as the monotremes and marsupials. Our book is necessary as we grapple with evolution of the immune system and it is also on target and unique, as we struggle to intensify the need for use of alternative, inexpensive, non-controversial models to decipher basic questions of immunity. This last concern is prompted by strident but perhaps relevant activities of animal rights activists. In other words, are we able to understand equally well the intricacies of the immune system by choosing ectotherms to answer certain basic questions concerning immunity? We think that there are certain problems/solutions for which these animals can be used appropriately.

The greatest achievement which produced a conceptual and functional bifurcation in the world of immunology came on the scene when Metchnikoff discovered phagocytosis in invertebrates and established, as it were, the universal macrophage. Immunology grew by leaps after this discovery and has maintained a two-pronged approach—cellular and humoral, thymus and bone marrow/bursa of Fabricius, T-cell and B-cell, Ig receptor and TCR. The book is cellular and tissue in its flavor and yet we have enlivened the text by presenting that which is more functional and sometimes molecular. We are organismic biologists without flinching, yet we recognize the importance of cellular biology and emerging approaches to our field through the molecular techniques. We hope to have presented a synthesis in the context of this sub-discipline of comparative immunology as presented in ten chapters.

In Chapter 1 we explore the main objective, i.e. to present the structure and, to some extent, the function of the immune system in vertebrates, emphasizing conditions in fish, amphibians, reptiles, birds and certain exotic mammals such as monotremes. In many instances, the condition in mammals and humans has been used as the structural basis for making comparisons; however, when certain organs are unique they will be described as such without reference to any non-existing mammalian counterpart. Early views on the immune system were relatively restricted to the lymphatic system composed of: (1) a system of vessels containing lymph, in which many of the same plasma proteins (e.g. gamma globulins) are found, as well as large numbers of cells, mainly lymphocytes; (2) scattered masses of lymphoid tissue associated with these vessels. Since proteins and lymphocytes can circulate freely within the blood, thereby gaining access to connective tissues and hemopoietic sites such as the bone marrow, a new term—the lymphomyeloid complex—is now commonly used. Yet, we employ the term immune system as it is understood today with respect to its cells, tissues, organs and various products such as antibodies and lymphokines.

As we learned early in our first exposure to biology, cells are the fundamental units of all life with respect to structure and function. In Chapter 2 we emphasize that cells of the immune system are not different in basic structure from any other cells, despite the wealth of information that tends to focus more on function than on structure. There is a trend, however, which is now shifting this course to balance newer facts gained by acquisition of information (which may be) peculiar to cells of the immune system.

Chapter 3 deals with bone marrow, which gives rise to stem cells that can differentiate into erythrocytes, granulocytes, thrombocytes (involved in clotting), monocytes (macrophages), plasma cells and lymphocytes. Before their appearance in adult marrow, they originated from embryonic cells which then become precursor stem cells. An actively hemopoietic bone marrow arose in evolution for the first time in the lungless salamander of the family Plethodontidae. The bone marrow of ectothermic vertebrates has not been fully investigated, which accounts for scanty results pertinent to immune responses. Almost all terrestrial vertebrates possess hemopoietic bone marrow. Beginning with amphibians, this specialized site of hemocytopoiesis becomes progressively differentiated during evolution. The obvious questions that arise are: why only terrestrial vertebrates? why inside bone marrow compartments? One simplistic interpretation is related to the tetrapod condition and the development of long, hollow bones. However, this does not explain the presence of bone marrow or its equivalents in sites other than in long bones.

There is also no explanation for the absence of marrow in fishes and other lower forms where abundant osteologic organization occurs. Hemopoietic bone marrow-like microenvironments are well developed in Osteichthyes, Chondrichthyes and Cyclostomata, located in organs such as the esophageal wall, kidneys, supraneural organs, spleen, Leydig organ and liver. However, adult amphibians and all higher forms show a shift in such hemopoietic sites corresponding to increased development of bone marrow. Whatever the condition, probably due to the external and internal environments, all vertebrates possess sites where stem cells and blood cells, including immunocompetent cells, are generated. These immunocytes circulate freely, gaining access to the immune system, where they generate responses after specific stimulation via antigen – receptor interactions.

Birds occupy a central place in Chapter 4. Since the bursa of Fabricius— a lymphoepithelial organ located in the distal side of the cloaca— is unique to them, its immunological role was firmly established after it was demonstrated that a deficiency occurs in antibody formation in chickens whose bursa had been removed at or prior to hatching. In fact, without this discovery all of immunology, not just comparative immunology, might have been detained and not developed as one of the pre-eminent fields it is today. Actually the bursa seems to function as a central or peripheral lymphoid organ during distinct life stages. During embryonic periods and the first few weeks post-hatching, the bursa is a central organ involved in the generation of immunological diversity. After seeding immunocompetent cells to peripheral lymphoid organs, i.e. spleen, primitive lymph nodes, cecal tonsils, Harderian glands, etc., the bursa functions as a peripheral lymphoid organ for local antibody production.

Chapter 5 treats the thymus, an organ unique to vertebrates, and its importance to evolution of adaptive immunity. Apart from little anatomical differences and the number of pharyngeal pouches that contribute to its ontogenetic formation, there is no special histological variation of thymic organization in all vertebrates except for Hassall's corpuscles in ectotherms. Therefore, a thymus gland which produces lymphocytes occurs in all gnathostomous vertebrates. By contrast, cyclostomes (myxinoids and lampreys) apparently do not possess a thymus or any morphofunctional equivalent.

This chapter presents current evidence on the structure of the vertebrate thymus with special emphasis on certain cell types, mainly non-lymphoid components, and their possible role in thymic functions. The functional role of the thymus in immune reactions of ectothermic vertebrates will be emphasized in fish (mainly teleosts), amphibians and reptiles. Although some histophysiological variations will be emphasized, information on variations which affect the thymus and other lymphoid organs of ectothermic vertebrates and their relationships with exogenous and endogenous regulatory mechanisms is presented in other chapters.

Chapter 6 is lengthy because of the unique situation of the spleen. The spleen is a large blood-filtering organ which evolved an increasingly important role throughout phylogeny by generating both T and B immune responses. Erythropoiesis, granulopoiesis and/or thrombopoiesis also occur in the spleen of some vertebrates. During vertebrate phylogeny, the spleen undergoes anatomical, histological and functional variations which reflect evolutionary strategies that have diversified and specialized splenic functions. In this regard, the roles played by distinct splenic cell compartments in immune reactions seem to be of differential importance in various vertebrate groups.

Thus, the presence or absence of sharply delimited white pulp, germinal centers and marginal zones and the possibility to differentiate T and B areas are important stages in defining the histophysiological evolution of the vertebrate spleen.

We will focus special attention on its role in the trapping and processing of antigen, the structural changes after antigenic stimulation and modifications which have occurred in its vascularization patterns that support splenic efficiency in immune reactions. Because, in contrast to other lymphomyeloid organs, the spleen is so intimately associated with the circulatory system, its gross morphology will be presented in some depth. For it is via the blood, perhaps in all species, that most antigens can be trapped and processed for antibody formation.

Chapter 7 is shorter since the situation with respect to lymph nodes or their precursors is different. During the evolution of the circulatory system, as blood pressure increased, more liquids and plasma proteins escaped from blood capillaries into the interstitial fluid that was then returned to them by veins. To accommodate this condition a separate lymphatic system evolved. The lymphatic system plays a role in returning fluid and plasma proteins from tissues to the main portion of the circulatory system. Since foreign, antigenic material which is potentially pathogenic may enter, both the circulatory and lymphatic systems simultaneously evolved organs associated with the immune system, the spleen and lymph nodes which can therefore filter blood and lymph.

A good deal of attention has been focused recently on other peripheral centers where immune reactions may be initiated. In mammals, gut-associated lymphoid tissues (GALT), bronchial lymphoid aggregates (BALT) and lymphoid tissue contained in other mucosal organs, such as urinary and genital tracts, mammary glands and salivary glands, constitute an integrated, mucosal associated lymphoid system. It is unclear if indeed a similar system occurs in ectothermic vertebrates, but some evidence suggests that, at least from a morphological viewpoint, non-mammalian vertebrates contain lymphoid tissues equivalent to those found in the mammalian mucosae.

In Chapter 8 we review the phylogeny of GALT with special attention given to that of reptiles as well as to the structure of avian cecal tonsils. No references on the organization of BALT are available but a dense lymphoid aggregate in the connective tissue layer between the epithelium and the tracheal cartilage of the snapping turtle *Chelydra serpentina* has been described. Some few accumulations of small lymphocytes are commonly found in the reptilian and anuran lung. Finally, we will describe other diffuse lymphoid aggregations, mainly lymphoid tissue, in the avian pineal system and Harderian gland.

In previous chapters we presented those most relevant aspects concerning the histophysiology of lymphoid organs. That coverage is clearly an oversimplification since these organs undergo seasonal variations which affect their structure and function. We have known for many years that there are influences such as low temperature, stress or pollution which affect fish immunoreactivity but the underlying mechanisms are essentially unknown.

In Chapter 9 we present information on seasonal variations which affect the immune system of ectothermic vertebrates. Three basic categories emerge: (1) different vertebrate classes or species undergo similar immune changes during distinct annual seasons; (2) individual genetic features might be important in explaining variable results (although there is minimal if any exhaustive evidence); (3) different causative agents, such as temperature, photoperiod, and/or internal, homeostatic mediators—hormones, neuromodulators, neuropeptides, etc., may be involved.

An integrative hypothesis concerning seasonal mechanisms involved in the regulation of ectothermic vertebrate immune responsiveness is difficult to formulate. From the current available information we conclude in Chapter 10 that immunity in ectotherms is dramatically influenced by ambient factors. It is necessary to describe immunological responses in ectotherms in the context of defined seasonal and other environmental factors that are properly coordinated with age, sex, light, antigen dose regimen, etc. Lack of adherence to these variables only complicates the variety of interpretations concerning immune responses in ectothermic vertebrates. In our minds, the area of research where the ectotherms will prove to be ever so useful concerns the points raised in this chapter and of course they impinge on information presented in the entire book.

A.G. Zapata
E.L. Cooper

Acknowledgements

Writing this book has been a memorable adventure prompted by friendship and uninhibited by national and cultural differences. It has been a long time since the comprehensive developments in comparative (ectothermic vertebrates) immunology have been assembled together in a single volume that combines cells, tissues, organs and physiology. Several endeavors sparked our interest in writing. First, the compelling desire to present the field as we see it inspired us to undertake the project. Comparative immunology, not by any means restricted to this text, is a recognized discipline supported by an international society (International Society of Developmental and Comparative Immunology), a journal (*Developmental and Comparative Immunology*), and global affiliations with the International Union of Immunological Societies and the International Union of Biological Societies. As you know, one of us has been instrumental in increasing visibility while engineering these various connective links, whereas the other has pioneered in the very essence of the text— microscopy, particularly at the electron microscopic level. We have cited the results of experimental immunology from our many friends and colleagues to add the workings of the immune system, which prompted the title histophysiology. Their works are amply covered, as you will view in the list of references.

At times, the writing was exceptionally challenging, with an occasional doubt about completing the book. After all, we both teach, are involved in numerous university activities and, most importantly, must meet deadlines as we seek financial support for our research laboratories, our graduate students and visiting scholars. Thanks to modern communications systems (tele-phone, Fax and airmail) we were able to stay in contact despite our professional and personal moves.

Both of us were together, mostly in Spain (Leon and Madrid) when Zapata held the chair in Leon and subsequently when he assumed the chair at Universidad Complutense. Both of us have held prestigious fellowships from Japan, where some of the writing was done— Zapata in Niigata with Professor Y. Honma; and Cooper, Senior Fellow, Japan Society for the Promotion of Science with Professor Susumu Tomonaga. A good deal of writing was also done while Cooper held a Senior Fulbright Fellowship to do research and lecturing at Cairo University in Egypt with Professor Rashika El Ridi. During the initial stages of writing Zapata journeyed to Cairo to lecture and to write. In fact, we did some of the writing while on board one of the popular Nile cruises with family and friends, allowing us at the same time to enjoy the richness of Egypt's past. What a way to write a text!

We teach the general aspects of histology, favoring, of course, the immune system, but almost never delving into the present intricacies of comparative histophysiology, obviously our favorite topic. We have tried to present form and function, integrating the present information at least up to the very last day before printing. Any missing information is due to publication deadlines; however, we hope that the field will grow sufficiently, and there is every indication that it will, to warrant a revision.

When a book is written, the authors cannot lay claim to having done all the work, for the help, inspiration and the actual compilation of the factual information rests with our ancestors, active colleagues and students, vigorous mentors, our own most immediate technical assistants, friends, and sometimes our families. That the facts are accurately presented is, of course, our responsibility.

Much typing was done in Cairo, Egypt, and we thank the staff at International Business Associates, under the direction of Mr W. Harrison. Mrs T. Fujikura did an exceptional job typing and setting up the new computer system while Cooper was a guest in the laboratory of Professor S. Tomonaga, Japan. Barbara Mersini, of the UCLA Dental School word-processing office, helped to get us started and we acknowledge her assistance. The final putting together would not have been possible without the hints, cues and advice on how to use the personal computer provided by UCLA graduate student Michael Suzuki. The bulk of word processing, reference checking and mounting of photographs was the responsibility of Valerie Williamson (UCLA) who took time out for several months from a career in advertising to assist us. She deserves enormous expressions of gratitude for bringing us to the deadline date for initial submission of the manuscript. At UCLA, we would also like to acknowledge the assistance of Jim Parker, Department of Anatomy and Cell Biology, for the photographic documentation of the photomicrographs. For clarity, Professor Susumu Tomonaga, Yamaguchi University, Ube, Japan read earlier versions of several chapters. To him we express appreciation.

Surely, we have acknowledged the research of our friends and colleagues whose work we have cited, without which the text would not have been possible. Both of us owe special thanks, however, to investigators who have increased the breadth of ideas we have covered by spending time in our laboratories. These include at UCLA over the years, Drs B. Baculi (Philippines), F. Boctor (Egypt), M. Boysenko (USA), B.A. Brown (USA), E.E. Eipert (USA), M. Faisal (Egypt), F. Garcia-Herrera (Mexico), M.H. Ghoneum (Egypt), M. Kalina (Israel), A.E. Klempau (Chile), R.L. Lallone (USA), M.L. Mandell (USA), M.H. Mansour (Egypt), E.J. Moticka (USA), J.A. Ramirez (Mexico), A.L. Reddy (USA), H.B. Riviere (USA), I.A. Sadek (Egypt), D.W. Schaeffer (USA), C.T. Smith (Chile), S. Tochinai (Japan), S. Tomonaga (Japan) and R.K. Wright (USA). The members of the Spanish Comparative Immunology group from the Complutense and Leon Universities in Spain include F. Alvarez, C.F. Ardavin, M.G. Barrutia, J. Fonfria, A. Fernandez, E. Garrido, R.P. Gomariz, P.G. Herradón, P. Herraez, J. Leceta, P. López Fierro, B. Razquin, M.T. Solas, M. Torroba and A. Villena.

Our wives (Conchita and Hélène) and children (Guillermo, Ricardo, Astrid and Amaury) experienced some mild discomfort (perhaps a bit of loneliness) due to our absences and lack of patience. We thank them for their endurance when our duty to writing sometimes compromised time with them. We hope especially for the sake of our children and our future students that they will see the value in scholarly pursuits and will in time forgive these intrusions, particularly at the time of deadlines. Will they be so inspired in this age of swiftness?

This book would not have been possible without the initial interest and encouragement of Michael Dixon. Patricia Sharp was an ever-present catalyst and Lesley Winchester saw the reaction through! Mr Iqbal Grewal, UCLA, assisted in preparing the index. To them we extend our heartiest expressions of appreciation.

1

Development, Structure and Organization of the Immune System

INTRODUCTION

Is Comparative Histology of the Immune System Important?

The main objective of our book is to present the structure and, to some extent, the function of the immune system in vertebrates including mammals but emphasizing conditions in fish, amphibians, reptiles, birds and certain primitive mammals. The evolution of vertebrates is depicted in Figure 1.1. In many instances we have used the condition in mammals and humans as the structural basis for making comparisons; however, when certain organs are unique they will be described as such without reference to any non-existing mammalian counterpart. Early views on the immune system were relatively restricted to the lymphatic system composed of: (1) a system of vessels containing lymph, in which many of the same plasma proteins (e.g. gamma globulins) are found, as well as large numbers of cells, mainly lymphocytes; (2) scattered masses of lymphoid tissue associated with these vessels. Since proteins and lymphocytes can freely circulate within the blood, thereby gaining access to connective tissues and blood cell forming sites such as the bone marrow, a new term, the lymphomyeloid complex, was proposed by Yoffey and Courtice (1970). Nevertheless we employ the term immune system as it is understood today with respect to its cells, tissues, organs and various products such as antibodies and lymphokines.

The explosion of information defining functions of the immune system, the interrelatedness of its components via highly migratory cells and diffusible products, and its vulnerability to both the internal milieu (e.g. hormones) and the external environment (season, temperature) makes it an irrefutably fascinating but complex system whose evolutionary development stimulates constant examination. As an introduction, and in simple terms, the cells are lymphocytes, monocytes and granulocytes which originate from the bone marrow, the source of stem or progenitor cells. Like the marrow, the thymus is a primary organ that receives cells destined to become T-lymphocytes. B-lymphocytes complete their development in the bone marrow or in the bursa of Fabricius of birds. The spleen and lymph nodes represent secondary organs of the immune system which filter blood and lymph respectively and, during phagocytosis, are able to trap foreign or non-self material and to get rid of it. Other lymphoid aggregations occur all over the body, generally embedded in connective tissue beneath epithelial surfaces, i.e. tonsils, Peyer's patches, appendix, which are in association with the intestine or gut-associated lymphoid tissue (GALT) and non-named aggregates in association with the bronchi of lungs (BALT).

The purpose of this chapter will be first to draw attention to the early discoveries of lymphatic vessels and lymph nodes which formed the basis for delineating the immune system, and second to reveal the

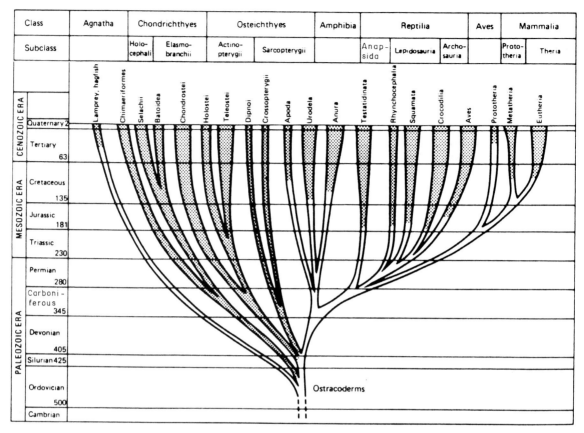

Figure 1.1 Evolutionary tree of vertebrates. Numbers indicate age in millions of years. (From *Natural History of the Major Histocompatibility Complex*, by J. Klein. Copyright © 1986 John Wiley & Sons Inc., reproduced by permission.)

evolutionary trend toward functional dissociation of hemopoietic capacities from those related to immunological reactions. We must emphasize at the outset that lymphatic vessels have been tapped repeatedly in mammals, revealing the presence of lymphocytes; to our knowledge this has not been done in primitive vertebrates. Thus, the immune system in these species is known to be linked more by means of the circulatory system than by the lymphatic system.

Who Started It?

The earliest history concerning the immune system began with observations of lymphatics (lacteals) in the small intestine as early as 300 BC by Herophilas and Erasistratus in the Alexandrian Medical School. The history has been amply reviewed in Battezzati and Donini (1972) and Rusznyak *et al.* (1967). Galen

doubted that lacteals were different from arteries, but this view was later dispelled during the Renaissance when Gasparo Asellius, Professor of Anatomy and Surgery in Pavia, described in 1627 the lymphatic vessels in the mesentery of a well-fed dog. Asellius observed that after pricking the lacteals, scattered over the whole mesentery and intestine, a white liquid leaked out. Later in 1651 Jean Pecquet, a physician of Montpellier, described the thoracic duct through which the 'liquor of the milkie veins' finally 'throws itself headlong into the whirlpool of the heart'. Shortly thereafter Rudbeck, Professor of Anatomy in Uppsala, described 'vasa serosa' in the liver. Almost simultaneously in 1653, Bartolinus, Professor of Anatomy in Copenhagen, found these serous vessels in many parts of the body and referred to them as lymphatics.

In 1661 in Bologna, Malpighi first saw capillaries in the lung of the frog and thus discovered the connection between the arteries and the veins. Some years later, van Leeuwenhoek carefully described the capillaries of fishes and other animals and suggested that these vessels might be the way by which elements from the blood would pass through the thin walls, thus furnishing the body with a continuous supply of nutrients. By the end of the seventeenth century, the gross anatomy and principles of the physiology of blood circulation including microcirculation were known. During the eighteenth century, Hunter, Cruikshank and Hewson proposed that lymphatic vessels are the absorbing vessels. Later, Hewson in 1774 made extensive dissections of the lymphatic system in fishes, birds and mammals and described in all of them a system of lacteals and lymphatics with their common trunk, the thoracic duct. He noted that lymph glands were absent in fishes and in the turtle, few in number in birds, and well developed in mammals. Hewson also observed the presence of globules (lymphocytes) in lymph and thought they were derived from the lymph glands from which they exit and then enter the blood via lymph channels.

Debate followed these observations, especially with respect to the manner by which lymph is formed, one school arguing that it is a filtrate of blood and the other that it is a secretion. Starling was the first to recognize a fundamental principle underlying lymph formation, i.e. the relationship between the hydrostatic pressure of the blood in the capillaries and the colloid osmotic pressure of the plasma proteins. Later, it was Drinker and Yoffey, in their book *Lymphatics, Lymph and Lymphoid Tissue* published in 1941, who proposed that 'the lymphatic system has evolved in the animal kingdom by physiological necessity and the probabilities are that the main factor has been the need for a specialized mechanism to return to the bloodstream blood proteins which have leaked from the blood capillaries'. We also know now that lymph vessels provide channels by which lymphocytes can move throughout the entire body. In fact, it is known that lymphocytes, traveling through lymphatic vessels, may vary in their phenotypic characteristics when compared with those that circulate in blood vessels. From the nineteenth century up to about 1940, the comparative histology of the immune system received a fair amount of attention (Cooper, 1976a). In closely paralleling the youthful vigor of modern immunology, the relatively young comparative immunology can now be linked with a comparative analysis of cells, tissues and organs of the immune system.

PHYLOGENY

Although the capillaries of lymphatic vessels and blood vessels are often in close proximity in the connective tissues and the lymph enters the venous circulation via the thoracic lymphatic duct, a fundamental separation of the two systems occurred during evolution. If we think of diploblastic metazoans that live in the sea, such as sponges and coelenterates, there is no blood circulation. The internal milieu of their cells is sea water, identical to that of the external milieu. Later in phylogeny the need for greater activity develops, requiring a system of tubes that carried a pigment capable of transporting oxygen. To do this more effectively and evenly a pumping device, the heart, developed and the circulating medium began to contain increasing amounts of protein. A rise in the pressure within the circulation would increase the escape of fluid from the small vessels. However, this escape is prevented by a corresponding increase in the concentration of proteins whose osmotic action opposes the capillary blood pressure. With these modifications, cells of the body were housed in a milieu different from that which surrounds it on the outside, necessitating a mechanism other than the blood vascular system for clearing the tissues of substances not readily absorbed by the blood.

This early interest in circulation of blood and lymph provided a firm basis for observations on the presence of lymph nodes. It was later that functional dissociation was discovered with respect to morphology, widening the knowledge of components of the immune system. In cartilaginous fishes there are vessels which contain blood and lymph in various proportions, but in teleost fishes the lymphatic system is differentiated from the blood vascular system. There are two groups of lymphatic vessels: a parietal group consisting of longitudinal superficial vessels along the course of which there are lymph sinuses, and deeper longitudinal lymphatics, the spinal and subvertebral trunks which represent the counterpart of the thoracic duct in mammals. There are no valves in the course of the vessels although valves are present at the lymphaticovenous junctions. Lymph enters the venous system at several of these junctions, but lymph hearts are only rarely observed. A median lymph heart in the tail propels lymph into the caudal vein through a valvular aperture.

In amphibians and reptiles, the general structure and arrangement of the longitudinal lymphatic vessels are similar to those in fishes. The superficial lymph sinuses which are dilatations of the lateral longitudinal vessels are usually more voluminous than in fishes or reptiles. The lymph sinuses accumulate a considerable amount of lymph from time to time. They are usually emptied suddenly by body movement, although lymph hearts do ensure a continual flow of lymph from the lymphatic vessels to the veins. In snakes, some of the longitudinal lymphatic vessels are perivascular, following the main arteries and veins and their branches, and the vessel associated with the aorta enlarges into a sac-like structure in the lower part of the abdominal cavity. In addition to these vessels, there are two elongated vertebral channels extending the entire length of the vertebral column into which lymph drains at each segment from the network of small vessels in the skin and muscle. Lymph from both sets of longitudinal vessels empties into the jugular sac at the base of the heart. This sac in turn is connected by two sphincter-like openings with the jugular veins. Posteriorly the vertebral vessels open into two lymph hearts which in turn open into the renal portal veins.

Lymph hearts are more numerous and highly developed in the amphibia. A pair of lymph hearts is found in each body segment in the most primitive amphibians, the apodans, thus in some species over 200 hearts may be present. In urodeles such as salamanders and newts, the paired segmental lymph hearts are located on each side of the trunk between the pectoral and pelvic girdles. The largest are the most anterior and posterior pairs situated at the levels of the anterior and posterior limbs. In anuran amphibians such as frogs and toads, usually only the anterior and posterior pairs remain. As we progress from the primitive to the more advanced amphibia, the number of lymph hearts recedes so that it decreases dramatically in the amniotes (reptiles, birds and mammals). All reptiles possess a well-developed pair of functioning posterior lymph hearts. In some birds such as the emu, cassowary and ostrich, aquatic birds such as ducks, geese and swans, as well as the swamp birds (herons and storks) the posterior lymph hearts persist through life. In chickens, lymph hearts are present only in the embryo and they regress before adult life. In mammals, there are no lymph hearts, even in the embryo.

With respect to lymph nodes, the precise group in evolution where they appear first is somewhat controversial. Most investigations have agreed that lymph nodes first appeared in birds but are present in only a few species, and when compared to those which are highly developed in mammals the structure is relatively simple. When examined in water, marsh and shore birds, two pairs have been observed. The larger pairs are the cervicothoracic nodes at the thoracic inlet. The second or lumbar pairs occur in the abdomen, first above the genital glands on either side of the abdominal aorta. The paucity or absence of lymph nodes in birds need not imply a deficiency of lymphoid tissue but it only means that the locations are different from those of mammals. For example, aggregations have been found in the walls of lymph vessels.

The source of most controversy centers around the anuran amphibians that have been studied most with respect to lymph 'nodes' and which possess a larval stage with a full complement of organs of the immune system. Anuran amphibians are in a unique position in evolution for they have structural and functional similarities to fishes, reptiles, birds and mammals. With regard to organs of the immune system the tadpole most closely resembles those of fish. Evolutionary precursors of the entire array of lymphoid and myeloid organs in mammals are first apparent in amphibians. These are the thymus, spleen and extralymphoid organs suggestive of mammalian hemal nodes; bone marrow also appears. Although the adult and larval lymph glands are similar structurally to the pronephros of fish, their homology to lymph nodes is questionable. Second, it is not entirely clear if these amphibian organs filter blood exclusively or lymph.

FUNCTIONAL DISSOCIATION WITHIN THE IMMUNE SYSTEM

One of the most obvious trends in the evolution of the immune system is the increasing complexity of hemopoietic and immunological components (Figure 1.2). Although there are variations, the best example is in the bone marrow and lymph nodes—bone marrow remaining essentially a source of stem cells, that give rise to all the blood cells, both myeloid with no role in

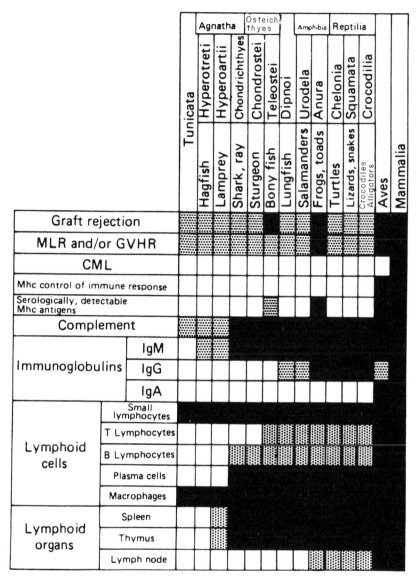

Figure 1.2 Evolution of immunologically important traits among Chordata. Solid boxes indicate presence of typical traits and stippled boxes presence of atypical or not fully developed traits; open boxes indicate either absence of traits or absence of knowledge about these traits in the indicated groups. (From *Natural History of the Major Histocompatibility Complex*, by J. Klein. Copyright © 1986 John Wiley & Sons Inc., reproduced by permission.)

immunological reactions, and lymphoid, entirely of immune function. Lymph nodes function exclusively as organs devoted to immune responses. The spleen during early stages is also primarily hemopoietic but later in ontogeny and phylogeny it acquires the addi-

tional role in immune reactions. It must be pointed out that these are trends and that dissociation either with respect to cells and/or effector activity must be viewed with caution within all the vertebrates, especially concerning sites like bone marrow. For example, we now know that cells housed in the bone marrow, in addition to hemopoiesis, do possess very important immune potentials.

Clearly, in mammals the microenvironment of the marrow is sufficient to support the maximum development of antibody-producing B-lymphocyte precursors equivalent to what must take place in birds in the bursa of Fabricius. There seems to be a similar situation in most anuran amphibians. The tissues which form the immune system are present throughout the vertebrate series but they are subject to great variation both in their location and their cellular composition since they undergo considerable evolutionary changes. Wherever they occur, they form mixed cell populations in which lymphocytes are intermingled, to a greater or lesser extent, with a number of other cell types. A cellular reticulum provides support for both granular and non-granular leukocytes in its interstices in several tissues and organs in association with the epithelium of the urinary, respiratory, reproductive and digestive systems and in the skull. There seems to be little or no penetration by cells in the blood or lymph into the nervous system.

CELLULAR MIGRATIONS AND CENTRAL VERSUS PERIPHERAL REGIONS

Clearly, blood vessels and lymph vessels provide a continuous network that is pervasive, allowing easy migrations, connections and therefore communication between cells of the blood and lymph (Figure 1.3). If we refer to compartments, there must first be a source of stem cells, the marrow or its equivalent, second, an inductive environment, the bone marrow in mammals and the bursa of Fabricius in birds and the thymus in birds and mammals; these are primary or central regions. The peripheral region or second level includes the spleen, lymph nodes and other secondary structures such as GALT and BALT. It is here that antigen signals are received and that the lymphocytes effect responses. By means of cell surface receptors, lymphocytes effect those responses that have been induced in them by specific contact with the antigen which fits the receptor properly, thus triggering a response. This occurs for both T- and B-lymphocytes, as has been worked out and delineated in birds and mammals. Whether these same levels and compart-

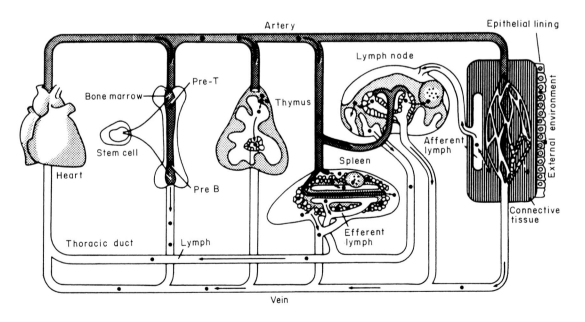

Figure 1.3 Circulation of lymphocytes. (From *Natural History of the Major Histocompatibility Complex*, by J. Klein. Copyright © 1986 John Wiley & Sons Inc., reproduced by permission.)

ments more or less exist in fishes, amphibians and reptiles awaits further critical analyses even though we know that the cells, tissues, equivalent organs and functions are present.

GENERAL FEATURES OF THE IMMUNE SYSTEM IN FISH, AMPHIBIANS, REPTILES, BIRDS AND MAMMALS

Lymphoid organs are central to the immune system in generating cells that affect integrated cellular and humoral immunity. These are the thymus, spleen, lymph nodes and various aggregations in mammals. In addition, these same organs and the bursa of Fabricius occur in birds. Among the fish, amphibians and reptiles, the thymus and spleen are present but there are several additional lymphomyeloid organs. These are well defined particularly in the anuran amphibians, and include the larval lymph gland, jugular, procoracoid and properiardial bodies of adults. Bone marrow, although primarily myeloid, is significant also for lymphopoiesis in the development of immune competence in all groups where it is present; it is absent in fishes, apodan, urodele (except family Plethodontidae) and larval anuran amphibians. Obviously, bone marrow function must therefore be affected by other structure(s).

Lymphoid organs generate lymphocytes. Small lymphocytes are cells $5-8$ μm in diameter, with a relatively large nucleus rich in densely aggregated chromatin granules and a thin cytoplasmic rim. Medium lymphocytes are $8-10$ μm in diameter, with a more abundant cytoplasm than the small type and less compact chromatin arrangement in the nucleus. Immature plasma cells are $12-15$ μm in diameter, with an eccentric nucleus that contains diffusely dispersed chromatin granules and one or two nucleoli; the cytoplasm is basophilic, with a clear area along one side of the nucleus. A mature plasma cell ranges from 8 to 14 μm in diameter, with an eccentric nucleus; it possesses the characteristic cartwheel arrangement of the chromatin and one or two small nucleoli. The cytoplasm is markedly basophilic and relatively more abundant than the immature types. Mature plasma cells also possess the characteristic clear area adjacent to the nucleus in the area of the cytocentrum. Often mature plasma cells show two nuclei.

Stem or blast cells are large cells, $15-20$ μm in diameter, with intensely basophilic cytoplasm and a voluminous nucleus; a stem cell contains relatively scanty chromatin and multiple large nucleoli. It closely resembles the stem cell that gives rise to myeloid types in the marrow. Reticular cells are also large, $15-25$ μm in diameter, with an irregular outline, an oval-shaped nucleus that contains scanty chromatin and abundant non-basophilic cytoplasm, sometimes with a foamy appearance. Finally, granulocytes are cells with a kidney-shaped or lobulated nucleus and a cytoplasm crowded with distinct acidophilic granules.

Bone marrow gives rise to stem cells that can differentiate into erythrocytes, granulocytes, thrombocytes (involved in clotting), monocytes, plasma cells and lymphocytes. Before stem cells first appear in adult marrow they originated from the yolk sac in the embryo or fetus. Stem cells, destined to participate chiefly in cellular immune reactions, are thought to pass through the thymus, where in the thymic environment they receive the necessary 'education' for becoming thymus-derived T-cells. Stem cells that will differentiate into antibody-secreting B-cells must receive further information by passing through the equivalent of the avian bursa of Fabricius. Thus, the immune system of fishes, amphibians, reptiles, birds and mammals in general is distributed throughout the body and is ubiquitous but basically a two-compartment system. To delineate such a precise bipartite system in fishes, amphibians and reptiles still requires more clarification.

How immunocompetent cells are identified is equally as important as how they function. Both the two cell types (T- and B-cells) participate in two distinct kinds of immune reactions. First, tissue antigens such as foreign tissue grafts elicit T-cell reactions or cell-mediated responses. It is not clear if antigen recognition occurs by means of cell surface antibody as receptors for detecting self versus non-self. Second, soluble large-protein antigens stimulate the humoral response. This occurs by activation of B-cells, which become antibody-secreting plasma cells.

During ontogeny most organs of the immune system originated embryologically from either endoderm (thymus, bursa of Fabricius) or mesoderm (spleen); none are derived from ectoderm. Regardless of origin, the epithelium provides the first line of defense, and if broken the underlying lymphocytes react second.

Fichtelius (1970) suggests that the immune system evolved with the invertebrate's ability to react to non-self, or antigens on either their external or internal epithelial surfaces. According to this view, the coelom separates the outer body wall from that of the gastro-intestinal tract, leaving the potential immunologically competent coelomocytes capable of reacting immediately to antigenic insult. Thus we can accept that lymphocytes, closely associated with the epithelium, particularly in all vertebrates, receive signals and from there effect the instructions in other sites. Analyzing lymphoepithelial relationships is important to understanding the development of immunity.

Fange (1966) considers the anterior kidney or pronephros, an epithelial derivative common to all vertebrate excretory systems, to be an evolutionary precursor of certain lymphoid structures. In addition to the excretory system the digestive system, derived from endoderm, contributed to the differentiation of immunocompetent cells and tissues. However, in most animals digestion and immunity evolved and became separate structural and functional systems. For example, vertebrates possess both the Kupffer or phagocytic cells of the liver and macrophages of the lymphomyeloid organs. As there are many features of primitive vertebrates not fully examined, there is an enormous need for further investigation into the sources of lymphoid cell precursors in phylogeny with respect to the immune system, the details of which will be emphasized in succeeding chapters.

WHAT HAPPENS DURING AN IMMUNE RESPONSE?

Introduction

In phylogeny, all animals respond to self and non-self, and within certain taxonomic groups the development of this response can be followed in ontogeny. When immunologically competent cells, whether *in vivo* or *in vitro*, are confronted with foreign antigens which pose a threat to survival, cells of the immune system recognize the differences and such antigens are destroyed. There are complex host regulatory influences that affect the efficiency of antigen disposal, but the basic control is at the genetic level. It is programmed within the genes by the variable structure of cell surface

receptors of immunocompetent cells, which antigens they will respond to, even those from close relatives. Histocompatibility genes determine how animals react to closely related cell and tissue antigens. These genes are controlled by the major histocompatibility complex or MHC, a complex locus that is described in chickens, mostly murine mammals (H-2) and humans (HLA). Homology probably exists in *Xenopus* and strong evidence is emerging in tunicates.

Assuming maximum recognition of such foreign antigens, events occur leading to the destruction of foreign cells or tissue transplants. These involve primarily the activities of various immune cells. For an immune response to occur, specific activation of T- or B-lymphocytes must take place via cell surface receptors, and one can distinguish phenotypic characteristic of both these cell types (Table 1.1). Most circulating lymphocytes are inactive (G_0 phase) cells which can be activated if they are suitably stimulated, either by antigen or by non-specific mitogens (Figure 1.4). Most antigens require a pre-treatment by macrophages before being able to activate lymphocytes, although phytomitogens like PHA can do so without the help of macrophages. Lymphocytes which have been triggered by a mitogenic stimulus are transformed into highly active cells which initiate various mediators of immunity; i.e. antibodies, if they are B-lymphocytes. It is well established both *in vitro* and *in vivo* that macrophages are needed for the induction, as well as expression, of immunological reactions.

A Typical T-lymphocyte-mediated Reaction—Graft Rejection

What happens if a tissue graft represents the source of antigen? A technically successful graft acts as a trigger that sets the mechanism of the immune system in motion; later the graft is destroyed. Briefly, this involves the host's recognition of the foreign transplant by T-lymphocytes and phagocytic cells producing a pronounced inflammatory reaction; finally, graft destruction is probably effected by a combination of unknown cell activities and their products, lymphokines, and perhaps even antibody. After an encounter with a graft, followed by its destruction, lymphocytes are capable of reproducing themselves and they, or their offspring, will respond to a second encounter with the same antigen that evoked the first

Table 1.1 Distinguishing properties of T- and B-cells

Properties	T-Cells	B-Cells
Surface properties		
T-cell-specific alloantigens and xenoantigens	+	−
B-cell-specific alloantigens and xenoantigens	−	+
Readily detectable Ig	−	+
Receptor for C3 complement component	−	+
Receptor for Ig Fc region	−	+
Receptor for SRBC	+	−
Negative charge	+	−
Adherence to artificial surfaces	−	+
Retained on antigen-coated columns	−	+
Retained on allogeneic monolayers	+	−
Migration and anatomical distribution		
Germinal centers and lymphoid follicles	−	+
Lymph node interfollicular cortex and paracortex; spleen periarteriolar sheath; interfollicular areas in Peyer's patches	+	−
Rapid recirculation from blood to lymph	+	−
Functional properties		
Killing of target cells	+	−
Antibody-forming cell precursors	−	+
Regulator cells in antibody- and cell-mediated immunological responses	+	−
Carrier specificity	+	−
Hapten specificity	−	+
Activated or tolerized at lower antigen concentrations	+	−
Proliferative response in mixed lymphocyte reaction	+	−
Proliferative response to phytohem-agglutinin and Con A	+	−
Proliferative response to endotoxin	−	+

Source: modified from I. Goldschneider and R. W. Barton, in G. Poste and G. L. Nicholson (Eds), *The Cell Surface in Animal Embryogenesis and Development*, pp. 599–695, Elsevier/North-Holland, Amsterdam, 1976, by permission.

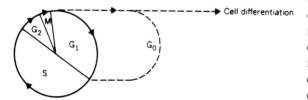

Figure 1.4 Cell cycle of a stem cell. G_0, G_1, G_2, M and S are phases of the cell cycle. (From *Immunology: The Science of Self–Nonself Discrimination*, by J. Klein. Copyright © 1982 John Wiley & Sons Inc., reproduced by permission.)

response; this is anamnesis, or memory. When animals respond to the first graft and finally destroy it, they are then usually capable, within certain time limits, of responding to that same antigen faster than they did upon first contact. Immune cells 'remember' they have 'seen' the antigen previously and they can therefore respond quicker, obviating the need for restimulating a new population of cells initially by antigen. A first graft is referred to as the first-set graft and a second from the same donor is the second-set graft. This aspect of the immune response is specific and serves to distinguish it from non-specific host mechanisms that involve phagocytosis by granular leukocytes such as neutrophils.

Immunological memory may now be viewed in broader, less strict terms because of new available information from studies of a number of animal groups. In the traditional sense, if an experimenter wants to test whether the host developed memory to a first-set transplant, it is necessary to wait a short period after the rejection of the first graft before transplanting the second one. In most animals that have been studied a great deal (e.g. mouse strains) and that differ at strong histocompatibility loci (H-loci), rejection of first-set grafts is rapid or acute and that of a second graft is even faster than the first. There are certain mouse strains and certain primitive vertebrates, notably apodan and urodele amphibians, however, where the time of second-set graft destruction is longer than the time required for rejection of the first graft. According to one interpretation, hosts that show faster rejections of second-set grafts than first-set grafts have developed positive memory, and those with longer rejection times negative memory. Actually both kinds of memory responses are represented throughout the animal kingdom in various phyla.

The graft rejection response is specific. In addition to first- and second-set grafts from the same donor, one can simultaneously test the capacity of a host to respond specifically to another graft, independent in origin from either of the other two grafts. Such a graft is often referred to as the third-party graft, and its destruction usually occurs at a time independent of either the first or the second graft. In the absence of specificity, a host would not be able to distinguish so sharply between antigens from any of the three grafts. Another test, cellular in nature, is useful for showing incompatibility between a host and several potential donors and is performed in the following way. Lymphocytes from an intended host are injected subcutaneously into a panel of recipients, one of which will be the donor. Of the four, the one that gives the minimal skin response is the best donor. Actually, the fact that a given host will not destroy an autograft but will reject a graft derived from a different but closely related donor is evidence for the earliest known specificity, even without a test from a third independent graft. Differentiating between self and non-self is specific.

A foreign graft heals initially, is temporarily recognized as self, and is nourished as if it were an autograft. However, the persistent immune surveillance system of every animal host recognizes the graft site to effect its destruction. Along with the molecular events accompanying graft rejection (i.e. lymphokines) in any animal, there are also external, often quantifiable, visible signs of graft destruction; the survival of pigment cells in invertebrates, fishes, amphibians and reptiles is the gross, easily observable criterion of graft viability. In birds and in mammals, it is the condition of the feathers and hair. Once mammalian and avian grafts are destroyed they are movable as a cicatrix, but in the primitive vertebrates grafts are gradually resorbed by the host; certain reptiles may be an exception. Except for the higher teleosts and mammals, graft rejection responses are chronic, i.e. slower than the acute response which is found throughout the animal kingdom, and may represent an evolutionary relic. A preponderance of primitive animals possess this characteristic.

B-Lymphocytes and Synthesis of Immunoglobulins

Introduction

The most unique feature of vertebrate immunity is the ability to synthesize antibodies in response to antigenic stimulation. This uniqueness is particularly noteworthy from two points of view: whereas invertebrates occur in larger number than vertebrates that often occupy the same environmental niches, the antibody-synthesizing capacity appears to be strictly limited to vertebrates. Secondly, the exquisite specificity that governs each antibody produced in response to countless numbers of antigens is phenomenal due to the

highly variable region of the Ig molecule that acts as a receptor for antigen. Antibodies or immunoglobulins are among the most interesting products of differentiated cells. This claim is based on two fundamental properties related to antibody synthesis.

First is the exquisite specificity of the host response, both to the antigen that induces the antibody and to the final antibody that sequesters the inducing antigen. Second, the cells of the immune system, once primed by a given antigen, are, upon second challenge, fully capable of responding in a specific, heightened manner due to the production of memory cells. Thus the cells or their descendants 'remember' that they have 'seen' the antigen previously and the entire sequence of events requires no renewal. Once differentiation of the primed cell proceeds, the cell 'knows' and is therefore ready for a more rapid second encounter with the same antigen, and except for closely related antigens there is almost no cross-reactivity. The simplest process by which antigen induces the formation of antibody is analogous in many respects to a stimulus—response situation. For example, the antigen acts as a stimulus, and immune cells of varying kinds give a response. In fact, in any stimulus—response system (especially obvious in animal sense organs) there must first be receptor cells (e.g. taste, smell, sight, hearing) that pulse the environment for the correct stimuli. So, too, must the receptor cell of the immune system sense appropriate antigens. Since the immune response is multifaceted, one can expect to define the entire series of events at various points in the immune response continuum. Although there are still unclear areas concerning the precise role of certain cells, we are safe in assuming that most B-lymphocytes and plasma cells synthesize and secrete antibody, which, except for cell-bound antibody, is released into the serum.

There is still controversy regarding the role of phagocytosis by macrophages in the scheme of antibody synthesis. If we assume that lymphocytes sense antigen, then a second appropriately equipped cell, the phagocytic cell, must be ready to trap and degrade the antigen, receive information and somehow communicate it to the effector cell, another lymphocyte or plasma cell that finally synthesizes and secretes the antibody. We know the respective functions for each cell type, but the crucial findings and interpretations will unite isolated observations to form a chain of events from contact with antigen to antibody synthesis.

Antigen Trapping

Because macrophages are strategically located throughout the body, they are able to make contact with and to capture antigen. Phagocytosis, although mainly non-specific, represents one facet of the immune response found throughout the animal kingdom; to it are gradually added, in evolution, several other immunocyte types with varied functional roles, notably antibody synthesis. Any vertebrate, for example, is amply equipped, by means of the various cells, tissues and organs throughout the entire body, for capturing and trapping antigen. The blood and lymph circulate throughout the body, and it, like other tissues, contains numerous cell types, at least two of which—the monocytes and neutrophils—function primarily in phagocytosis. Regardless of the level of phylogeny, all vertebrates and invertebrates possess an array of phagocytic cells, thereby fulfilling the basic primeval necessity for a system capable of eliminating antigen. This portion of the immune response fits broadly into the inductive period. In addition to phagocytosis, pinocytosis is as efficient in leading to removal of soluble antigens. During the first hour antigen is eliminated from the blood, and if we searched from this time on through the fourth to the seventh day we would find the antigen localized in the cells and tissues.

Antigen is broken down or degraded by enzymatic hydrolysis and digestion during the inductive period. Therefore this period requires that several factors operate to insure optimum degradation. Certainly a host animal must possess the necessary enzymes to react with an antigen. Presumably under the usual circumstances, i.e. when an animal is confronted by an antigen in nature, it is equipped with the required enzyme for antigen degradation. This may not be the case, however, in experimental conditions where various animals are often bombarded with an array of antigens, e.g. synthetic haptens for which they may not possess the required enzymes since many antigens are unnatural. The final phase of antigen removal, should it occur at all, may require extensive time, from weeks or months to years. However, there is a second major burst of antigen elimination different from the first and reflecting antigen removal from the blood. This period of antigen removal is partly due to the combination of newly formed antibody molecules with the antigen, promoting a second burst of phagocytic activity, diges-

tion, and antigen removal. Antigen—antibody complexes are easier to phagocytose.

The Immunoglobulins

Immunoglobulins (antibodies) are a group of structurally related proteins produced by plasma cells, secreted into the serum or tissue fluids, and characterized by certain physicochemical and biological properties. Most immunoglobulins are associated with the gamma globulin fraction of serum. They are called gamma globulins because they migrate more slowly toward the anode in an electric field at pH 8.6; this was different from the groups of faster proteins, termed the alpha and beta globulins, that migrated toward the cathode. Immunoglobulins of mammals can be divided into five major classes, usually called IgM, IgG, IgA, IgD and IgE, which differ physicochemically and immunologically. All vertebrates synthesize immunoglobulins resembling the IgM class. Concentrated studies of crossoptygerian fishes, ancestors of the urodele amphibians and a species more primitive than the anurans, suggest that IgG immunoglobulins probably first evolved in anuran amphibians. Those vertebrates considered morphylogenetically advanced than amphibians possess multiple classes of immunoglobulins that resemble IgM, IgG and possibly other classes of antibodies of mammals. As in other fundamental aspects oimmunity, the structural properties of mammalian immunoglobulin molecules serve as convenient models for comparative studies.

ENVIRONMENT AND THE IMMUNE SYSTEM

In 1976 it was proposed, without direct evidence, that the endocrine system exerts a powerful influence on the tadpole's immune system since all other organ systems are similarly affected (Cooper, 1976b). Clearly, the thymus and spleen remain, but the lymph gland disappears and the jugular body and bone marrow appear. At least in one experiment, frogs immunized before metamorphosis showed weakened antibody responses when compared with either unimmunized or immunized tadpoles (Moticka et al., 1973). The question of hormones affecting the immune system should now be viewed in relation to other potent influences such as light, seasons and temperature. Only among reptiles is information accumulating showing the effects of seasons on the immune system (Hussein *et al.*, 1978; Leceta and Zapata, 1985). At least in frogs as early as 1926, Von Braumuhl described seasonal changes in the thymus of *Rana esculenta*, showing clearly the decline and rejuvenation of thymocytes from summer to summer; there are no studies, however, published to date which deal with function of the immune system in relation to seasons of the year, although experimentally induced hibernation effects over two seasons have been analyzed (Wright and Cooper, unpublished). There is mounting evidence that the environment (external or internal) is an important variable when considering an animal's immune response. Studies on fish include the effects of season, sexual maturity, the pineal gland and photoperiod on the involution of the thymus (see Tamura, 1978 for review). In amphibians there have been studies related to season

and hematological changes in *Rana pipiens* (Wright and Cooper, unpublished). In birds, seasonal change and environmental factors have been considered in relation to immunity, and in mammals the relationship between the immune system and the endocrine system has been emphasized.

In a recent preliminary study, Garrido and Zapata (personal communication) have compared the spleen and thymus from frogs (*Rana ridibunda*) left for 35 days in darkness. The thymus seemed to show a decrease in medullary lymphocytes with an increase in numbers of epithelial cysts. In the spleen, however, T-dependent areas surrounding central arteries were depleted of lymphocytes, changes more evident after 42 days in darkness, emphasizing that the immune system is vulnerable to the influence of external factors such as light and season. The neuroendocrine system is thus affected and, in turn, the immune system (Figure 1.5).

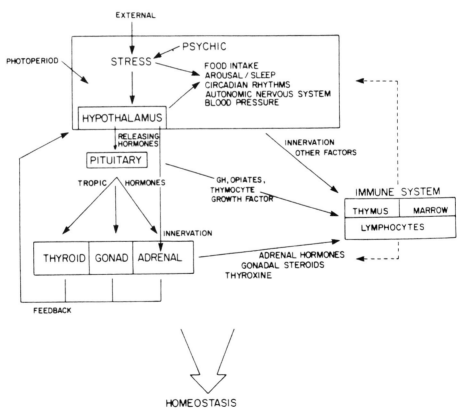

Figure 1.5 A schematic diagram of possible interrelations between the integrative systems involved in the maintenance of homeostasis. (From *Stress, Immunity, and Aging*, by E.L. Cooper (ed.), 1984. Reproduced by permission of Marcel Dekker Inc.)

FINAL COMMENT

It is impossible to make a comparative study of the vertebrates or the invertebrates without formulating some general concept of the nature of evolutionary processes. Most structural changes in the organs of the immune system and the functional changes in the immune system were probably adaptive modifications to a variety of environments and modes of life. Clearly there is not sufficient information from functional comparative studies of diverse immune systems to warrant even a hazardous guess as to the nature of the pressures that brought about these evolutionary adaptations. Nevertheless the varied modifications which vertebrate immune organs have undergone and the varied immune functions which they have assumed have, of course, come about as the result of evolution. As a physiological event, the immune response, a product of cells, tissues and organs of the immune system, is unique. It represents a condition found throughout the animal kingdom, but is probably the least reported of all the functional organ systems, especially in its comparative aspects. Respiration, digestion and reproduction are examples of areas in physiology that are fully treated. Although the situation is changing rapidly, immunity still has not been viewed as essential as the other functional systems of living organisms.

The immune system is also unique because specificity is one of its chief hallmarks. Where antibody is involved, the response is specific. There are, however, non-specific immune responses such as phagocytosis that are important in every animal's immunological armamentarium. Every individual is unique because of its peculiar and specific self or antigenic make-up. Furthermore, every individual, particularly a vertebrate, is amply equipped with cells or their progenitors that are capable of responses to an infinite array of foreign material. Depending on the antigen and the organism, one can expect cell-mediated immune reactions, humoral immune responses, or both responses integrated together. All animals are able to recognize and distinguish between self and non-self components. At every evolutionary level the immune response is essential to the well-being of an organism. Without it, each living creature would be preyed upon by a variety of external harmful pathogens—viruses, bacteria and fungi—and by internal parasites. Indeed, cancer, the most potent internal, detrimental threat, is now promi-

nent as a disease that may develop because of a weakened immune system, and up to now invasive neoplasms are known to occur in fishes, amphibians, reptiles, birds and mammals. The role of the immune surveillance system, explained clearly by Burnet (1970), has been extended far beyond the mere development of antibodies to a given antigen. Indeed, this recognition of foreign cells that may become neoplastic is the one feature common to all immune systems regardless of their level of phylogeny.

REFERENCES

Asellius G (1627). *De Lacteibus sive Lacteis Venis, Quarto Vasorum Mesaroicum Genere novo invento*. J.B. Bidellium: Mediolani.

Bartolinus T (1653). *Dubia anatomica de lacteis thoracicis...Publice proposita*. Copenhagen: Melch., Martzan.

Battezzati M and Donini I (1972). *The Lymphatic System*. John Wiley & Sons: New York.

Burnet FM (1970). *Immunological Surveillance*. Pergamon Press: New York.

Cooper EL (1976a). *Comparative Immunology*. Prentice Hall: Englewood Cliffs, New Jersey.

Cooper EL (1976b). Immunity mechanisms. In Lofts B (Ed), *Physiology of the Amphibia*. Vol III. Academic Press: New York. pp 163–272.

Cruikshank V (1790). *The Anatomy of the Absorbing Vessels of the Human Body*. London.

Drinker CK and Yoffey JM (1941). *Lymphatics, Lymph and Lymphoid Tissue; Their Physiological and Clinical Significance*. Harvard University Press: Cambridge, Mass.

Fange R (1966). Comparative aspects of excretory and lymphoid. In Smith R, Miescher P and Good R (Eds), *Phylogeny of Immunity*. University of Florida Press: Gainesville. pp 142 ff.

Fichtelius KE (1970). Cellular aspects of the phylogeny of immunity. *Lymphology* 3: 50–59.

Hewson W (1774). A description of the lymphatic system in the human subject and in other animals. In Gulliver G (Ed), *The Works of William Hewson*. Sydenham Society: London, 1846.

Hunter W (1784). Two introductory lectures to his last course of anatomical lectures at his theatre in Windmill, London.

Hussein MF, Badir N, El Ridi R and Akef M (1978). Differential effect on seasonal variation on the lymphoid tissue of the lizard *Chalcides ocellatus*. *Dev Comp Immunol* 2: 297–309.

Leceta J and Zapata A (1985). Seasonal changes in the thymus and spleen of the turtle, *Mauremys caspica*. A morphometrical, light microscopical study. *Dev Comp Immunol* 9: 653–668.

Malpighi M (1661). De pulmonibus. Observations anatomical. Bologna. Cited in J.F. Fulton's *Selected Readings in the History of Physiology* pp 61−67. Thomas: Springfield, Ill., 1930.

Moticka EJ, Brown BA and Cooper EL (1973). Immunoglobulin synthesis in bullfrog larvae. *J Immunol* **110**: 855−861.

Pecquet J (1651). Experimenta nova anatomica, quibus incognitum chyli receptaculum et ab eo per thoracem in ramos usque subclavios vasa lactea detegunter. Seb. and Gab. Cramoisey: Paris.

Rudbeck O (1653). Nova exercitatio anatomica exhibens Ductus Hepaticos Aquosos et Vasa Glandularum Serosa nunc primum in venta aeneisque figuris delineata. Arosiae. Euchar, Lauringerus.

Rusznyak I, Foldi M and Szabo G (1967). In Youlten L (Ed), *Lymphatics and Lymph Circulation*. Pergamon Press: London.

Tamura E (1978). Studies on the morphology of the thymus in some Japanese fishes. Sado Marine Biological Station (Japan).

Von Braumuhl A (1926). Uber einige myelolymphoide und lymphoepitheliale. Organe der anuren. *A Mikrosk Anat Forsch* **4**: 635−688.

Yoffey JM and Courtice FC (1970). *Lymphatics, Lymph and the Lymphomyeloid Complex*. Academic Press: New York. p 942.

2

Cells of the Immune System

INTRODUCTION

As we learned early in our first exposure to biology, cells are the fundamental units of all life with respect to structure and function. This central place occupied by the cell applies equally to unicellular protozoans and multicellular metazoans. In fact, the recognition of cells as being fundamental was clearly enunciated as early as the late 1830s by Schleiden and Schwann, who proposed the cell theory. Since that time, largely due to unparalleled technical advances in microscopy, coupled with the machinery and expertise derived from other fields such as chemistry and physics, we know an infinite amount about cell structure and function. All activities of any cell are controlled by the nucleus, which houses the genetic material that dictates properly coded functions. The entire cell, of course, is composed of protoplasm which contains organelles and the nucleoplasm which fills the nucleus.

Hardly amorphous, protoplasm is enclosed within the plasmalemma or plasma membrane. The plasma membrane, probably the most important of all cell membranes, is just one of several others that are fundamental components of all the cell's organelles responsible for various activities. One can thus envision an infinite continuum of connecting membranes comprising the cell. The details of membrane structure and function are described in numerous histology and biochemistry textbooks; thus this very complicated topic, although worthy of description, will not be presented. We wish to emphasize, however, that cells of the immune system are not different in basic structure from any other cells, despite the wealth of information that tends to focus more on function than on structure. There is a trend, however, which is now shifting this course to balance out the acquisition of information relative to structure and function of immune cells.

MONOCYTES AND MACROPHAGES

Historical Work

We begin a description of the immune system with monocytes and macrophages since these cells have functional counterparts throughout the animal kingdom. Their wide distribution represents a constant reminder of the immune system's phylogenetic ancestry with the most primitive phagocytic cell, the amoeba. Secondly, although we consider macrophages to be relatively simple and non-specific functionally, they have reached high functional development in vertebrates. Thirdly, present in several organ systems, monocytes and macrophages handle or process antigen, and they therefore play an indirect role in antibody synthesis. Finally, monocytes and macrophages participate in cell-mediated immune reactions. Taken together, their activities are of great importance to the body's defense against foreign infectious material. Metchnikoff fully realized the capabilities of these cells and, in a series of brilliant comparative and descriptive studies, he related the phagocytic function of metazoan amoebocytes to vertebrate macrophages. The applications of his work concerned host-defense reactions to infectious agents and other materials that cause inflammation. Later, during the first quarter of the twentieth century, certain cytochemical procedures extended and facilitated the recognition that phagocytic cells such as monocytes and macrophages were of widespread occurrence.

Monocytes

Monocytes comprise 3−8% of the leukocytes of normal blood in humans and appear to be rather infrequent in a cursory examination of stained blood smears. Monocyte structure is distinctive, however, so that they can be readily distinguished without difficulty, even though the uninitiated eye might confuse monocytes with large lymphocytes. Monocytes measure 12−15 μm in diameter when suspended in fluid, where they assume a more or less spherical shape; when placed in flat vessels they adapt easily, readily adhere, and flatten. They often appear larger, 20 μm, when flattened in dried stained blood smears, and at least one cytoplasmic component is always obvious— vacuoles involved in phagocytosis (Figure 2.1).

The nucleus usually shows a characteristic indented or horseshoe shape, although nuclei are ovoid or indented. The chromatin appears granular, hence it is less condensed than that of lymphocyte nuclei. In many respects the cytoplasm resembles that of lymphocytes, except that the cytoplasm of monocytes is more abundant. It is pale blue-gray in color with the usual blood cell stains, and it contains fine azurophilic granules, which are lysosomes equipped with acid phosphatase and other enzymes such as peroxidase necessary for destroying phagocytosed material. Analysis of fine structure also reveals many small mitochondria with typical cristae; mitochondria are more abundant than in lymphocytes and granulocytes. The well-developed Golgi apparatus, located near the point where the nucleus is usually indented, consists of stacks of smooth-surfaced lamellae vesicles. The endoplasmic reticulum consists of numerous vesicular structures scattered throughout the cytoplasm that contain associated ribosomes.

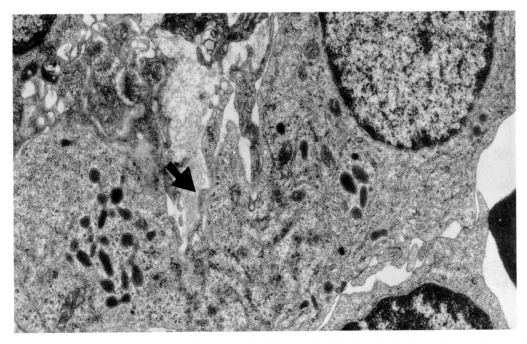

Figure 2.1 Monocyte in the blood sinusoid of the red pulp of the natterjack *Bufo calamita*. Note the granular population occurring in the cytoplasm. A portion of the cytoplasm is shown squeezing through the sinusoidal wall ($\times$ 14525).

Macrophages

Structure

Tissue macrophages differ markedly from monocytes and exhibit a much greater morphological heterogeneity. The nucleus varies in size and shape and often multinucleated forms can be observed. Macrophages can vary from 15 to 80 μm and because of their size they are literally termed 'Big Eater'. When stained by Wright's or Giemsa methods they show moderate cytoplasmic basophilia with varying numbers of azurophil granules and remnants of ingested debris. Particulate materials are especially useful for demonstrating macrophages after phagocytosis. Macrophages, after being confronted with simple preparations such as carbon particles or even minute particles of iron dust, will rapidly ingest them. Phagocytosis of iron offers the additional advantage of making them attractive to magnets, and when applied they can be removed easily after ingesting iron dust.

The endoplasmic reticulum is often segregated in the periphery of the cytoplasm and not associated with the Golgi apparatus. The area of the Golgi is enlarged, demonstrating aggregations of smooth-surfaced vesicles and flattened sacs. Many membrane-bound granules are either scattered throughout the cytoplasm or arranged around the centrosomes. These granules show great variability in size, shape, internal structure and electron density. Some appear to have a homogeneous matrix, others appear to be multi-vesiculated, and still others are composed of concentric layers of osmiophilic membranes known as myelin figures. Typical mitochondria are abundant and are usually found on the side of the nucleus opposite from that of the centrosphere, giving the cell a polarized appearance. With the scanning electron microscope (SEM), important for demonstrating three-dimensional surfaces, macrophages exhibit great structural variations. The membranes of macrophages are ruffled and long filopodial extensions create intercommunications between them.

Found everywhere macrophages provide, as do lymphocytes and granulocytes, an ever-present protective mechanism against invading pathogens. Peritoneal macrophages are easily obtained from experimental animals by douching the peritoneum (Figure 2.2). They vary little in either structure or bio-chemical and physiological requirements in different animals (mice, hamsters, chickens, rats, guinea-pigs). Alveolar macrophages (from the lungs) show several major morphological differences when compared to peritoneal macrophages of germ-free rats (gnotobiotes—animals born and living in entirely sterile conditions).

In lymphoid organs we find macrophages. These include the spleen, lymph nodes, thymus and organs associated with the gastrointestinal (GI) and/or respiratory tract such as the tonsils. Although splenic macrophages are structurally similar to peritoneal macrophages, they may occasionally be larger because of their functional peculiarities. The spleen is an efficient blood-filtering organ; thus, its macrophages remove effete erythrocytes, and they are also in the position to trap antigen. Splenic macrophages may reach the size of $20-30\ \mu$m in diameter or even larger. Lymph node macrophages appear in at least two varieties. Typical macrophages, the first type, are located in many sites and are especially concentrated in the lumen of medullary sinuses and within the germinal centers of lymph nodes (Figure 2.3). The second group, not strictly macrophages by terminology, is composed of reticular cells that have long dendritic processes capable of retaining foreign material on their surfaces, especially antigen that has been introduced experimentally. Tonsil macrophages are similar to lymph node macrophages and are especially prominent in patients with chronic tonsillitis. Thymic macrophages, which are also similar to lymph node macrophages, were once unknown. However, only recently their importance has been greatly appreciated when we consider the amount of cell death that occurs in the thymus. It is the thymic macrophages that remove those thymocytes that have died despite the large amount of cell reproduction which has occurred.

Two other principal macrophages are important in the body: the liver macrophage, known as the Kupffer cell; and the macrophages of the central nervous system, the microglial cells. So prominent are liver macrophages that they constitute a substantial portion of the liver's entire cellular volume. Considering that after the skin the liver is one of the body's largest organs, the liver macrophages constitute a formidable number of cells capable of phagocytosis. Microglial cells of the central nervous system are considered to be phagocytic, but only under conditions of trauma. In

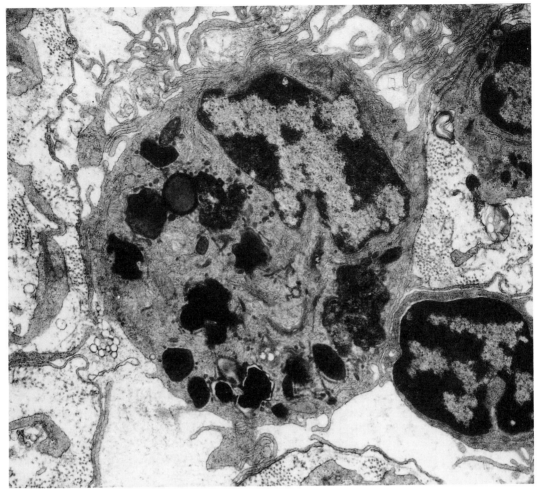

Figure 2.2 Macrophage containing melanin granules in the connective tissue of *Petromyzon marinus* (× 15300).

such cases they become typical amoeboid phagocytic cells capable of ingesting dyes that have been injected intravenously.

Origin of Monocytes and Macrophages

Life history studies of mononuclear phagocytes reveal that they develop in the bone marrow from promonocytes. Monocytes are then transported to the circulating blood and eventually end up as tissue macrophages (Figure 2.2). This same developmental pathway applies equally to peritoneal macrophages, Kupffer cells, alveolar macrophages and skin macrophages, as determined by labeling studies in mice. The turnover time of tissue macrophages appears to be several months. Stages in the life history of mononuclear phagocytes differ from those of neutrophils, which are granulocytes, phagocytic and also originate in bone marrow. Newly differentiated monocytes appear almost immediately in the peripheral blood, but neutrophils remain in the bone marrow for some days. Monocytes remain in the blood only a day or so and in the tissues for a few months, whereas neutrophils remain in both sites for a few days.

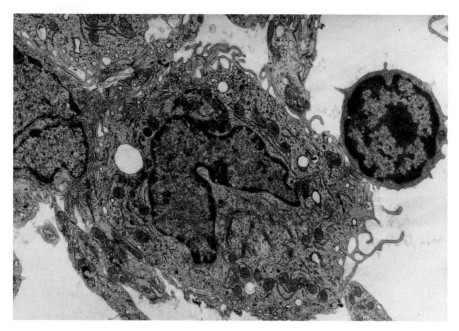

Figure 2.3 Macrophage of the medullary sinus of a rat lymph node. The cell shows abundant finger-like processes on its surface suggesting activation. Note lymphocyte on the right ($\times$ 3850).

The Macrophages of Anuran Amphibians

This chapter has dealt mostly with mammalian macrophages and, to a limited extent, fish macrophages. Now we shall turn to a representative vertebrate to gain an appreciation of the universality of macrophages. Amphibians occupy a critical position in the evolution of terrestrial vertebrates, and the larvae of frogs resemble fish when certain aspects of their anatomy and physiology are considered. The bullfrog tadpole possesses in its branchial region, in close connection with the gills, a lymphomyeloid organ (LMO) that contains lymphocytes and macrophages; sinusoids through which blood flows are lined by macrophages characterized by effective phagocytic properties attributed to its macrophages. If tadpoles are injected intraperitoneally with colloidal carbon, the bright red pear-shaped lymph gland becomes heavily blackened within a few hours. As an indicator of its role in specific immune responses, tadpoles whose lymph glands are removed prior to immunization with BSA (a soluble protein antigen) are incapable of synthesizing antibodies to it.

After metamorphosis the lymph gland disappears, and the frog develops three similar but different organs in the neck region: (1) the paired jugular bodies near the thyroid gland and jugular veins; (2) the paired prepericardial bodies near the heart; and (3) the paired procoracoid bodies anterior to the coracoid bone. The larval lymph gland and the adult organs possess two types of macrophages. The three organs in the adult frog are lymphocytopoietic (sites for the development of lymphocytes); however, they resemble mammalian hemal nodes or spleen that filter blood instead of lymph, and they also serve as graveyards for dead cells, as does the spleen. Where primitive vertebrate macrophages originate is unknown, but presumably from the marrow in terrestrial species.

GRANULOCYTES

Introduction

Blood which transports antibodies contains two major cell types: erythrocytes, or red blood cells, and leukocytes, or white blood cells. For purposes of studying the immune system the leukocytes are central.

Leukocytes are composed of granular cells called granulocytes, because the cytoplasm possesses characteristic granules, and non-granular cells, either lymphocytes or monocytes, that possess no distinguishing cytoplasmic granules. Granulocytes are, in turn, classified into three types according to the staining property of their cytoplasmic granules. With Giemsa or Wright's stain for blood, granules stain reddish (eosinophils), bluish (basophils), or take up little or no stain, thus appearing unlike either of the other two, essentially neutral (neutrophils). As basic immunological research has progressed, the function of each granulocyte has become somewhat clearer. They share at least one common function, that of phagocytosis, but each one possesses its own unique function.

Neutrophils

Structure

Neutrophils, often referred to as polymorphonuclear leukocytes (PMN) or heterophils are the most numerous of the granulocytes, constituting 60−70% of the total number; in absolute numbers they range from 3000 to 6000 per cubic millimeter. An individual containing 5 liters of blood possesses 15−30 billion circulating PMN. Neutrophils, like other granulocytes, develop in the bone marrow and are released into the bloodstream. Mature neutrophils are highly motile, show amoeboid activity, and measure between 10 and 12 μm in diameter. The nucleus is in the form of

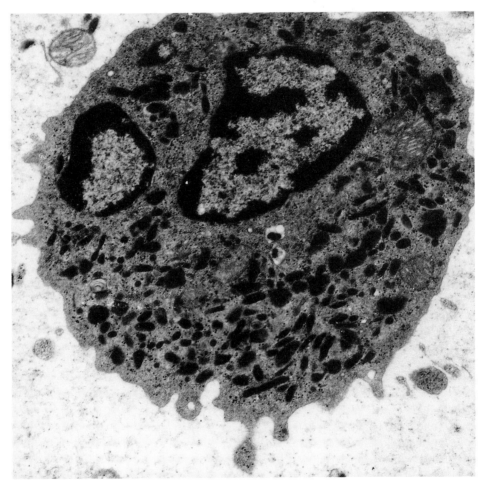

Figure 2.4 Neutrophil in a blood sinusoid of *Petromyzon marinus*. Note the presence of small aggregates of glycogen in the cytoplasm ($\times$ 15 000).

lobes, often from one to five, that appear to be connected by delicate strands. Densely packed, coarse chromatin that stains deep blue to purple comprises the nuclear material. In electron micrographs the nucleus appears to possess fewer lobes because the sections are usually thin. The lobes have condensed chromatin distributed along the inner surface of the nuclear envelope.

Mature neutrophils show cytoplasmic granules which are difficult to see in light microscopic preparations; often they show up only as lilac in color, and occasionally larger granules appear that are reddish-purple. By means of the electron microscope, however, the cytoplasmic organelles are more obvious. There are a few mitochondria, a small Golgi apparatus, and often scattered glycogen particles (Figure 2.4), 50–200 per cell. By newer techniques, the presence and functions of numerous specific cytoplasmic gran-

ules can be verified. Neutrophils can be disrupted in sucrose or in potassium chloride solutions, centrifuged differentially to yield undamaged cytoplasmic granules free from other formed cellular elements. These granules disrupt or lyse at pH 5 or lower, after alternate freezing and thawing or treatment with saponin. Following chemical analysis these granules show large quantities of protein with only trace amounts of lipids and nucleic acids. Studies of disrupted neutrophil granules reveal various digestive enzymes associated with or contained within them (Figure 2.5). Neutrophil granules resemble in physical and chemical properties cytoplasmic organelles called lysosomes. In addition to acid hydrolases, neutrophil granules contain the anti-bacterial substances phagocytin and lysozyme.

The neutrophil utilizes glucose as an energy source and stores a reserve supply in the form of glycogen in the cytoplasm. Even if neutrophils are allowed to use

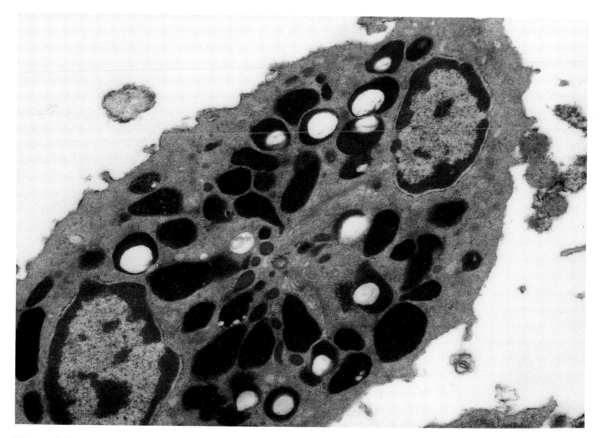

Figure 2.5 Mature bone marrow neutrophil in *Lacerta hispanica*. Some granules show electron-lucent holes (× 9000).

[14]C-labeled glucose, clearly they possess and utilize extensively the hexosemonophosphate shunt for degradation of sugar. The hexosemonophosphate shunt involves reactions by which glucose is metabolized in the absence of oxygen. They are identical to those by which glucose is metabolized in the presence of oxygen except for the last step, the pyruvic acid stage. In the absence of oxygen, pyruvic acid is converted to lactic acid, which accumulates. In the presence of oxygen, pyruvic acid is metabolized to acetyl coenzyme A, carbon dioxide and water via the Krebs citric acid cycle. During phagocytosis the rates of glucose uptake, of glycogen breakdown, of lactic acid production, and of hexosemonophosphate shunt activity increase markedly in neutrophils, indicating that glycolysis provides the energy for phagocytosis. Neutrophils show active metabolism of lipids, particularly neutral lipids and phosphatides, components that increase markedly during phagocytosis. Accelerated lipid metabolism accompanying phagocytosis may be based on specific events such as synthesis of new cell membranes.

Function

Neutrophils are important in inflammation, a process set in motion when living tissue is affected by injurious agents. Certain injurious agents include bacteria, viruses, protozoa, or other kinds of pathogenic organisms. Inflammation can also be caused by other external agents such as heat, radiation, cold or chemicals, and by certain substances. Once an inflammatory response is initiated, neutrophil functions involve a sequence of steps that consist of: (1) the attachment to capillary endothelium in the area; (2) locomotion; (3) emigration through the vessel wall into the tissues; (4) attraction by chemotaxis to an intruding microbe; (5) engulfment of the invading bacteria by phagocytosis; (6) degranulation of the invading bacteria or egestion of the foreign matter. Inflammation can be described as being chronic, acute or subacute. First the vascular system becomes involved, resulting in the distension of blood vessels, causing leakage of plasma by exudation into the adjacent intercellular substance. Almost as soon as blood flow slows down and exudation is complete, neutrophils stick to the lining endothelium of venules. Under experimental conditions their natural tendency to stick has been verified,

as they will stick to foreign surfaces such as glass or to one another to form clumps. It appears that divalent cations are required and, at least in some situations, plasma proteins, particularly fibrinogen, seem to play an important role.

After sticking to the lining of blood vessels, it appears that many neutrophils actually migrate by means of their pseudopodia through vessel walls, thereby entering the intercellular substance. Neutrophils are able to slither about on blood vessel walls and through them into loose connective tissues, or on foreign surfaces such as glass under experimental conditions. They usually do not move for long distances in a straight line, but tend to change direction approximately every 20 μm by sending out a new pseudopodium in random fashion. The rate of neutrophil locomotion depends on the physical and chemical nature of the environment. When conditions are ideal, it has been estimated that neutrophils can travel 35 – 40 μm per minute.

Eosinophils

Structure

Eosinophils are the second most numerous granulocyte in human blood, constituting 1 – 3%. In absolute figures 150 – 450 per cubic milliliter of blood is considered a normal concentration. Eosinophils were recognized as a distinct cell type in blood and tissues approximately 100 years ago. The cytoplasm of eosinophils has a somewhat irregular outline, caused by the presence of occasional pseudopodia. The cytoplasm is further characterized by the presence of granules that are colored red or orange in well-stained blood films (Figure 2.6). Poorly stained films show the granules as pink or reddish. The granules are numerous, large and refractile, making them easier to observe, since the cell seems to be literally packed with them; this contrasts with a few mitochondria and poorly developed endoplasmic reticulum. With the electron microscope the granules appear to be membrane-bound. They are dense and measure 0.5 – 1 μm in diameter. In immature eosinophils the granules are composed of a homogeneous material of considerable density, but in mature cells some of them contain still denser bodies in the more central region. These are actually crystalline in structure and may appear as

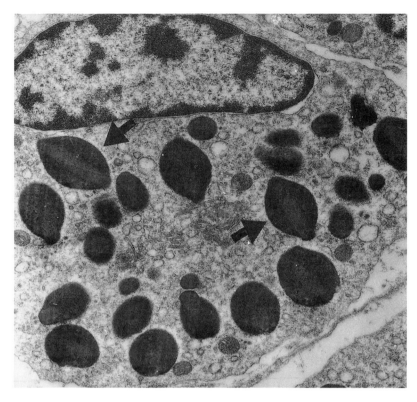

Figure 2.6 Mature eosinophil in the Leydig organ of the skate *Raja clavata*. Granules contain an electron-lucent bar-shaped core (× 12 000).

rough squares or rectangles (Figure 2.7). These granules contain large amounts of a stable peroxidase and most, but not all, of the enzymes present in neutrophils: oxidases, catalase, proteinases, phosphatases and lipase. Eosinophils also possess lysosomes. There is little or no information on the metabolism of eosinophils, mainly because immunologists have been unable to obtain large purified quantities of them free from other cell types. Perhaps adequate quantities could be obtained in instances of extreme eosinophilia, as during parasitic infections.

Function

Eosinophils, like neutrophils, can also function once they leave the bloodstream and enter the tissues. They are normally found in the lining of the intestine, in the lungs, in the dermis of the skin, in tissues of the external genitalia and other parts of the reproductive system (e.g. uterus). Eosinophils differ from neutrophils in that they are not actively phagocytic of bacteria, nor are they as motile. They are found in higher quantities in individuals infected with parasites. Eosinophils have been recognized for a long time as being involved in anaphylactic phenomena; they are numerous in the tissues that are the sites of allergic reactions. Eosinophils are also attracted to various sites that contain antigen–antibody complexes that have been injected experimentally; it is believed that eosinophils phagocytose such complexes. It is difficult to characterize eosinophil granules, since the cells are almost impossible to isolate from other types of blood leukocytes; as in the case of neutrophils it is most difficult to obtain the cell without at the same time releasing intact granules (Figure 2.8). In several successful studies using the eosinophils of animals, certain characteristics have been better understood. For example, isolated granules can be disrupted by freezing and thawing, by

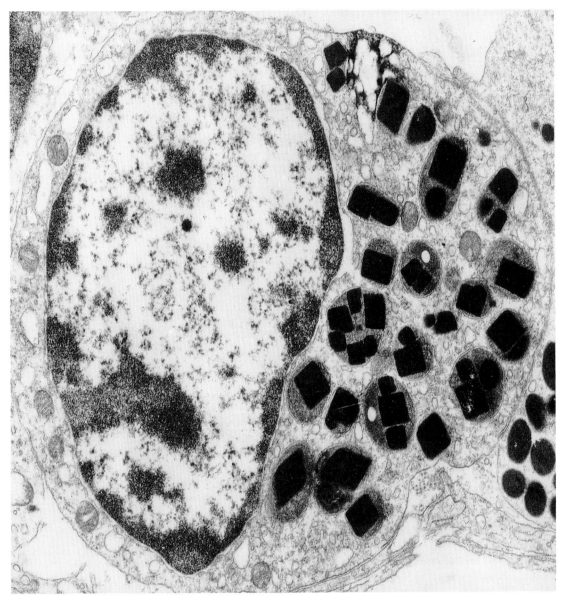

Figure 2.7 Mature eosinophil in the ovary of the torpedo ray *Torpedo marmorata*. Note the crystalline bodies present in each cytoplasmic granule (× 10500). (From *Dev Comp Immunol* 5: 43, 1981, reproduced by permission.)

exposure to weak acid, or by treatment with surface-active agents which liberate large amounts of protein. These proteins include various enzymes such as cathepsin, β-glucuronidase, arylsulfatase, nucleases, phosphatase and peroxidase, localized to a high degree in the granules.

In many respects the physiological behavior of eosinophils closely resembles that of neutrophils. Eosinophils in the blood sometimes stick to the inner surface of blood vessels (vascular endothelium) and emigrate into tissues by sliding through intercellular spaces. Phagocytosis, too, is similar to that seen in

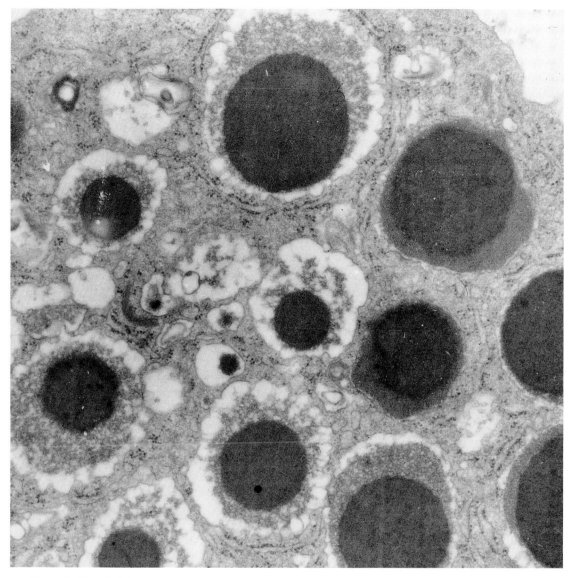

Figure 2.8 Detail of the contents of the cytoplasmic granules of an eosinophil of *Chimera monstrosa* (× 38 700).

neutrophils. Under appropriate circumstances eosinophils ingest objects by a process that involves morphological phenomena comparable to those observed in phagocytosis by neutrophils. Coating, or opsonization, of a doomed particle with antibody appears to facilitate engulfment. After phagocytosis degranulation occurs. Granules which break are always situated adjacent to the object being engulfed or next to a clear zone that remains after a granule has ruptured.

Degranulation may thus be based on membrane fusion and emptying of granule contents into the phagocytic vacuole, as is the case in neutrophils. Presumably, when granules rupture, liberation and activation of hydrolytic enzymes occurs, and the engulfed matter is eventually digested.

Although the numbers of eosinophils increase during certain parasitic infections, the precise function of eosinophils is still not clear. One unique approach has been developed that shows considerable promise. It is a monospecific rabbit antimouse eosinophil serum (AES) used to study the roles of eosinophils in a mouse model of schistosomiasis. Schistosomiasis is the most important helminth infection of man, frequently associated with peripheral eosinophilia and large numbers of eosinophils in the granulomatous lesions developing around parasite eggs trapped in tissues. When the schistosomula or immature worms migrate from the lungs to the liver, there is a mild transient eosinophilia, but soon after the onset of egg-laying by mature schistosomes there is an important and prolonged increase in eosinophils.

Basophils

Structure

Basophils constitute the least numerous of the granulocytes in humans. They comprise only about $0.5-1.0\%$ of the blood leukocytes, making them difficult to find in blood smears (Figure 2.9). Like eosinophils, the difficulty in obtaining large quantities presents a formidable problem for continued research on the functions of basophils. Despite their low numbers, making them difficult to study, the development of improved isolation procedures shows great promise for providing increased cell numbers for various

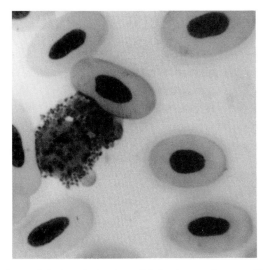

Figure 2.9 Circulating basophil in the apodan caecilian *Ichthyophis kohtasensis* ($\times$ 1425).

analyses. By a combination of procedures, basophils can be obtained from the blood (mean purity 62%) and bone marrow (mean purity 38%).

Basophils usually measure $10-12$ μm in diameter, about the same size as neutrophils. Almost half of the cell consists of nucleus, which is irregular and often segmented. The basophil nucleus stains much less intensely than do the nuclei of either the neutrophil or the eosinophil. In blood smears the appearance of the nucleus is overshadowed by large, dark blue-staining cytoplasmic granules. Basophil granules are similar to those of mast cells and, like them, contain histamine and heparin. By means of the electron microscope the granules have been shown to be membrane-bound.

Function

Despite low numbers of basophils for experimental purposes it has been learned that basophils are phagocytic and probably contain about half of the histamine present in the blood (Figure 2.10). Basophils, like eosinophils, tend to leave the bloodstream under the influence of certain adrenal gland hormones. They are also involved in allergic and inflammatory phenomena. Another important function is their relationship to IgE. Circulating IgE (involved in allergy) becomes readily attached to the surface of basophils. Thus, when a basophil with surface Ig from an allergic individual and the allergen (antigen) that induced IgE antibody production by plasma cells come in contact, release of granules has been observed to occur in some instances. Histamine, one of the substances that is released during degranulation, affects blood vessels like those substances liberated from mast cells. Such a reaction, if of great magnitude, involves entire systems (circulatory, respiratory, muscular) and can result in vascular collapse and death.

Mast Cells

Structure

Mast cells contain prominent nuclei which are round or oval in shape and are generally not lobulated; occasionally kidney- and horseshoe-shaped nuclei occur. Nuclear chromatin shows a wide variety of patterns; the chromatin is often marginated and the nuclear membrane well stained. One, two or more

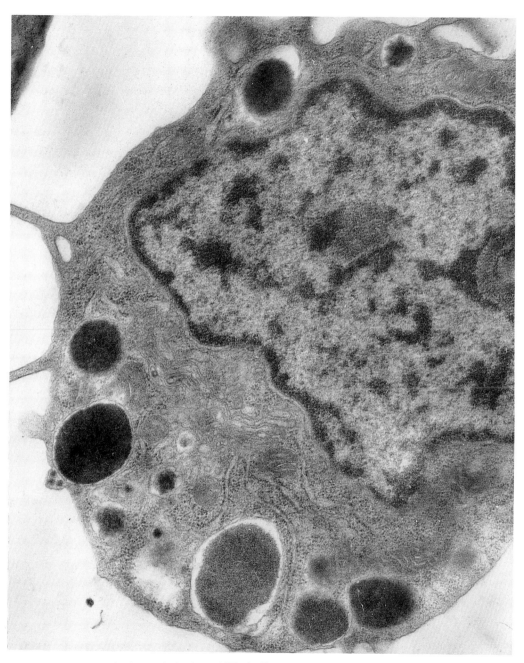

Figure 2.10 Circulating basophil in the lizard *Psomodromus algirus* ($\times$ 21 000).

well-defined nucleoli are generally present. The main feature of the cytoplasm is its great content of large granules around 0.5 μm in diameter, each of which is membrane bound. Mast cell granules vary, some appearing solid and dense, others appearing less electron-dense and having a finely granular texture. The endoplasmic reticulum is not very prominent in mast cells but the Golgi apparatus is well developed. Secretory vesicles containing electron-dense material bud off from Golgi saccules, and thus probably play an important role in the synthesis of sulfated mucopolysaccharides. The mitochondria of mast cells are relatively inconspicuous.

Function

Mast cells contain sulfated mucopolysaccharides, substances responsible for their peculiar staining reaction known as metachromasia. Mast cells contain heparin, which prevents blood coagulation, and histamine, a base derived from the amino acid histidine, which exerts a profound effect on smooth muscle which causes it to contract. In most species histamine also causes blood capillaries to dilate and to leak plasma. Histamine release is related to antigens in the following way. The first dose of antigen administered to a guinea-pig leads to the formation of specific antibodies by plasma cells. Some of these antibodies become attached to mast cells. If a second dose of antigen is given it circulates in the blood and quickly makes contact with the specific antibody complex. Antigen – antibody complexes that form on mast cells cause the cells to release their granules, which when released at the same time as histamine leads to anaphylaxis. Although of great clinical importance to humans because of allergy, histamine and mast cells are certainly known to occur in ectothermic vertebrates, and similar kinds of physiological responses to antigen have been observed as well.

LYMPHOCYTES AND PLASMA CELLS

Lymphocytes

Structure

Lymphocytes are involved in cellular and in humoral immunity. Early microscopists recognized lymphocytes in histological sections; they now can be removed from the body, cultivated *in vitro* and subjected to intensified analysis. Indeed, the growth of information in modern immunology results in part from innovative methods of studying and treating these cells as if they were microorganisms. Immunologists in some respects are at a point in dealing with isolated lymphocytes where early microbiologists once were experimenting with various microbes. Although lymphocytes are grouped into two broad functional classes, T and B, there are numerous aspects of their characters that still remain to be deciphered. Belonging to the broad category of non-granular, or agranular, leukocytes, they range from 20 to 30% in a normal blood smear, and in absolute numbers they represent approximately 2000 per cubic milliliter of blood. There are three sizes of lymphocytes—small, medium and large—and to distinguish between them one need only compare relative amounts of nucleus and cytoplasm. Small lymphocytes appear to be dominated by nucleus, and in blood smears they are also easy to distinguish by measuring them against erythrocytes; both are approximately 7 – 8 μm. Larger lymphocytes measure up to 12 μm and the cytoplasm is more abundant, but the basophilia is less intense than in small lymphocytes (Figure 2.11).

Viewed with the electron microscope the cytoplasm contains only a few mitochondria, suggesting a low metabolic rate. Occasionally centrioles are obvious and the Golgi apparatus is situated to their outer side. Endoplasmic reticulum is scarce, but free ribosomes are present in sufficient numbers to account for cytoplasmic basophilia easily observed in blood smears. The rather unspectacular picture of the small lymphocyte's cytoarchitecture is in marked contrast to that of a blast cell, which the small lymphocyte will become after being triggered by an antigen or a mitogen—substances used extensively to stimulate lymphocytes. Then a small lymphocyte loses its specialization, becomes enlarged and undergoes a change in cytoarchitecture. When this occurs the cytoplasm then possesses large quantities of free ribosomes.

By light microscopy these cells are increasingly basophilic and more easily stained by pyronin, and are thus called pyroninophilic cells. Not only does the endoplasmic reticulum increase in size, but also the irregular nucleus of the small lymphocyte then

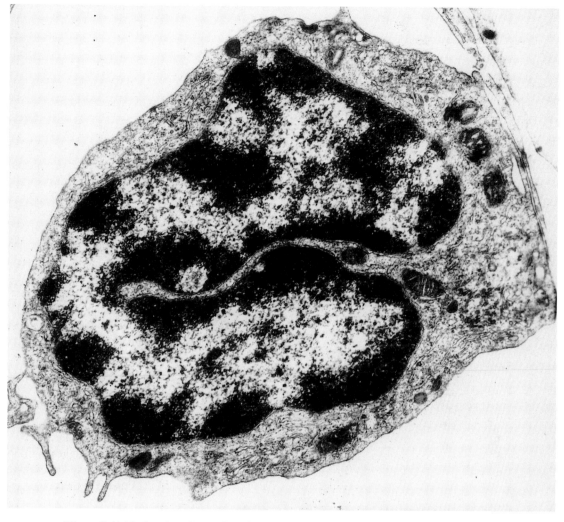

Figure 2.11 Medium lymphocyte in a blood sinus of the bone marrow of *Rana perezi* (× 20 000).

becomes regular and round and relatively small in relation to the surrounding cytoplasm, where the number of organelles such as the Golgi apparatus, mitochondria and lysosomes have also increased. Other organelles, the polyribosomes, increase in number and become associated with membranes forming an extensive network of endoplasmic reticulum, especially in plasmablasts—a sign of synthesis and then secretion of proteins, specifically immunoglobulins.

Function

T-Lymphocytes. It was debatable whether T-lymphocytes had a surface Ig that acts as a receptor for antigen, which led to the erroneus view that T-lymphocytes were incapable of antigen recognition. This is not the case since cellular immunity is mediated by T-lymphocytes that obviously must be able to recognize antigen often in combination with self major histocompatibility (MHC) determinants. Thus, T-lymphocytes

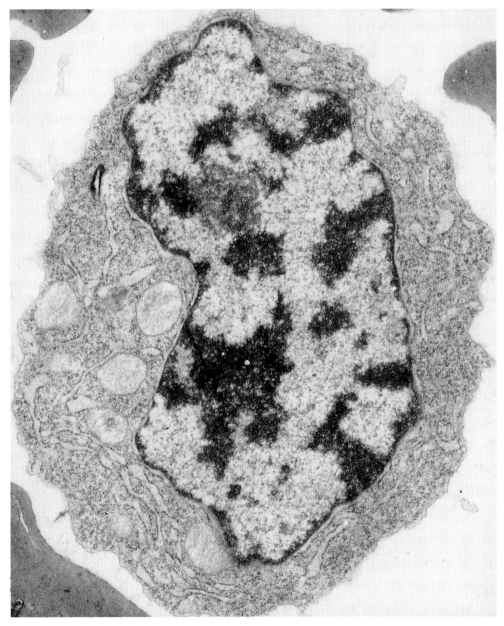

Figure 2.12 Circulating developing plasma cell in the anadromous sea lamprey *Petromyzon marinus*. Note the few flattened cisternae of rough endoplasmic reticulum (× 21 800). (From *Acta Zool Stockh* **69**: 23, 1988, reproduced by permission.)

are able to distinguish specifically between various antigens just as are B-lymphocytes, and therefore T-cells would be expected to possess some definable recognition unit or surface receptor. However, the search for Ig on T-lymphocytes has been negative and frustrating. Thymocytes or peripheral T-cells are negative when examined by immunofluorescence and radioautography, even after using antibodies raised in rabbits, chickens or rats against mouse Ig or Fab fragments. Antibodies, therefore, do not seem to recognize antigenic determinants on the surface of most T-cells. There are several explanations, although recent research using cDNA clones reveals a protein having extensive homology to Ig chains which is specific for T-cell membranes. Clearly the T-cell receptor is not classical Ig.

B-Lymphocytes. The direct demonstration of Ig on lymphocytes, as mentioned previously, involves incubation of viable lymphocytes in a suspension with fluorescent or radioiodinated anti-Ig antibodies. After being well washed, the treated cells are examined under the fluorescence microscope or by radioautography, techniques that clearly discriminate between two lymphocyte populations: a positive one and a negative one. The proportion of Ig-positive lymphocytes varies among different lymphoid tissues: in the spleen it is about $45-60\%$; in lymph nodes $10-30\%$; in peripheral blood $10-25\%$; and in thymus less than 1%. This finding tends to confirm that the majority of Ig-bearing lymphocytes are of the B variety and not of the T variety. In mice this is substantiated still further by the production of Ig-bearing lymphocytes in thymectomized adult mice in which syngeneic bone marrow cells have been transplanted. Thymectomized mice have lymphocytes that bear surface Ig equal to those of non-thymectomized, control mice treated in the same way. Lymphocytes that also possess the alloantigen theta (Thy-l), a specific marker for T-cells, are negative for surface immunoglobulin. Finally, mice with thymic aplasia, a condition that renders them congenitally deficient in T-cells, have the same number of lymphocytes with surface Ig as do normal mice.

Plasma Cells

Structure

Early investigations in 1948 and 1955 revealed that plasma cells synthesize antibodies. Since they synthe-

size proteins, in the form of Ig, their cytoarchitecture is geared for this synthetic process. In ordinary histological preparations plasma cells are generally rounded when lying free in tissues; however, if they are pressed upon by other cells, their outlines may appear angular (Figure 2.12). The cytoplasm is plentiful and the round nucleus is situated eccentrically. The chromatin of the nucleus is usually condensed. Most often the chromatin is arranged in dense-staining flakes distributed just like the spokes of a wheel or like the characters on a clock face. The usual 'clock face' appearance of plasma cells has become a rather common way of identifying them. The cytoplasm is usually strongly basophilic except in an area near the nucleus, called the perinuclear clear zone or the Golgi region; the centrioles also occupy the same position. The pronounced basophilia is due to large concentrations of RNA.

The cytoplasm of plasma cells shows a great specialization for the synthesis of Ig and its final secretion. Crammed with rough-surfaced cisternae of endoplasmic reticulum which may be flattened or somewhat dilated, the cytoplasm when cut at appropriate angles reveals the ribosomes on the endoplasmic reticulum arranged in the form of spirals (Figure 2.12); these are polyribosomal units.

The Golgi apparatus, usually large in plasma cells, is located near the nucleus in a region where the centrioles are also found. The Golgi apparatus consists of three usual components which are: (1) flattened, smooth-surfaced vesicles consisting of (2) transfer and (3) secretory vesicles. The carbohydrate of Ig is thought first to be added in the rough endoplasmic reticulum; the remainder of it is added in the Golgi apparatus and then it is secreted. Secretory vesicles probably originate in a manner typical of other secretory cells. Secretion first accumulates at the edge of a flattened saccule where a localized, expanded, vesicular structure is formed that then buds off from the edge of the flattened vesicle to become a free secretory vesicle (Figure 2.13). Final secretion is also typical; secretory vesicles reach and deliver their contents through the cell surface as in other typical secretory cells.

Function

Ig or antibodies are among the chief protein products of the immune system. Like other proteins, they are

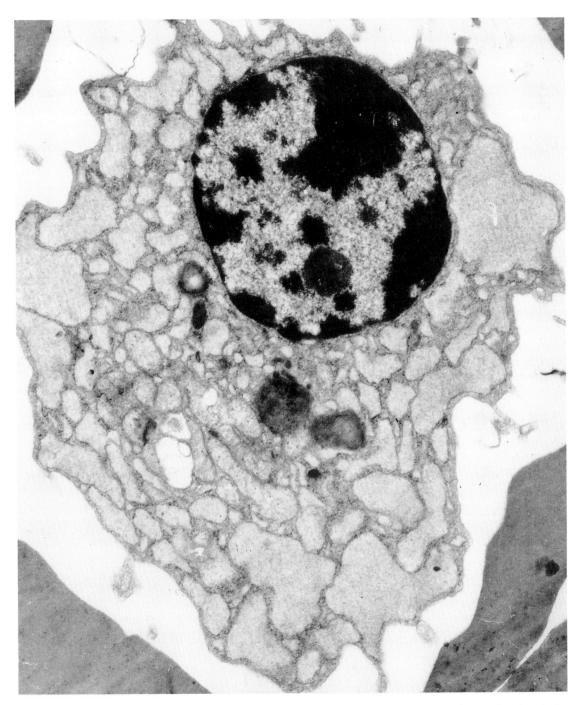

Figure 2.13 Mature circulating plasma cell showing numerous profiles of dilated cisternae of rough endoplasmic reticulum in *Petromyzon marinus* (× 35 000).

synthesized by specialized cells, the plasma cells. Plasma cells, or stimulated B-cells, synthesize Ig and are scattered throughout the body, notably in the spleen, lymph nodes and bone marrow. Although each plasma cell probably synthesizes only one class or subclass of heavy chain and one type of light chain, the actual number of cells producing each class or subclass of Ig may be proportional to the percentage of each Ig class within the body. Ig is synthesized by ribosomes associated with the endoplasmic reticulum and then localized between its membranes. Heavy and light chains are synthesized separately and combined prior to release, and carbohydrate is added last. The completed molecule is thought then to be transported to the Golgi complex, where more carbohydrate is added. Presumably Ig is retained in secretory vesicles prior to secretion.

FURTHER READING

Al-Adhami MA and Kunz YW (1977). Ontogenesis of haematopoietic sites in *Brachydania rerio* (Hamilton-Buchanan) (Teleostei). *Dev Growth and Diff* **19**: 171–179.

Bruning H, Cochran MD, Suhar T, Brown RD and Armentrout RW (1981). Early events in the development of the immune system of *Xenopus laevis*: characterization of lymphocytes in two-day-old embryos. *Dev Comp Immunol* **5**: 607–616.

Clem LW, Sizemore RC, Ellsaesser CF and Miller NW (1985). Monocytes as accessory cells in fish immune responses. *Dev Comp Immunol* **9**: 803–809.

Cormier F, de Paz P and Dieterlen-Lievre H. (1986). *In vitro* detection of cells with monocytic potentiality in the wall of the chick embryo aorta. *Dev Biol* **118**: 167–175.

Deparis P and Jaylet A (1984). The role of endoderm in blood cell ontogeny in the newt *Pleurodeles waltlii*. *J Embryol Exp Morph* **81**: 37–47.

El Deeb S, Zada S and El Ridi R (1985). Ontogeny of hemopoietic and lymphopoietic tissues in the lizard *Chalcides ocellatus* (Reptilia, Saura, Scincidae). *J Morph* **185**: 241–253.

El Deeb S, El Ridi R, and Zada S (1986). The development of lymphocytes with T- or B-membrane determinants in the lizard embryo. *Dev Comp Immunol* **10**: 353–364.

Ellsaesser CF, Miller NW, Cuchens MA, Lobb CJ and Clem LW (1985). Analysis of channel catfish peripheral blood leucocytes by bright-field microscopy and flow cytometry. *Trans Am Fish Soc* **114**: 279–285.

Ferguson HW (1976). The ultrastructure of plaice *Pleuronectes platessa* leucocytes. *J Fish Biol* **8**: 139–142.

Flajnik MF, Horan PK and Cohen N (1984). A flow cytometric analysis of the embryonic origin of lymphocytes in diploid/triploid chimeric *Xenopus laevis*. *Dev Biol* **104**: 247–254.

Hine PM and Wain JM (1987). Composition and ultrastructure of elasmobranch granulocytes I. Dogfishes (Squaliformes). *J Fish Biol* **30**: 547–556.

Hunt TC and Rowley AF (1986). Studies on the reticulo-endothelial system of the dogfish, *Scyliorhinus canicula*. Endocytic activity of fixed cells in the gills and peripheral blood leucocytes. *Cell Tissue Res* **244**: 215–226.

Hyder SL, Cayer ML and Pettey CL (1983). Cell types in peripheral blood of the nurse shark: an approach to structure and function. *Tissue and Cell* **15**: 437–455.

Ishizehi K, Nawa T, Tachibana T, Sakakura Y and Iida S (1984). Hemopoietic sites and development of eosinophil granulocytes in the loach, *Misgurnus anguillicaudatus*. *Cell Tissue Res* **235**: 419–426.

Maeno M, Tochinai S and Katagiri Ch (1985a). Differential participation of ventral and dorsolateral mesoderms in the hemopoiesis of *Xenopus*, as revealed in diploid–triploid or interspecific chimeras. *Dev Biol* **110**: 503–508.

Maeno M, Todate A and Katagiri C (1985b). The localization of precursor cells for larval and adult hemopoietic cells of *Xenopus laevis* in two regions of embryos. *Dev Growth Diff* **27**: 137–148.

Mainwaring G and Rowley AF (1985a). Separation of leucocytes in the dogfish *Scyliorhinus canicula* using density gradient centrifugation and differential adhesion to glass coverslips. *Cell Tissue Res* **241**: 283–290.

Mainwaring G and Rowley AF (1985b). Studies on granulocyte heterogeneity in elasmobranchs. *Fish Immunology*. Academic Press: London.

Morrow WJ and Pulsford A (1980). Identification of peripheral blood leucocytes of the dogfish *Scyliorhinus canicula* L. by electron microscopy. *J Fish Biol* **17**: 461–475.

Nakamura H and Shimozawa A (1984). Light and electron microscopic studies on the leucocytes of the medaka. *Medaka* **2**: 15–21.

Parish N, Wrathmell A, Hart S and Harris JE (1986a). Phagocytic cells in the peripheral blood of the dogfish *Scyliorhinus canicula* L. I. *In vitro* studies. *Acta Zool* **67**: 215–224.

Parish N, Wrathmell A, Hart S and Harris JE (1986b). Phagocytic cells in the peripheral blood of the dogfish *Scyliorhinus canicula* L. II. *In vivo* studies. *Acta Zool* **67**: 225–234.

Parish N, Wrathmell A, Hart S and Harris JE (1986c). The leucocytes of the elasmobranch *Scyliorhinus canicula* . I. A morphological study. *J Fish Biol* **28**: 545–561.

Peault BM, Thiery J-P and Le Douarin NM (1983). Surface marker for hemopoietic and endothelial cell lineages in quail that is defined by a monoclonal antibody. *Proc Natl*

Acad Sci USA **80**: 2976–2980.

Rowley A and Page M (1985). Ultrastructural, cytochemical and functional studies on the eosinophilic granulocytes of larval lampreys. *Cell Tissue Res* **240**: 705–709.

Smith PB and Turpen JB (1985). Hemopoietic differentiation potential of cultured lateral plate mesoderm explanted from *Rana pipiens* embryos at successive developmental stages. *Differentiation* **28**: 244–249.

Turpen JB and Smith PB (1985). Dorsal lateral plate mesoderm influences proliferation and differentiation of hemopoietic stem cells derived from ventral lateral plate mesoderm during early development of *Xenopus laevis* embryos. *J Leuk Biol* **38**: 415–427.

Zapata A (1980). Splenic erythropoiesis and thrombopoiesis in elasmobranchs: an ultrastructural study. *Acta Zool* **61**: 59–64.

3

The Bone Marrow and Its Equivalents

INTRODUCTION

Bone marrow gives rise to stem cells that can differentiate into erythrocytes, granulocytes, thrombocytes (involved in clotting), monocytes (macrophages), plasma cells and lymphocytes. Before their appearance in adult marrow, they originated from embryonic cells which then become precursor stem cells. Stem cells, destined to participate chiefly in cellular immune reactions, pass through the thymus, where they receive the necessary 'education' for becoming thymus-derived T-cells. Stem cells that will differentiate into antibody-secreting B-cells, in the case of mammals, remain in the marrow's environment or, in the case of birds, they must receive further information by passing through the bursa of Fabricius. Thus, via lymph and blood, cells of the immune system—of birds, mammals and probably that of fishes, amphibians and reptiles—are distributed throughout the body, are ubiquitous, and comprise a two-part functional system. Such a precise bipartite system in fishes, amphibians and reptiles requires further clarification. The ways by which immunocompetent cells are identified are as important as their function. Both cell types (T- and B-lymphocytes) participate in two distinct kinds of immune reactions. First, tissue antigens such as foreign tissue grafts elicit T-cell reactions or cell-mediated responses. Antigen recognition surely occurs by means of cell surface receptors that can detect self versus non-self. Second, soluble or particulate antigens stimulate antibody synthesis or the humoral response which occurs by activation of B-cells or antibody-secreting cells.

Most organs of the immune system originated embryologically from either endoderm (thymus, bursa of Fabricius) or mesoderm (spleen); none are derived exclusively from ectoderm. Regardless of origin, the epithelium provides the first line of defense, a function strengthened by the granulocytes, macrophages and lymphocytes found in the underlying connective tissue. Perhaps lymphocytes, in close association with the epithelium, particularly in vertebrates, receive signals and execute the instructions away from there in other sites. This lymphoepithelial relationship is important to the study of the development of immunity. Fange (1966) considers the anterior kidney (or pronephros, an epithelial derivative common to all vertebrate excretory systems) to be an evolutionary precursor of certain lymphoid structures. In addition to the excretory system, the digestive system, which is derived from endoderm, contributed to the differentiation of immunocompetent cells and tissues. In most animals, though, digestion and immunity evolved to become separate structural and functional systems. Vertebrates, for example, possess both the Kupffer or phagocytic cells of the liver and the macrophages of the lymphomyeloid organs. As there are many features of primitive vertebrates that have not been fully examined, there is an enormous need in studies of phylogeny for further investigation into the sources of lymphoid cell precursors from bone marrow or its equivalents (Table 3.1).

Table 3.1 Precursors of bone marrow or its equivalents

Cyclostomes

Myxinoids	PRONEPHROS, INTESTINAL LYMPHOID HEMOPOIETIC AGGREGATES
Lampreys	TYPHLOSOLE, NEPHRIC FOLD, SUPRANEURAL BODY

Chondrichthyes

Holocephali	ORBITAL and SUBCRANIAL LYMPHOHEMOPOIETIC TISSUE
Elasmobranchii	EPIGONAL and LEYDIG'S ORGANS. MENINGEAL TISSUE (*Dasyatis akajei*)

Osteichthyes

Crossopterygii	?
Dipnoi	SPIRAL VALVE, KIDNEY, GONADS
Chondrostei	CRANIAL CAVITY, HEART, KIDNEY
Holostei	CRANIAL CAVITY, HEART, KIDNEY, GONADS
Polypteriformes	?
Teleostei	KIDNEY

Amphibians

Apodans	LIVER, LYMPHOID – HEMOPOIETIC AGGREGATES IN KIDNEY (?)
Urodelans	Appearance of bone marrow in family Plethodontidae. LIVER, LYMPHOID – HEMOPOIETIC AGGREGATES IN KIDNEY (pronephros and mesonephros) (Family Protidae)
	Primitive families: MENINGEAL LYMPHOHEMOPOIETIC AGGREGATES (*Megalobathracus japonicus*)
Anurans	Embryonic and larval PRONEPHROS and MESONEPHROS

THE BONE MARROW IN LOWER VERTEBRATES

Multipotential stem cells are concentrated in the bone marrow cavity, where they differentiate into every hemopoietic cell line. An actively hemopoietic bone marrow arose in evolution for the first time in the lungless salamander of the family Plethodontidae. The bone marrow of ectothermic vertebrates has not been fully investigated and what scanty information there is related only to each hemopoietic function, which thus accounts for the lack of results which pertain to immune responses. From its appearance, the histological organization of the bone marrow is similar in all vertebrate classes. Seasonal variations in the same species and differences between various species of anuran amphibians and reptiles have revealed that granulopoiesis, erythropoiesis or thrombopoiesis occurs exclusively in bone marrow. Yet Campbell (1970) and Curtis *et al.* (1979) reported the absence of erythropoietic activity in bone marrow in *Rana pipiens* and *Plethodon glutinosus*. However, the bone marrow of *Bufo calamita* contains numerous erythroblasts, at least during certain months of the year (Zapata, unpublished). A similar seasonal dependence has been suggested for bone marrow in species of hibernating Plethodontidae (Curtis *et al.*, 1979).

In the lizard *Phrynosoma solare* the spleen is the primary blood-forming organ, but in most lizards the bone marrow is the main source of hemopoietic cells. In turtles there is an almost equal division of erythropoiesis between the spleen and bone marrow (Jordan, 1938). Thus, reptiles seem to represent a transitional group between amphibians, where the spleen is mainly erythropoietic, and adult birds, where bone marrow is practically the only blood-forming organ (Le Douarin, 1966). However, in other vertebrates, such as agnathan and gnathostomatous fishes, apodans, primitive urodeles and larval anurans, there is no bone marrow but equivalents do exist. These include the kidney, intestine, liver, gonads, pericranium, etc. By contrast, the intra- or extravascular formation of erythrocytes in bone marrow of lower vertebrates is a point of disagreement, a fact possibly related to the role played by cellular microenvironments in governing blood cell differentiation. In amphibians and reptiles, erythropoiesis occurs in the lumens of marrow sinuses (Campbell, 1970; Curtis *et al.*, 1979; Zapata *et al.*, 1981a). In some birds, erythropoiesis has been reported as an intravascular process, but in others erythrocyte formation occurs in cell cords as in mammalian bone marrow (Zapata and Fonfria, unpublished results).

HISTOLOGICAL ORGANIZATION OF THE BONE MARROW

The Stroma (Cell Microenvironmental Components)

Bone marrow is found, to some extent, in all bones but mainly in long ones (Figure 3.1). Pneumatic bones of birds are an exception, however, since islands of bone marrow occur in the spicules of medullary bones, a region that has become important for some vertebrates such as turtles and snakes. The cell microenvironment which governs differentiation of blood cells is formed by stromal cells and blood sinusoids. The histology of this cell microenvironment in bone marrow is similar in all vertebrates; it consists mainly of reticular cells and endothelial cells which line the blood sinusoids. The bone marrow vasculature, studied in three amphibian species, has shown an increasing progression toward the mammalian pattern (Tanaka, 1976).

Bone marrow adipose cells appear before independent, true hematopoietic activity. The first primitive locus of marrow hemopoiesis occurs in the subostium, where granulopoiesis begins; it appears simultaneously during the development of primitive sinusoids.

The basic organization of marrow vasculature is established in advanced anurans, but not in *Xenopus*, when the central vein develops. Therefore, perhaps the appearance of this basic, vascular pattern is necessary in order to produce an adequate environment for hemopoietic activity. In any case, numerous enlarged blood sinusoids are the major components of vertebrate bone marrow. Blood sinusoidal walls are formed by electron-dense endothelial cells which are joined together by tight and gap junctions (Figure 3.2). These cells, apart from playing a mechanical role, are typical cellular components of bone marrow necessary for its endocytic function. Although vertebrate marrow has macrophages and reticular cells with endocytic capabilities, the endothelial lining cells represent the major cell type which removes foreign material from the circulation. As a consequence, endothelial lining cells contain cytoplasmic lysosomes, phagosomes and coated vesicles (Figure 3.2). While a basement membrane has been described beneath sinusoidal endothelial cells in bone marrow of rats, mice and guinea pigs (Weiss, 1965; Campbell, 1972), it is apparently not associated with the endothelium in bone marrow of frogs (Campbell, 1970), reptiles (Zapata *et al.*, 1981a), chickens or pigeons (Campbell, 1967). Nevertheless, the basement membrane is generally considered to be absent between endothelial cells and adventitial cells (de Bruyn *et al.*, 1971).

The stroma of bone marrow in all vertebrates contains a tridimensional sponge-like meshwork formed by the processes of reticular cells (Figure 3.3). In reptiles and mammals, the reticular cell processes constitute a discontinuous layer of adventitial cells beneath the sinusoidal lining cells. A considerable proportion of the vascular endothelium is covered by adventitial cells which are integral components of the sinusoidal walls (Tavassoli, 1977; Hoshi and Weiss, 1978; Zapata *et al.*, 1981a). This partial layer has not been described in avian bone marrow (Campbell, 1967). The morphology of reticular cells in *Lacerta hispanica* is similar to that described in other vertebrates (Campbell, 1970, 1972; Biermann and Graf von Keyserlingk, 1978; Hoshi and Weiss, 1978). These

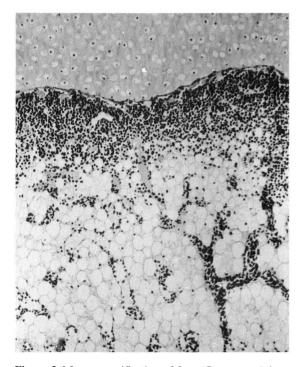

Figure 3.1 Low magnification of frog (*Rana perezi*) bone marrow. Note lymphomyeloid cells beneath the cartilage and between adipose cells (× 190).

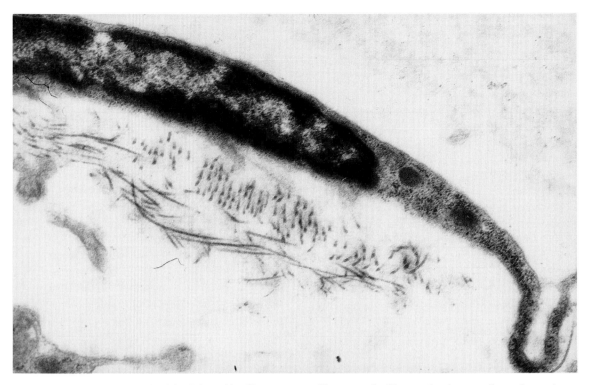

Figure 3.2 Endothelial cell lining blood sinusoids of bone marrow (*Rana perezi*). Observe the absence of a continuous basement membrane beneath the endothelium and collagenous fibers in the stroma ($\times$ 31500).

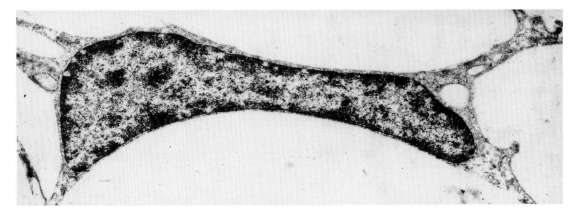

Figure 3.3 Adventitial reticular cell (*Rana perezi*) in a sponge-like network supporting the lymphohemopoietic masses. Note its irregular shape and numerous cell processes ($\times$ 22 800).

cells are lighter staining than endothelial cells and appear to be ramified wherever developing hemopoietic cells are located. Reticular cells have been considered to be fibroblasts, despite their ultrastructure and intimate association with reticular fibers (Hoshi and Weiss, 1978).

In *Lacerta hispanica*, many observations suggest a functional relationship between reticular cells and developing blood cell elements. These relationships may constitute an important element in the hemopoietic microenvironment, inducing the differentiation of stem cells into a particular cell line and trapping human fetal marrow stem cells from blood (Chen and Weiss, 1975). No other type of supporting cells has been found in bone marrow of non-mammalian vertebrates, although in bone marrow of the spotless starling, *Sturnus unicolor*, reticular cells sometimes contain lipid droplets and crystalline inclusions. Weiss (1981) suggested that reticular cells which resemble those of mammalian bone marrow tend to accumulate fat and will become adipocytes. In contrast, when hemopoiesis is intense, other branched cells appear in close association with hemopoietic cells of mammalian bone marrow (Weiss, 1981). Nevertheless, branched cells are not associated with reticular fibers nor are they phagocytic, suggesting a type of macrophage. Although reticular cells function mainly by supporting the freely developing lymphohemopoietic cells, some investigators have considered the possibility that they secrete short-range regulatory factors. In this regard, the importance of interactions between developing hemopoietic and stromal cells in the differentiation of various blood cell lines has been demonstrated *in vivo* and *in vitro*. Dexter (1981) and Westen and Bainton (1979) have described two types of reticular cells: a fibroblast related to the granulocytic precursor and a macrophage type which may be associated with erythroid differentiation.

The Parenchyma (Free Cells)

In addition to the phagocytic role played by endothelial lining cells, numerous free macrophages occur in the stroma, but to a lesser extent they are found in the lumen of blood sinusoids (Figure 3.4). Together with macrophages, lymphocytes and plasma cells are always present in vertebrate bone marrow, mixed in the parenchyma with other developing and mature blood cells (Figure 3.5). Despite the presence of lymphocytes, lymphocytopoiesis in bone marrow appears to be rather variable, mainly in birds, an observation which is controversial although numerous dense lymphoid nodules with germinal centers which contain large and medium lymphocytes have been described in young and adult chicken bone marrow (Taliaferro and Taliaferro, 1955; Zapata and Fonfria, unpublished results). In contrast, no nodules have been found in marrow of adult chickens (Campbell, 1967). To explain this discrepancy, attention has been focused on the possibility that these nodules are abnormal, ectopic lymphoid aggregates (Lucas and Jamroz, 1961). Nevertheless, the morphology of lymphoid cells is similar to that found in lymphoid organs of all other vertebrates. Small lymphocytes exhibit a high nucleocytoplasmic ratio, abundant condensed chromatin arranged peripherally and scanty numbers of cytoplasmic organelles such as mitochondria and granules (Figure 3.6). Plasma cells with dilated cisternae of rough endoplasmic reticulum, typical of ectothermic vertebrates, have been found in amphibian and reptilian bone marrow (Campbell, 1970; Curtis *et al.*, 1979; Zapata *et al.*, 1981a) (Figure 3.7), but developing, immature plasma cells were found only in lizard bone marrow (Zapata *et al.*, 1981a). Immune function of bone marrow in ectothermic vertebrates will be described later.

BONE MARROW AS IMMUNE ORGAN

Antibody Synthesis

As source of immunologically competent cells, the bone marrow has only been examined in anuran amphibians and not to any great extent in reptiles and birds. In the anurans, it is not clear if lymphocytes are equivalent to mammalian T- and B-lymphocytes, yet experimental results show functional, cellular equivalents. Plasma cells and large pyroninophilic cells appear in the marrow of ranid frogs after immunization with BSA (Cowden and Dyer, 1971) or with sheep erythrocytes (SRBC) (Minagawa *et al.*, 1975). As a major lymphoid organ, adult frog bone marrow (*Rana pipiens* and *Rana catesbeiana*) contains leukocytes equivalent, in number, to those present in the spleen. As in the spleen, a high percentage of leukocytes are

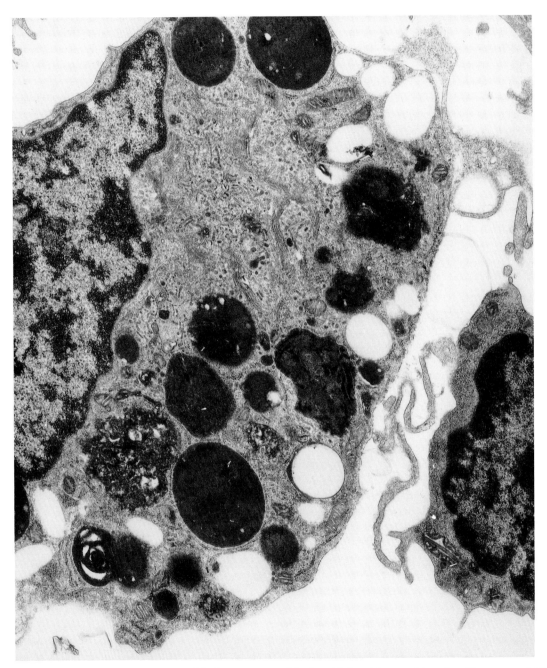

Figure 3.4 Free macrophage in the stroma of the bone marrow of the Spanish lizard *Lacerta hispanica*. There are numerous cell projections and dense bodies present in the cytoplasm. The cell is in the process of phagocytosing debris ($\times$ 31 500).

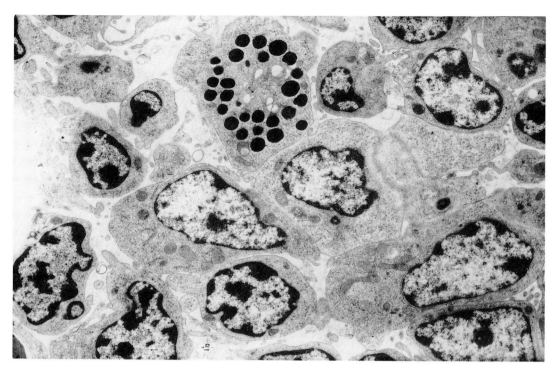

Figure 3.5 Low magnification of a cell core of the bone marrow in the starling *Sturnus unicolor*, showing abundant myeloblasts, mature granulocytes and small lymphocytes arranged between processes of reticular cells (× 6000).

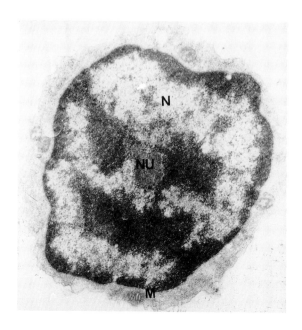

Figure 3.6 Small lymphocyte in the bone marrow of *Rana perezi*. Note the high nucleo-cytoplasmic ratio, the patent nucleolus and abundant condensed chromatin (× 10 400).

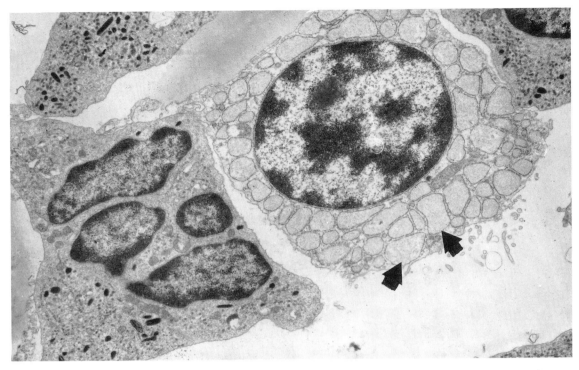

Figure 3.7 Mature plasma cells between granulocytes in the bone marrow of *Rana perezi*. Within the cytoplasm there are numerous dilated cisternae of rough endoplasmic reticulum (× 13 400).

identified morphologically as lymphocytes and the bulk of these can be categorized as small or medium ones. In young frogs (*Rana catesbeiana*) the ratio of marrow to splenic leukocytes is considerably greater than in adults and in certain limited comparisons a high percentage of lymphocytes is found.

A comparison of adult marrow and spleen anti-TNP (trinitrophenyl) plaque-forming cell responses at various days early during antibody response indicates that in most frogs marrow normally produces a higher total primary response (Eipert *et al.*, 1979). Moreover, this heightened marrow reactivity also occurs during *in vitro* proliferative reactions in response to both B- and T-mitogens (Eipert *et al.*, 1977). Comparisons of relative spleen and marrow cell responsiveness in *Rana catesbeiana* to *in vitro* mitogen activation have been made. The degree of responsiveness to Con A, PHA and LPS by bone marrow cells has been demonstrated in spleen cells. Spleen cells were, in fact, virtually inert and different culture conditions indicate that bone marrow responses were not selected by a variable due to culture conditions. After assessing blastogenesis

and total cell recovery following culture, failure to be stimulated and/or poor growth, rather than failure to incorporate [^{3}H] thymidine, accounted for inert splenic responses. In contrast, functionally mature T- and B-lymphocytes have not been demonstrated in *Xenopus* marrow using the mitogens Con A and PHA, which are specific for T-cells, and the B-cell mitogen PPD (Green and Cohen, 1979). Using dextran sulfate, precursor B-cells were not identified in toadlet marrow or liver although such cells were found in the spleen.

Role in Cell-mediated Immunity

The structure of *Rana pipiens* bone marrow suggests the presence of stem cells and differentiating lymphocytes together with various stages of neutrophilic and eosinophilic precursor cells. To investigate the presence of hemopoietic stem cells or mature functional lymphocytes, Cooper and Schaefer (1970) quantified circulating leukocytes of peripheral blood and analyzed the effect of cobalt-60 gamma radiation at 5000 R on the survival of skin allografts in adult leopard frogs, *Rana pipiens*. Autografts healed and the median survival time (MST) of allografts was 14.25 ± 1.5 days. No graft rejection was observed in total body irradiated frogs at the time they died, at the earliest, on the seventh day post-grafting, and the latest on the 20th day. By contrast, skin allografts in the partially irradiated and shielded (marrow-protected) group were rejected almost as rapidly (within two days) as those observed in normal unirradiated controls. The mean percentage of lymphocytes in peripheral blood declined sharply, but less so in the partially shielded group. Little change was observed in the percentage of basophils, eosinophils or monocytes, but neutrophil numbers seemed to rise, which suggests an increase in bacterial infections. In addition, of most importance, bone marrow was sufficient to maintain life itself.

Reconstitution by Bone Marrow

In irradiated frogs bone marrow can restore the graft rejection capacity, a T-cell function. Frog marrow lymphocytes are also able to develop plaque-forming cells (PFC) against a T-independent antigen. For these two contrasting mechanisms of immune reactions, investigations were necessary to further clarify the marrow's immune capabilities by performing PFC assays against SRBC, a well-known T-dependent antigen. Adult *Rana pipiens* were subjected to total body irradiation or partially irradiated, with one hind leg shielded at 5000 R and immunized intraperitoneally with 0.1 ml of SRBC (50%). Cells from spleen and bone marrow from the shielded and irradiated legs were assayed at 7, 14 and 21 days post-irradiation for PFC using a modified Jerne technique.

Control frogs developed responses showing slightly higher PFC counts in bone marrow than in spleen. Total body irradiated frogs were unable to react against SRBC, which resulted in no PFC. Groups of irradiated and shielded frogs had impaired immune responses at 7 days but some were always present. At 14 days, their responses were slightly recovered, but at 21 days PFC were present in spleen and bone marrow, well above background levels. Total body irradiated frogs died before the 20th day and never recovered immune responses, whereas irradiated and shielded frogs survived until 21 days without high mortality. Thus, bone marrow-derived cells, more effective than those

of the spleen, reconstituted the immune response to SRBC, as was observed in response to skin allografts, at least up to 21 days. Moreover, frog marrow is an important source of cells capable of responding to Con A and producing PFC against SRBC. We suggest that bone marrow is a source of stem cells and mature T- and B-lymphocytes which can recirculate within the immune system.

BONE MARROW EQUIVALENTS IN CYCLOSTOMES

The Pronephros of Hagfish

Structure

Since lymphoid cells have been found in all living vertebrates from cyclostomes to humans, comparative immunologists have attempted to define the possible morphofunctional equivalents of bone marrow in those primitive vertebrates where it is absent. Hagfishes (myxinoids) and lampreys (petromyzontids) are the most primitive vertebrates. These fish are grouped within the Cyclostomata (Agnatha) although in almost all their organs they differ morphologically, which suggests distant relationships. The earliest experimental attempts to demonstrate immune reactivity were a failure, but when it was discovered that the conditions of husbandry must be excellent, Thoenes and Hildemann (1969) succeeded in demonstrating immune responses in hagfish. This was a critical observation, emphasizing the importance of persistence and precision in science.

The main lymphohemopoietic organs of adult hagfish are the pronephros and intestine since a thymus has not yet been discovered (see description later). The pronephros or head kidney is a complex structure which, according to an early immunobiologist, has lost its renal function (Price, 1910). Apart from acting as a possible source of endocrine activity (Idler and Burton, 1976) the chief function of the pronephros is lymphohemopoietic (Holmgren, 1950). The pronephros is a small paired organ suspended in the wall of the pericardial cavity, which, in turn, is part of the peritoneal cavity. The pronephros on the right is situated close to the portal heart, whereas the pronephros on the left side is adjacent to the atrium of the systemic heart.

According to Holmgren's observations, the pronephros is composed of three regions: tubuli, central mass and glomus (Figure 3.8). The tubuli are branched and consist of ciliated epithelial cells surrounded by blood vessels or sinuses. At one end the tubuli open into the pericardial (peritoneal) cavity by nephrostomes (peritoneal funnels). At the other end, instead of forming a urinary duct, the tubuli connect with an irregular cell mass, the central mass, which is suspended in the wall of the pronephric vein. The glomus is a tuft of arterial capillaries enclosed within a pocket of the pericardial wall. Such a structure is probably efficient in producing peritoneal fluid, not urine.

The structural organization of the pronephros indicates that the cilia of the tubuli transport fluid from the pericardial (peritoneal) cavity into the central mass by which it reaches the blood. Because the peritoneal cavity is open to the exterior through the porus abdominalis, the pronephric tubules, in fact, constitute a means of communication between the external environment and venous blood. Observations of living specimens show that carmine particles, etc., which have been injected into the peritoneal cavity, are carried into the blood by intense ciliary activity (Price, 1910; Fange, 1963). The pronephros may therefore serve to clean the peritoneal cavity of foreign

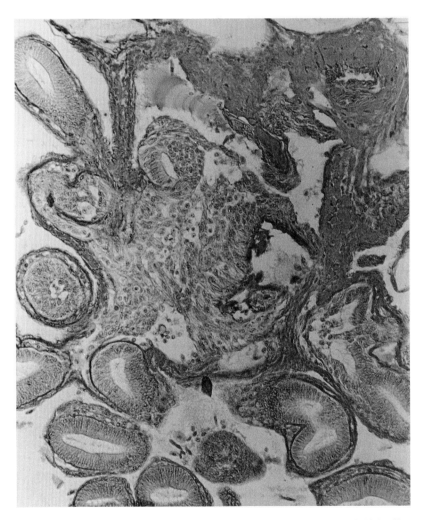

Figure 3.8 Pronephros of an adult Atlantic hagfish, *Myxine glutinosa*, showing ciliated epithelial cells of the tubules and

materials. Willmer (1960) suggested that the hagfish pronephros may function as a primitive lymph node. However, ultrastructural observations emphasize a possible relationship to bone marrow of higher vertebrates since the pronephros contains, together with filtering phagocytic cells, lymphocytes, plasma cells and other developing and mature blood cells, mainly erythroblasts. The pronephros thus resembles more closely the hemopoietic condition of bone marrow and not lymph nodes.

The central mass is composed mainly of lymphohemopoietic elements. According to some immunobiologists, the central mass is formed by transformation of cells in the basal portions of the pronephric tubules, which then lose their epithelial character. However, histological observations indicate that the central mass consists of both epithelial and lymphohemopoietic elements which are thin basal membranes. The epithelial cells form cords between blood capillaries. In special regions, between the epithelial components, lymphohemopoietic cells are predominant in the central mass. Among these are blast cells, lymphocyte-like cells, spindle cells and erythroid cells (Figure 3.9). A high mitotic activity in these areas indicates that the cell accumulations are foci, active in producing new blood cells. The central mass is supported by connective tissue consisting of ramifying fibroblasts, fibrocytes and collagenous bundles. Macrophages, together with connective tissue cells and collagenous fibers, form degenerate areas in which old, altered erythrocytes appear. The surface layer of the central mass is formed by mesothelial cells, which sometimes project into the venous lumen, suggesting that cells may be released from there.

Examinations of ultrathin sections by electron microscopy have revealed numerous, typical plasma cells within the central mass found in unimmunized *Myxine glutinosa* (Zapata *et al.*, 1984). Observing many plasma cells suggests a regional distribution of lymphohemopoietic tissue and of epithelial elements, which, in the central mass, appear to be true renal filtrating cells. The lymphohemopoietic masses consist principally of lymphoblasts, erythroblasts, mature erythrocytes, lymphocytes, plasma cells and macrophages, which are all supported by a network of myofibroblasts joined together by desmosomes and elastic sheaths that surround the free elements (Figure 3.9).

Moreover, epithelial components, consisting of podocytes, mesangial cells and epithelial cells, occur in the central mass and are similar to those of the parietal layer of Bowman's capsule of the higher vertebrate kidney.

Immune Function

We would like, lastly, to emphasize the presence of developing and mature plasma cells in the pronephric mass of unimmunized adult Atlantic hagfish, *Myxine glutinosa*, before confirming their universal presence in all other vertebrates (Zapata *et al.*, 1984). Previous attempts to demonstrate plasma cells in hagfish failed repeatedly, so that the humoral immune capacity was attributed to large lymphocytes and lymphoblasts of peripheral blood cells capable of synthesizing DNA and proliferating in response to the mitogen PHA (Tam *et al.*, 1977). Since the humoral immune system of *Eptatretus stoutii* is poorly developed, this suggested to some comparative immunologists that hagfish lack the humoral immune system equivalent to the usual B-lymphocyte − plasma cell system (Raison *et al.*, 1978).

As one explanation for this difference, it was suggested that Ig could exist in a membrane-bound state, functioning solely as a lymphocyte surface receptor; the presence of serum Ig could result from shedding of receptors rather than active secretion of Ig. Recent evidence, using a monoclonal antibody against serum Ig, confirms a high incidence (65%) of Ig-positive cells in blood leukocytes of *Eptatretus stoutii* (Raison and Hildemann, 1984), which suggests that at this evolutionary level the divergence between T and B lineages has not occurred. Lack of observed distinctions between these cells may have been due to the use of a monoclonal antibody which could not resolve possible similarities or cross-reactivities between the immune recognition unit or receptor of 'T'-cells and serum Ig.

The Intestine of Hagfish

Structure

The intestine forms a straight tube, without distinct divisions, whose submucosa is occupied mostly by large fat cells situated within reticular tissue; blood vessels pass between the fat cells as components of

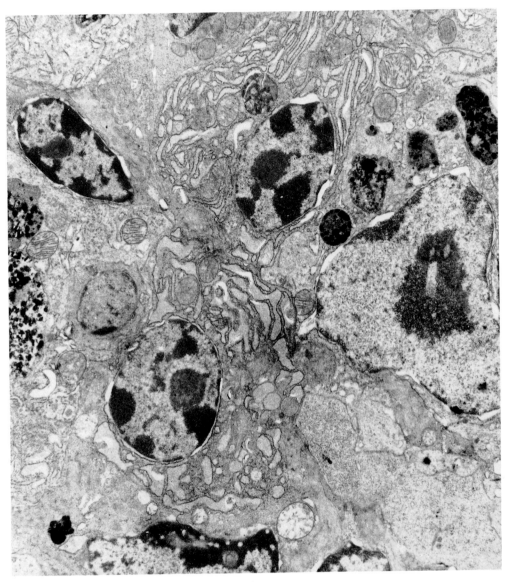

Figure 3.9 Lymphohemopoietic tissue of the pronephric central mass of an adult *Myxine glutinosa*. Lymphoblasts, small lymphocytes and other developing blood cells are arranged between processes of myofibroblastic cells and elastic sheaths (× 9500).

connective tissue. The blood supply originates from approximately 35 mesenteric arteries which split up into main branches at the surface of the intestine. Smaller arteries originate from these main branches and pass into the intestinal wall, forming a subepithelial network in contact with the mucosal epithelium. Richly branched small veins or sinusoids carry blood from subepithelial capillaries to the portal (supraintestinal) vein at the surface of the intestine (Grodzinski, 1926; Tanaka *et al.*, 1981). The veins in the submucosa are surrounded by lymphohemopoietic cell masses occupying about 10% of the intestinal wall's volume. Arteries supplying the subepithelial capillary network have been compared to penicillar arteries of the spleen (Jordan and Speidel, 1930), and the association of lymphohemopoietic cell masses with the portal vein system strongly resembles the organization of the vertebrate spleen. However, the view that hagfishes possess a primitive intestinal spleen (Tomonaga *et al.*, 1973) has been criticized by Tanaka *et al.* (1981) based on anatomical evidence. Likewise, according to their function and ultrastructural characteristics, the intestinal lymphohemopoietic masses of *Myxine glutinosa* resemble the bone marrow of higher vertebrates (Zapata *et al.*, in preparation).

Hemopoietic Function

Neutrophils in various stages of development comprise the most abundant cell population of the intestinal lymphohemopoietic tissue (Figure 3.10). Small, non-granulated cells probably derived from reticular cells have been proposed as precursors of granulocytes (Tomonaga *et al.*, 1973). Mitoses are common, indicating a high rate of new blood cell formation. Tanaka *et al.* (1981) observed, by electron microscopy, that mature granulocytes migrate through a barrier of endothelial cells similar to migrations in bone marrow of higher vertebrates. Some lymphocyte-like cells have been identified ultrastructurally (Zapata *et al.*,

1984) although Good *et al.* (1966) found no foci of lymphoid cells or plasma cells by light microscopy in the intestine of the pacific hagfish, *Eptatretus stoutii*.

This tissue may be characterized as myeloid (bone marrow-like) and mainly granulopoietic. However, several immunobiologists have claimed from light microscopic evidence that, within the intestinal lymphohemopoietic tissue, granulocytes, erythrocytes and various other types of non-granulated cells develop (Jordan and Speidel, 1930; Holmgren, 1950; Good *et al.*, 1966). In contrast, Tomonaga *et al.* (1973) and Tanaka *et al.* (1981) were unable to identify erythrocyte precursors, spindle cells (or thrombocytes) in the intestine. According to Jordan and Speidel (1930), undifferentiated lymphocytes or lymphoid hemoblasts are formed within the intestine, differentiating intravascularly into erythrocytes, spindle cells and/or thrombocytes. To reconcile these differences, Tomonaga *et al.* (1973) injected ^{59}Fe ferric salts into *Eptatretus burgeri* and examined sections of the intestine by autoradiography, but found no synthesis of hemoglobin. This negative finding seems to support the theory that erythrocytes differentiate outside the intestine, in the peripheral blood or in other loci, for instance in the pronephros, as was demonstrated by the ultrastructural studies of Zapata *et al.* (1984).

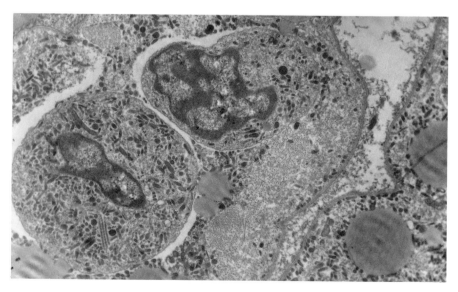

Figure 3.10 Developing blood cells, mainly neutrophilic granulocytes, which occur between adipose cells and large bundles of collagenous fibers in the intestinal lymphohemopoietic masses of *Myxine glutinosa* ($\times$ 3000).

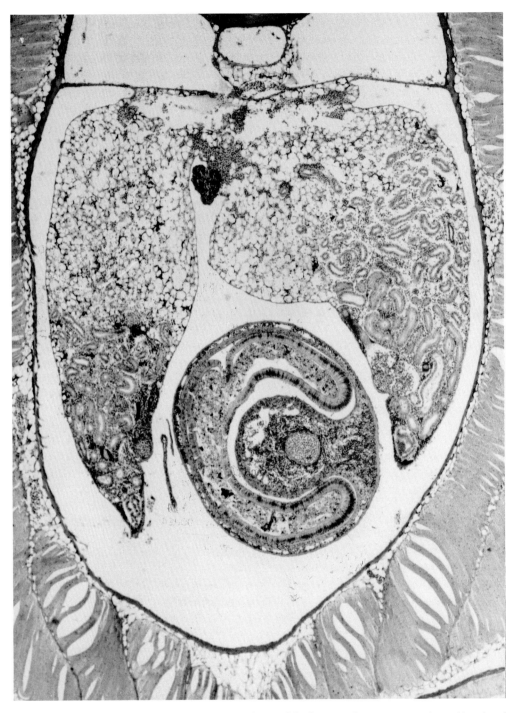

Figure 3.11 Nephric fold and typhlosole of an ammocoete larva of the lamprey *Petromyzon marinus*. Abundant lympho-hemopoietic tissue appears in the gut lamina propria between renal tubules and in adipose tissue associated with the opisthonephros (× 68). (From *Dev Comp Immunol* **11**: 79, 1987, reproduced by permission.)

The Typhlosole of Lampreys

Structure

Lampreys have a long and complex life cycle. During larval stages, ammocoetes remain buried in the river silt (Hardisty and Potter, 1971a). After metamorphosis, young adults migrate to the sea, where they parasitize teleost fish by attaching to the integument (Hardisty and Potter, 1971b; Potter and Huggins, 1973). During metamorphosis, ammocoetes undergo extensive changes affecting their anatomy, biochemistry and physiology. In addition to external changes such as the appearance of eyes and the oral disc, and modifications of the gill clefts (Youson and Potter, 1979), internal changes also occur, mostly as modifications in the branchial apparatus and intestine (Wright and Youson, 1976) and in the degeneration of the larval opisthonephros to form the adult kidney (Ooi and Youson, 1979; Youson and Ooi, 1979).

Lymphohemopoietic organs are also affected by extensive alterations during metamorphosis. In the ammocoetes, the main lymphohemopoietic organs are the typhlosole and the opisthonephros (Jordan and Speidel, 1930; Sterba, 1962; Percy and Potter, 1976; Ardavin et al., 1984). Modifications during metamorphosis, affecting the digestive apparatus, together with degeneration of the larval opisthonephros, cause loss of their lymphohemopoietic capacities, which then become located in the supraneural body, the principal lymphohemopoietic organ of the adult lamprey (Finstad et al., 1964; Percy and Potter, 1977; Ardavin et al., 1984). Therefore, as a result of these changes, lamprey lymphohemopoietic organs are excellent models for analyzing the importance of cell microenvironments which provide adequate conditions for hemopoiesis. After extensive research on the ultrastructural changes which occur throughout its life cycle in the hemopoietic organs of the anadromous sea lamprey, Petromyzon marinus, the lymphohemopoietic tissues have been considered equivalents of vertebrate bone marrow (Ardavin et al., 1984; Ardavin and Zapata, 1987).

In ammocoetes, the typhlosole, intertubular and adipose tissue of the nephric fold are the principal lymphohemopoietic organs (Figure 3.11) (Ardavin et al., 1984). The intestinal hemopoietic foci or typhlosole in cyclostomes are considered as primitive spleens (Tanaka et al., 1981). In contrast, ultrastructural similarities between cell microenvironments of these typhlosolar lymphohemopoietic foci and vertebrate bone marrow, and their common function as hemopoietic organs, lend support to the view of a similar morphofunctional capacity in both of them. The typhlosole in ammocoete larvae is formed by an invagination of the epithelium in the anterior gut, which extends from the end of the esophagus to the hind gut. The enlarged lamina propria is occupied by lymphohemopoietic tissue. The typhlosole is vascularized throughout its length by the mesentery or typhlosolar artery, which gives off arterioles dorsally that open into enlarged blood sinusoids, providing vascularization for the typhlosolar lymphohemopoietic tissue as in mammalian bone marrow (Percy and Potter, 1979; Ardavin and Zapata, 1987). By contrast, in the typhlosole of Entosphenus reissneri, the arterioles connect with peripheral venous capillaries which then empty into blood sinuses (Tanaka et al., 1981).

Lymphohemopoietic tissue of the typhlosole consists of mature and developing blood cells arranged without any defined pattern of organization between connective tissue elements of the stroma (Figure 3.12). In this locus, differentiation of erythrocytic, lymphocytic, monocytic and granulocytic lineages occurs. Although full development of each lineage is generally an extravascular phenomenon with migration of mature cells through the endothelial wall, sometimes immature blood cells, principally erythrocytic and granulocytic ones, cross the endothelia or remain inside blood sinuses, which suggests that the last phases of erythro-, granulo- and monocytopoiesis of Petromyzon marinus may occur in the bloodstream. A similar situation exists in the plasmacytic lineage since plasmablasts, proplasmacytes and mature plasma cells occur in both the typhlosolar lymphohemopoietic tissue and blood sinuses.

Reticular cells, forming the supporting apparatus of the typhlosolar lymphohemopoietic tissue, are irregular elements interposed between the developing lymphohemopoietic cells, whose processes constitute a tridimensional network. These reticular cells show an irregular shape, sometimes lobulated nuclei with numerous indentations and scant, condensed, peripherally arranged chromatin (Figure 3.13). On the surface, reticular cells are closely apposed to reticular

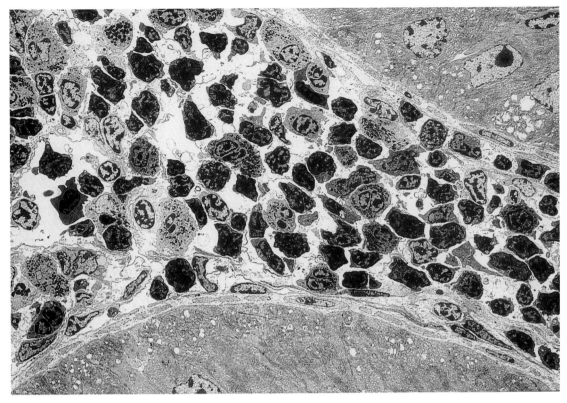

Figure 3.12 Cell components of the typhlosolar lymphohemopoietic tissue including developing and mature lymphocytes, plasma cells and myeloid cells (× 2185).

and collagenous fibers which are sometimes surrounded by these cell processes. In some instances, reticular cells, with a certain phagocytic capacity, occur also in the ammocoete's typhlosole. The endothelial lining cells of the typhlosolar blood sinuses are formed by elongated irregular cells without a continuous basement membrane. As in mammals, cells involved in phagocytosis are a matter of some controversy. For some immunobiologists, endothelial cells of the venous plexuses of these lymphohemopoietic foci of lower vertebrates are active in phagocytosis (Tanaka *et al.*, 1981; Zapata, 1979). Others consider, by contrast, that only free macrophages are capable of phagocytosis (Campbell, 1970; Curtis *et al.*, 1979).

The lymphohemopoietic tissue of the typhlosole undergoes substantial modifications throughout the lamprey's life cycle owing to morphofunctional variations which affect its digestive apparatus. The importance of cell microenvironments in phylogenetic relationships of the typhlosolar lymphohemopoietic tissue has been confirmed by the discovery of their role which determines the blood-forming capacity of the lamprey's life cycle. During the larval period, the typhlosole maintains lymphohemopoietic capacity despite a gradual increase in connective tissue (Percy and Potter, 1977; Tanaka *et al.*, 1981; Ardavin and Zapata, 1988). The feeding of adult lampreys requires a full transformation of the digestive apparatus during metamorphosis, including formation of the oral disc (Youson and Potter, 1979), transformation of the intestinal epithelium (Youson and Horbert, 1982), development of the intestinal villi (Youson and Connely, 1978) and an improved circulatory system (Percy and Potter, 1979). In the ammocoete's

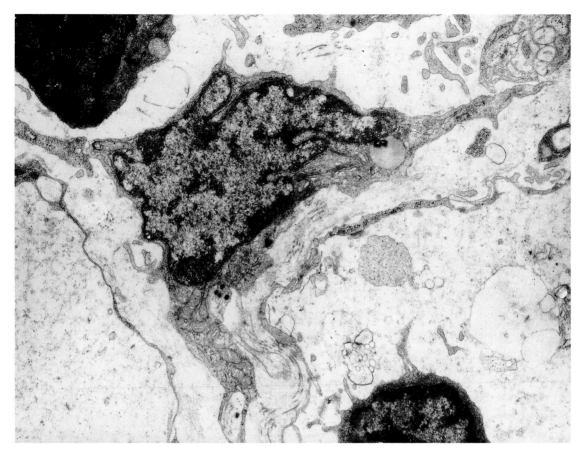

Figure 3.13 Reticular cell forming the supporting network of the typhlosolar lymphohemopoietic tissue. The morphology resembles that of stromal cells of higher vertebrate bone marrow. Note the association with reticular fibers and its long cytoplasmic processes ($\times$ 14700).

typhlosole, slow circulation in the blood sinuses causes low blood pressure, which is irrelevant to the sedentary life of ammocoetes. Adult lampreys, by contrast, need a more efficient blood supply, which is guaranteed by the formation of capillary plexuses in the intestinal villi and development of the typhlosolar vein (Percy and Potter, 1979).

During metamorphosis, there is a notable increase in connective tissue, with a consequent disappearance of the sinusoidal system which vascularizes the typhlosole. At the beginning of metamorphosis, the lymphohemopoietic tissue consists of mature blood cells and macrophages but not of blasts and immature blood cells (Figure 3.14). Therefore, the typhlosole loses its lymphohemopoietic capacity before the first

internal signs of metamorphosis appear, including the endostyle (Wright and Youson, 1976) and adenohypophysis (Leach, 1951; Thompson, 1971). This loss is a consequence of the modification which the typhlosolar cell microenvironment undergoes, and it consists basically in the development of connective tissue and disappearance of slow blood circulation. When metamorphosis ends, the intestine of *Petromyzon marinus* contains dense connective tissue without lymphohemopoiesis capacity (Percy and Potter, 1976; Tanaka *et al.*, 1981; Ardavin and Zapata, 1987). These metamorphic changes in the lamprey's typhlosole are similar to those which occur in the lymphohemopoietic masses of the intestine in myxinoids (Tomonaga *et al.*, 1973).

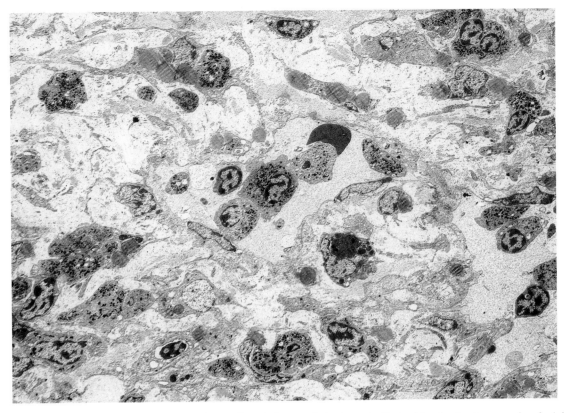

Figure 3.14 Ultrastructural evidence showing no lymphohemopoietic tissue in the typhlosolar lamina propria of adult lamprey. Increased connective tissue contains only macrophages and mature granulocytes and lymphocytes (× 2280).

Immune Function

Contacts between macrophages and lymphoid cells inside the typhlosolar sinuses, where there are also plasmablasts and plasma cells, are perhaps related to macrophage involvement in the trapping, processing and presentation of antigens, as well as in T−B-lymphocyte cooperation which is necessary for antibody synthesis. Little information is available about the role played by non-lymphoid cells in the lamprey's immune reactions. Polymorphonuclear leukocytes found in the brook lamprey, *Petromyzon reissneri*, appear to play an essential role as effectors in defense mechanisms against invading foreign microbes. Polymorphonuclear leukocytes show significantly enhanced phagocytic activity against SRBC *in vitro* provided they are first opsonized with the specific lamprey antibody against SRBC (Fujii, 1982). In addi-

tion to the typhlosole, macrophages have been observed to be involved in trapping carbon and bacteria in the cavernous bodies, kidneys and supraneural body of lampreys (Page and Rowley, 1984; Ardavin and Zapata, 1988).

The immune capacity of the typhlosole, analyzed ultrastructurally, reveals numerous mature and immature plasma cells (Zapata *et al.*, 1981b). Brook lampreys, *Petromyzon reissneri*, immunized with a large dose of SRBC, show antigen-binding cells in the typhlosole and blood after four days (Fujii *et al.*, 1979). In addition, the numbers of plasma cells have been shown to increase in the typhlosole, opisthonephros and supraneural body after repeated immunization with ovine erythrocytes (ORBC). Thus, the typhlosole of *Petromyzon marinus* is a lympho-hemopoietic organ which functions in hemopoiesis and in immune responses but it loses this capacity when the complex modifications of metamorphosis affect the idiosyncrasies of cell microenvironments.

The Opisthonephros of Lampreys

Structure

The nephric fold is formed anteriorly by the larval opisthonephros and posteriorly by nephrogenic tissue which will transform later, during metamorphosis, into the adult opisthonephros (Percy and Potter, 1976, 1977; Ardavin and Zapata, 1987). The larval opisthonephros consists of renal corpuscles and tubules surrounded by connective tissue which, extensively developed in the dorsal region, constitutes the opisthonephric adipose tissue (Youson, 1980). The nephric fold in ammocoetes contains lymphohemopoietic tissue arranged in the intertubular connective tissue (Sterba, 1962; Percy and Potter, 1976; Kilarski and Plytycz, 1981; Ardavin and Zapata, 1987) and in the adipose tissue constitutes the dorsal zone of the opisthonephros and the posterior region of the nephric fold (Percy and Potter, 1976; Ardavin and Zapata, 1987). In both regions, developing blood cells are housed in a connective tissue stroma which surrounds tubules or adipocytes and are separated from the intravascular space by an endothelium which lines the intertubular sinuses (Figure 3.15).

Sinusoidal endothelial cells and stromal reticular components are morphologically similar to those in the ammocoete typhlosole. The phagocytic capacity of endothelial cells is a matter of discussion. Phagocytic

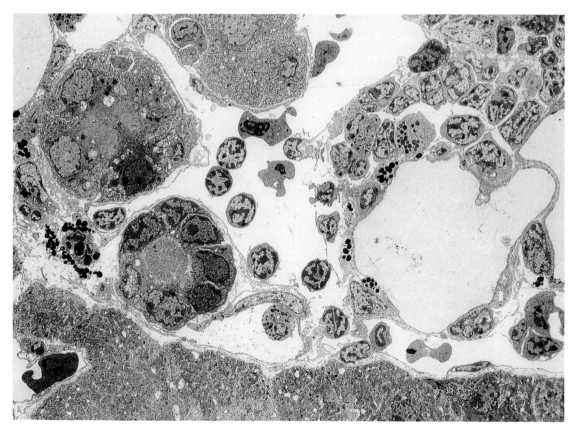

Figure 3.15 Lymphohemopoietic tissue consisting of developing and mature lymphocytes between the opisthonephric tubule of ammocoete larvae of *Petromyzon marinus* (× 240). (From *Dev Comp Immunol* **11**: 79, 1987, reproduced by permission.)

endothelial cells have been reported in myxinoids (Tanaka *et al.*, 1981), teleosts (Zapata, 1979) and birds (Campbell, 1967), while Campbell (1970) and Curtis *et al.* (1979) in amphibians, and Tavassoli and Shaklai (1979) in mammals considered them to be non-phagocytic. In agreement with our own results, the absence of a basement membrane beneath the sinusoidal endothelium has been reported in teleosts (Zapata, 1979), amphibians (Campbell, 1970; Curtis *et al.*, 1979) and mammals (Weiss, 1965).

Hemopoietic Function

The lymphohemopoietic tissue of the nephric fold of *Petromyzon marinus* contributes to the production and differentiation of erythrocytes, lymphocytes, monocytes and granulocytes (Ardavin *et al.*, 1984; Ardavin and Zapata, 1987). As in the typhlosole, the sinusoids of the lymphohemopoietic masses in the nephric fold contain numerous plasmablasts, immature and mature plasma cells and large macrophages, whose projections make contact with both the endothelial cells and circulating lymphoid elements. Abundant phagosomes, in the cytoplasm of these macrophages, suggest an important role in the elimination of senescent cells, mainly erythrocytes, as described for the spleen and bone marrow of mammals (Weiss and Greep, 1977).

In contrast, the possible role played by macrophages of the typhlosole has already been described. It is important, however, to point out the presence of engulfed pigment granules in the cytoplasm of the opisthonephric macrophages which are involved in erythrophagocytosis, although X-ray microanalysis has not revealed the presence of iron in these pigment inclusions (Page and Rowley, 1984). Moreover, since these cells were strongly acid-phosphatase positive, this suggests that they play some role in non-specific immune responses (Page and Rowley, 1984). In summary, the plasmacytopoietic capacity, revealed in the lymphohemopoietic tissue of the opisthonephros of *Petromyzon marinus*, and the presence of macrophages, represent morphological evidence for immunoreactivity in the opisthonephros of ammocoetes (of the brook lamprey, *Petromyzon reissneri*) especially after immunization with SRBC (Fujii *et al.*, 1979).

Changes in the lymphohemopoietic capacity of the opisthonephros are dependent, as in the typhlosole, on

profound modifications affecting lampreys during metamorphosis, especially on variations in its self-hemopoietic inductive microenvironment. For the larval period, the opisthonephros retains its lympho-hemopoietic nature, surely determined by such a suitable cell microenvironment, but during metamorphosis there is total degeneration of the larval opisthonephros, giving rise to the adult kidney from the nephrogenic tissue of the posterior nephric fold (Ooi and Youson, 1979). At the beginning of metamorphosis, the regressing larval opisthonephros shows much reduced blood sinuses, degenerated renal tubules with cytoplasmic dense bodies and vacuoles, and an enlarged basement membrane. At this time, the stroma of the opisthonephros contains more connective tissue, with abundant collagenous fibers and numerous pigment cells. As a consequence of changes in the stroma, and of vascularization, the organ then lacks its lymphohemopoietic potential. In the posterior portion of the nephric fold with nephrogenic capacity where the adult opisthonephros is being formed, there are, however, numerous developing blood cells in the associated adipose tissue.

At the end of metamorphosis, the recently formed opisthonephros has no lymphohemopoietic capacity (Percy and Potter, 1977; Ardavin and Zapata, 1987). Nevertheless, the opisthonephros of an old adult *Petromyzon marinus* constitutes an important hemopoietic locus which contains abundant developing blood cells that divide by mitosis (Figure 3.16) (Ardavin *et al.*, 1984; Ardavin and Zapata, 1987; Romer, 1971) despite previous conflicting reports (Percy and Potter, 1977). Accordingly, characteristics of the inductive microenvironment, stroma and enlarged blood sinusoids of the adult opisthonephros resemble those of the larval opisthonephros. Thus the condition in the opisthonephros of aging lampreys would indeed appear to be similar to that of the kidney of adult teleosts (Zapata, 1979), where the pronephros and the mesonephros are active lymphohemopoietic organs (see later descriptions). In summary, the opisthonephros and typhlosole are important foci in ammocoetes for the housing and differentiation of blood stem cells, a condition which resembles ultrastructurally that of the bone marrow of homothermic vertebrates or its equivalent in ectothermic vertebrates. When the inductive microenvironments become modified as a consequence of new needs

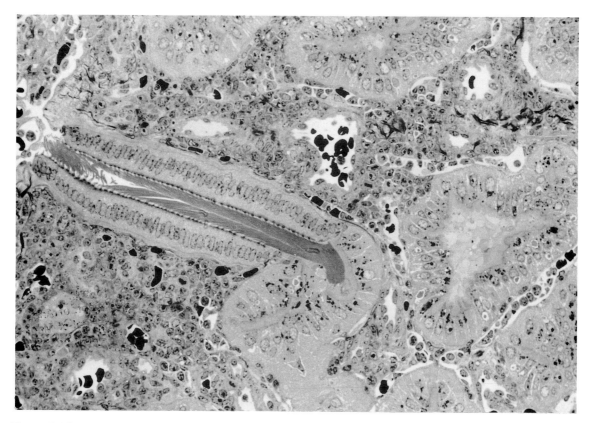

Figure 3.16 Abundant lymphohemopoietic tissue occurs between the renal components of adult opisthonephros of *Petromyzon marinus* (× 304). (From *Dev Comp Immunol* **11**: 79, 1987, reproduced by permission.)

imposed by metamorphosis, these organs transform, losing their lymphohemopoietic potential and the role they must play in the lamprey's immune responses, chiefly through loss of lymphocytes, macrophages and plasma cells.

The Supraneural Body of Lampreys

Structure

The supraneural body, classically proposed as the phylogenetic precursor of bone marrow, shows precisely the same histology as lymphohemopoietic tissue in the typhlosole and nephric fold. The supraneural body is a column of adipose tissue included in the fibrocartilaginous sheath dorsal to the nerve cord. Until premetamorphosis, the supraneural body is not lymphohemopoietic. In young adult lampreys (nearly

five years), numerous lymphohemopoietic aggregates appear in the supraneural body, which possesses the identical organization as that of adipose tissue associated with the larval nephric fold. In adult stages, the supraneural body represents the most important hemopoietic organ. It contains mature and developing blood cells of several lineages, including lymphocytes, plasma cells, abundant blasts and other cells in division distributed between connective tissue which contains bundles of collagenous fibers and adipose cells (Figure 3.17).

Immune Function

Although information about immune functions of the supraneural body is lacking, indirect evidence suggests a certain capacity for effecting immune responses. Thus, after repeated immunization with

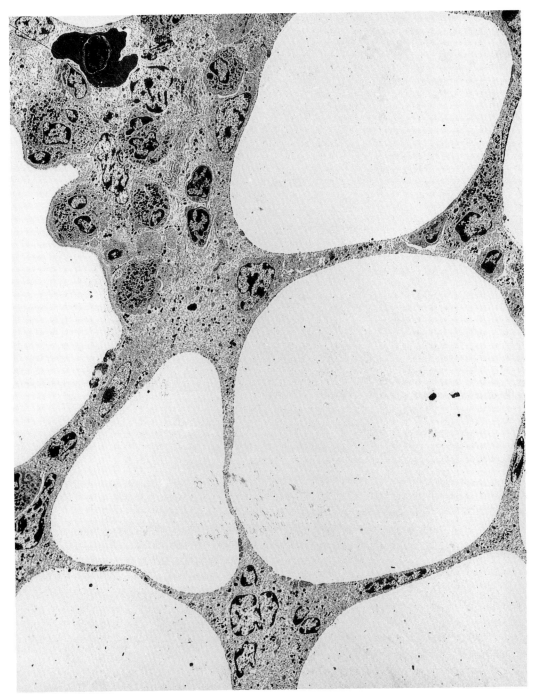

Figure 3.17 Small lymphocytes and developing and mature granulocytes appear between giant adipose cells and reticular cells in the supraneural body of adult lamprey, *Petromyzon marinus* (× 3600).

SRBC, increased numbers of plasma cells occur in supraneural bodies (Fujii, 1981) and antigenic stimulation with Bacillus Calmette-Guerin (BCG) in Freund's complete adjuvant induces proliferation of cells in it as measured by the *in vivo* uptake of tritiated thymidine (Finstad and Good, 1964). Moreover, antibody-producing cells have been localized by immunocytochemical techniques in the supraneural body of adult *Petromyzon marinus* previously immunized with human erythrocytes type O Rh $^+$ (Hagen *et al.*, 1983). Lymphohemopoietic activity of the supraneural body is the reverse of what has been observed in the typhlosole and nephric fold; however, the possible role played by the cell microenvironment is similar in both cases. During larval stages, the arterial pressure is insufficient to promote an adequate hemopoietic microenvironment of the supraneural body, but during metamorphosis growth of the heart, which produces increased blood pressure (Claridge and Potter, 1974), and lipid depletion, due to starvation of metamorphosing lampreys, increases fluid circulation in the adipose tissue of the supraneural body, thus favoring lymphohemopoiesis.

BONE MARROW EQUIVALENTS IN MODERN FISH

Introduction

Modern fish constitute an abundant group of vertebrates which can be divided into two main categories: Chondrichthyes, including Holocephali and Elasmobranchi, and Osteichthyes, which comprise Crossopterygii, Dipnoi, Chondrostei, Holostei, Polypteriformes and Teleostei. Although fish, except the teleosts and a few elasmobranchs, have not been investigated extensively from an immunological viewpoint, they do present many interesting peculiarities such as a myriad of lymphohemopoietic tissues located in diverse organs and with a common histological organization resembling the bone marrow of higher vertebrates.

Structure of Epigonal Leydig Organ in Chondrichthyes

Chondrichthyes comprise Holocephali (Chimaeriformes) and Elasmobranchii, representing the most primitive vertebrates with a clearly defined thymus. Nevertheless, important differences exist between the two groups which are reflected in their respective lymphohemopoietic tissues. Leydig (1851) described white, lobulated masses in the orbital and subcranial region of *Chimaera monstrosa* as lymph nodes without efferent ducts, but later these structures were identified as lymphoid or myeloid tissue (Leydig, 1857; Kolmer, 1923; Holmgren, 1942), an observation which has so far not received renewed attention. The cranial lymphohemopoietic tissue forms white masses in the orbit, in the preorbital canal of the cranial cartilage and in a depression in the basis cranii. The subcranial portion is covered ventrally by the pharyngeal mucosa, and caudally it surrounds a structure assumed to belong to the hypophyseal system (Fahrenholz, 1929; Fujita, 1963). Together with classical light microscopic observations (Fange and Sundell, 1969), recent ultrastructural evidence has confirmed the lymphohemopoietic capacity of this organ (Zapata *et al.*, in preparation), which relates it to the epigonal and Leydig organs of elasmobranchs.

The organ consists of ramified reticular cells which form a network where lymphocytes but principally granulocytes differentiate (Figure 3.18). Granulocytes comprise neutrophils and eosinophils. Neutrophils contain two different cytoplasmic granules whose functional relationships are difficult to understand. Eosinophils contain a single population of granules which consist of large electron-dense granules without crystalline inclusions. Numerous mature and immature plasma cells and some macrophages are also present. No further important lymphohemopoietic foci seem to occur in *Chimaera monstrosa*; however, according to Jacobshagen (1915), the intestinal spiral fold contains a rich infiltration of lymphocytes, suggesting a certain lymphocytopoietic capacity. In other regions, Citterio (1931) described erythropoiesis in the cardiac epithelium of larval ratfish. In contrast, no lymphohemopoiesis seems to occur in the urogenital system of chimeroids (Stanley, 1963) as has been reported in other cartilaginous fish. No information is available, at present, on the immune functions

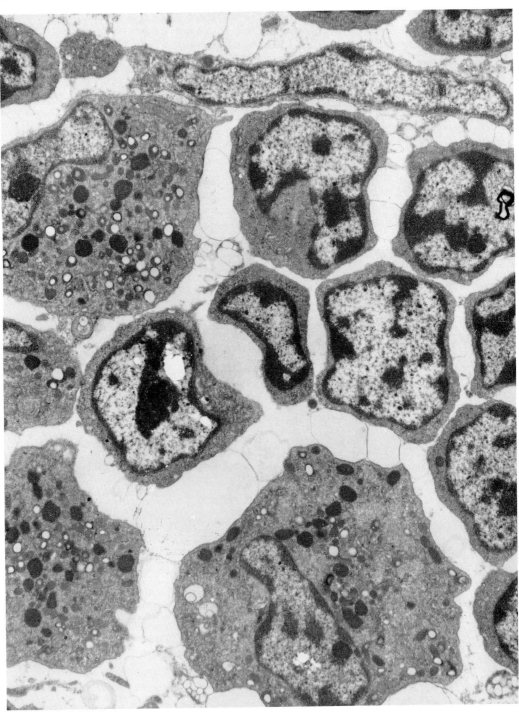

Figure 3.18 Lymphocytes and neutrophilic cells distributed between reticular cells in the lymphohemopoietic orbital organ of *Chimera monstrosa*. Note its resemblance to the histological organization of Leydig and epigonal organs of modern elasmobranchs ($\times$ 11560).

possibly played by the cranial organ of *Chimaera monstrosa*, although the presence of lymphocytes and mainly plasma cells suggest capacities that can effect immune responses.

The existence of lymphohemopoietic epigonal and Leydig organs has been known for some time. Many elasmobranchs possess both structures but others have only one of them (for review see Fange, 1982). In no elasmobranchs are both the epigonal and Leydig organs absent. The Leydig organ is a lymphohemopoietic structure located at dorsal and ventral positions in the gut submucosa, extending from the oral cavity to the stomach (Zapata, 1981a). The epigonal organs of rays (*Raja clavata* and *Torpedo marmorata*) occupy the parenchyma of the ovary (Figure 3.19) and testis, commencing from the connective tissue capsule and ending at the ovules and seminiferous tubules (Zapata, 1981a). In the dogfish, *Scyliorhinus canicula*, the epigonal organ forms an irregular mass in the mesenteric folds of the gonads. In young rays, the gonads are embedded in and partially covered by lymphohemopoietic tissue, whereas in sexually mature sharks

the size of the epigonal tissue decreases when compared to that of the ovary. In male dogfish the epigonal tissue is Y-shaped due to the presence of two testes (Fange and Pulsford, 1983).

Apart from their anatomical characteristics, these organs are histologically similar. Masses of maturing granulopoietic cells are distributed in a stroma which consists of fibroblasts, collagenous fibers and blood vessels, together with a variable amount of lymphocytes and plasma cells (Fange and Mattisson, 1981; Zapata, 1981a; Mattisson and Fange, 1982; Fange and Pulsford, 1983) (Figure 3.20). Evidently, the epigonal and Leydig organs of elasmobranchs are mainly granulocyte-producing tissues although, according to Matthews (1950), the Leydig organ of the basking shark, *Cetorhinus maxime*, is active in erythropoiesis; after splenectomy, there is evidence of compensatory erythropoiesis (Fange and Johansson-Sjobeck, 1975).

Supposed immune functions of these lymphohemopoietic organs are largely unknown. Tomonaga *et al.* (1984) have reported, using immunofluorescence, the presence of high-molecular-weight (HMW)

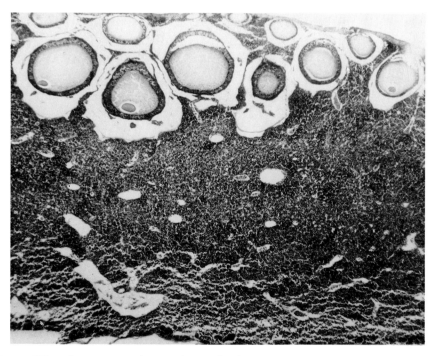

Figure 3.19 Ovary of *Torpedo marmorata*, the torpedo ray, showing lymphohemopoietic tissue arranged between developing oocytes (× 300). (From *Dev Comp Immunol* **5**: 43, 1981, reproduced by permission.)

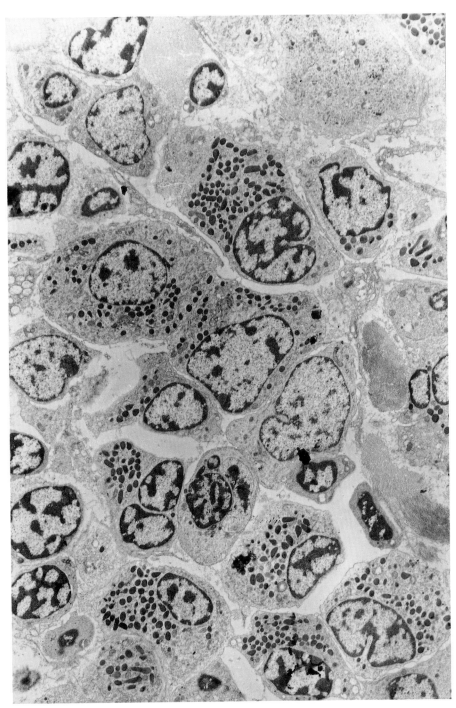

Figure 3.20 Lymphoblasts, small lymphocytes, developing and mature granulocytes occur between blood vessels and large bundles of collagenous fibers in the Leydig organ of *Torpedo marmorata* (× 2200).

and low-molecular-weight (LMW) Ig-positive cells in the Leydig organ of the ray, *Raja kenojei*. Due to abundant vascular sinusoids, these organs could actually filter antigenic material, house lymphocytes or provide an adequate microenvironment for differentiation of progenitors of antigen-responsive cells (Manning, 1984). The epigonal and Leydig organs are also rich in hydrolytic enzymes (acid phosphatase, glycosidases, chitinase) which are obvious candidates for participating in immunodefense reaction (Fange, 1982; Mattisson and Fange, 1982). There seems to be an absence of lymphohemopoietic tissue in the kidney of most elasmobranchs, although Maximow (1910) described it in *Acanthyas vulgaris*.

Structure and Function in Dipnoi

The lymphohemopoietic system of lungfish was investigated by Jordan and Speidel (1931) and more recently by Mimura and Mimura (1977), but available information on its immune capacity is lacking. Caudally to the spleen of *Protopterus ethiopicus*, granulopoietic tissue is developed within the spiral intestine, and similar tissue covers the kidney and gonads. In short, lympho- and erythropoiesis occur mainly in the spleen, and granulopoiesis in the kidney and gonads.

Structure and Function in Chondrosteans and Holosteans

Chondrosteans as well as holosteans, formerly considered together as the so-called ganoids, have two characteristic lymphohemopoietic tissues which closely resemble the bone marrow of higher vertebrates (Jordan, 1938; Good *et al.*, 1966). In both chondrosteans and holosteans, the main site of granulopoiesis is in the cranial cavity of the meninges. In young sturgeons, this tissue occupies the upper region of the medulla oblongata and the anterior portion of the spinal cord. Moreover, sturgeons and paddlefish have abundant lymphohemopoietic foci overlying the base of the heart which extends down over the atrium and ventricle. The histology of both lymphohemopoietic areas is similar, consisting of lobes of closely packed cells, granulocytes and lymphocytes separated by venous or lymphatic spaces. In both chondrosteans and

holosteans, the kidney is an important lymphohemopoietic organ, as in teleosts and in *Amia calva* there is granulopoietic tissue in the ovary like that described in elasmobranchs. Although immunological information is greater in this group than in other primitive fish, the role played by its lymphoid organs in immune reactions is unknown. Extensive immunization of paddlefish results in a marked increase of plasma cells in the spleen and in the pericardial hemopoietic tissue, without revealing information with respect to renal reactivity (Good *et al.*, 1966).

Morphology of the Pronephros in Teleosts

The kidney is an important lymphohemopoietic organ in teleosts. It appears as a sheet of tissue which extends in a dorsal position and is attached by connective tissue and mesothelium to the walls of the body cavity. The teleost kidney consists of two distinct segments: an anterior segment (the cephalic kidney) (Figure 3.21), and a second or middle and posterior segment (the trunk kidney). Both regions exhibit lymphohemopoietic capacity, which is greater in the cephalic kidney where the renal tubules have disappeared (Figure 3.21). However, the structure of lymphohemopoietic tissue is the same in both areas (Ellis and de Sousa, 1974; Zapata, 1979, 1981b). By electron microscopy, no clear demarcation between red and white pulp has been demonstrated as other comparative immunologists have described (Ellis and de Sousa, 1974; Sailendri and Muthukkaruppan, 1975a), although clumps of lymphoid cells tend to occupy defined areas (Zapata, 1979).

Renal lymphohemopoietic tissue is supported by a connective tissue capsule where pigment cells abound and by numerous ramified reticular cells which form a framework in the parenchyma (Figure 3.22). Certain reticular cells exhibit phagocytic capacity, as do endothelial cells which line blood sinusoids, an important function, necessary in the process of recognizing and processing antigens. Every line of hemopoietic differentiation has been observed in the teleost kidney, including the capacity for lympho- and plasmacytopoiesis (Smith *et al.*, 1970; Zapata, 1979, 1981b); pluripotent hemopoietic stem cells are also present (Al-Adhami and Kunz, 1976; Zapata, 1981b). Because of these characteristics, the teleost kidney has been compared to mammalian bone marrow, although

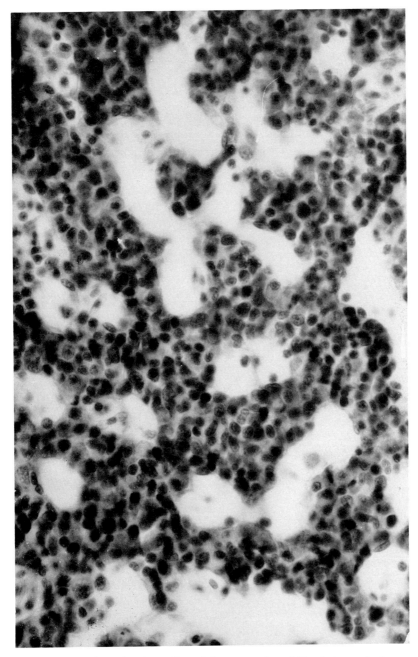

Figure 3.21 Lymphohemopoietic tissue forming cell cords between enlarged blood sinuses in the pronephros of *Rutilus rutilus*, a fresh-water teleost (× 250). (From *Dev Comp Immunol* **3**: 55, 1979, reproduced by permission.)

some investigators have claimed a resemblance to lymph nodes, which of course would demand a role in its immunological capacities. Nevertheless, both capacities, that of concentrating and differentiating hemopoietic stem cells and that of certain immune capacities, are compatible with the phylogenetic relationships of pronephros to bone marrow (Zapata, 1979).

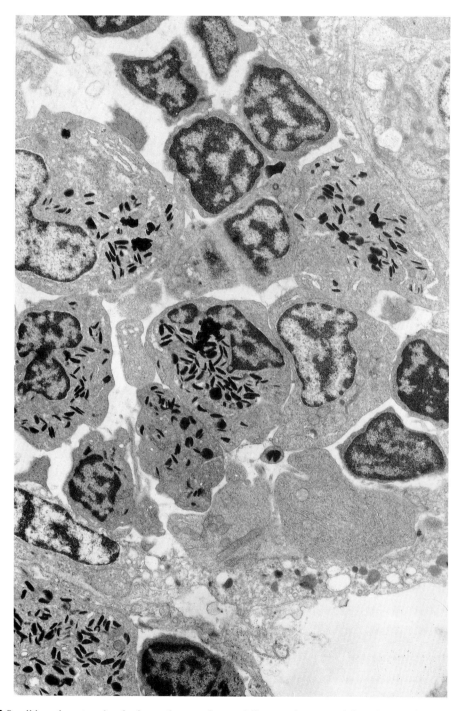

Figure 3.22 Small lymphocytes, developing and mature heterophilic granulocytes and thrombocytes in cell cords arranged between renal tubules and endothelial phagocytic cells in the mesonephros of *Gobio gobio* (× 5320).

Function of the Teleost Pronephros

During embryonic life, lymphocytes first appear in the thymus, but hemopoietic stem cells are already present in the kidney (Ellis, 1977; Grace and Manning, 1980). Cellular 'bridges' between the pronephros and thymus have been identified in *Salmo gairdneri* (Manning, 1981), although cell traffic between both organs has not been demonstrated conclusively. In general the teleost kidney is considered to be a postembryonic source of hemopoietic stem cells (Al-Adhami and Kunz, 1976). As reported in the spleen, antigen-binding cells and antibody-producing cells have been found in the lymphohemopoietic tissue of the teleost kidney (Anderson, 1978; Chiller *et al.*, 1969; Neale and Chavin, 1971; Pontius and Ambrosius, 1971; Ruben *et al.*, 1977; Sailendri and Muthukkaruppan, 1975b; Smith *et al.*, 1967; Warr and Marchalonis, 1977). In contrast, leukocytes of the pronephros from rainbow trout are stimulated by LPS, but not by Con A and PPD, whereas in blue gills pronephric lymphocytes can be stimulated by PHA, Con A and LPS (Cuchens *et al.*, 1976). Moreover, an antiserum against blue gill brain tissue plus complement killed 90% of pronephric lymphocytes (Cuchens and Clem, 1977). Surviving cells respond to LPS but not to PHA, whereas un- treated pronephric cells can be stimulated by both LPS and PHA, which suggests that T-lymphocytes are removed by this antiserum.

Pronephric lymphocytes as well as those from other sources can usually mount several immune responses *in vitro* with respect to mixed lymphocyte reactions (MLR) in *Salmo gairdneri*. Allogeneic combinations of leukocytes from peripheral blood (PBL) or pronephros of trouts can show marked proliferative responses, revealing maximum ones at 7 days for pronephric cells and 9 days for PBL (Etlinger *et al.*, 1976, 1977). McKinney *et al.* (1976) were unable, however, to induce MLR in teleosts of the family Lutjanidae. Regarding environmental effects, at least with respect to temperature, 12 of 15 random combi- nations of pronephric cells of *Lepomis macrochirus* were reactive at 32 °C but not at 22 °C (Cuchens and Clem, 1977). In another assay, to reveal cytotoxic responses, cells of the pronephros of *Ictalurus punctatus* can show higher non-specific cytotoxic activity than PBL (Graves *et al.*, 1984; Evans *et al.*, 1984).

Since lymphocytes are known to secrete factors which contain immunoreactive substances other than antibodies, further assays have been developed. For example, supernatants derived from cultures of pronephric leukocytes of *Cyprinus carpio*, activated by PHA, contain a growth factor which induces prolif- erative responses in purified lymphoblasts (Caspi and Avtalion, 1984), but this factor is not mitogenic if isolated from fresh leukocytes, and its activity is reduced by absorption with the supernatant of mitogen-activated lymphoblasts. Supernatants from MLR also induce specific proliferation of mitogen- activated lymphoblasts, suggesting the first appear- ance of lymphokines early during evolution.

Although antigen trapping by the immune system is presented in other chapters, it is important to consider briefly here how the teleost kidney traps antigen. Circulating non-antigenic particulate material is phagocytosed in the network of reticuloendothelial cells in pronephric lymphohemopoietic tissue. Pyroninophilic cells and/or macrophages seem to be involved rather than reticular fibers (Ellis, 1980; Secombes and Manning, 1980, 1982) and cells con- taining carbon particles often migrate to melano- macrophage centers of the kidney and spleen (Ellis *et al.*, 1976). After challenge with particulate antigen, using for instance *Aeromonas salmonicida*, specific fluorescence occurs in individual pyroninophilic cells scattered throughout the pronephric parenchyma (Secombes and Manning, 1980, 1982). After a second challenge with a soluble antigen such as human gamma globulin (HGG), the pronephros of *Cyprinus carpio* shows clusters of pyroninophilic cells that will trans- form eventually into areas which contain melanin (Secombes *et al.*, 1981). Thus antigen trapping appears to be more intra- than extracellular and direct relationships with Ig deposition cannot always be demonstrated.

The Liver and Pronephros in Amphibians

Amphibians without a functioning blood-forming bone marrow show active lymphohemopoiesis in the liver and kidney, principally during embryonic and larval life. In some primitive urodele species, such as the giant Japanese salamander, the meningeal region has been claimed to be a site of lymphopoiesis

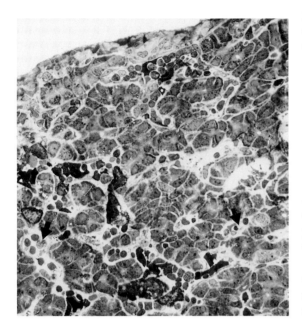

Figure 3.23 Lymphoid cells (see arrows) between hepatocytes in the liver of the apodan caecilian, *Ichthyophis kohtaoensis* (× 240). (From *Acta Zool Stockh* **63**: 11, 1982, reproduced by permission.)

(Cowden and Dyer, 1971). In adult Apoda (Figure 3.23) and Urodela lymphohemopoietic aggregates occur in the liver, scattered throughout the hepatic parenchyma (Figure 3.23) or they form a more or less continuous perihepatic layer. In these areas, developing and mature granulocytes, mainly neutrophils and eosinophils, as well as lymphocytes and plasma cells, are arranged between fibroblasts and bundles of collagenous fibers (Figure 3.24).

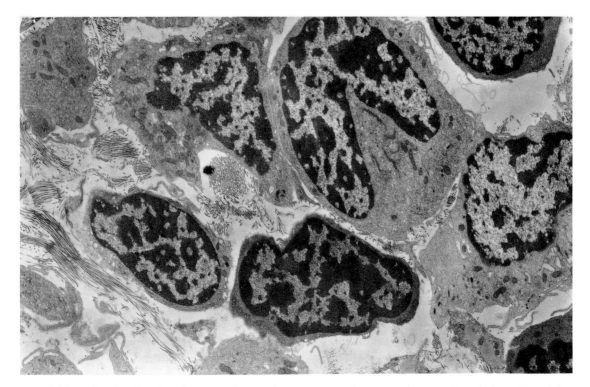

Figure 3.24 Small and medium lymphocytes and promyelocytes arranged between collagenous fibers in the perihepatic layer of *Pleurodeles waltlii* (× 2385).

The importance of the urodelan liver in the immune process was first pointed out by Cohen (1971), who demonstrated its capacity for immunosuppressive activity against allografts. Moreover, the injection of horse erythrocytes (HRBC) into neotenous adult *Ambystoma mexicanum* induces the appearance of specific rosette-forming cells (RFC) in the liver (Tahan and Jurd, 1981). Numerous developing and mature plasma cells have also been observed in the perihepatic layer of salamanders (Henry and Charlemagne, 1977; Zapata *et al.*, 1979), although antigenic stimulation resulted in no significant increase in their numbers (Henry and Charlemagne, 1977). Thus, the liver of urodeles and to some extent that of apodans has been considered equivalent to the avian bursa of Fabricius (Henry and Charlemagne, 1977) or to the mammalian bone marrow (Zapata *et al.*, 1979).

In some anurans, as in urodeles and apodans, lymphoid accumulations can also occur in the liver, mainly during embryonic and larval life and in the most primitive groups such as *Xenopus laevis* (Manning and Horton, 1969; Hadji-Azimi and Fischberg, 1967). The liver of *Xenopus laevis* is the site for development of B-cell lineages (Hadji-Azimi *et al.*, 1982). Surface cytoplasmic markers have aided in more precise identifications, for example cIg$^+$ sIg$^-$ pre-B-cells appear for the first time in the developmental stage 46, rise to a maximum level at stage 49, and begin to decrease in the liver at the same time as similar cells emerge in the spleen.

Adult embryonic and larval kidneys (pronephros and mesonephros) seem to be a source of lymphocytes and granulocytes in various urodeles (Figure 3.25) and anuran amphibians; these organs can participate in immune responses. Rosette-forming cells (RFC) occur in the kidney of *Nothopthalmus viridescens* after immunization with foreign erythrocytes, a process that can be induced *in situ* since RFC numbers are unaffected after splenectomy (Ruben *et al.*, 1973). A role for the kidney has also been suggested in apodans (Cooper, 1976). Extensive lymphohemopoietic tissue appears in the intertubular regions of the pronephros and mesonephros during larval life of *Rana pipiens* (Horton, 1971), *Alytes obstetricans* (du Pasquier, 1968) and *Rana perezi* (Zapata, unpublished), but not in *Xenopus laevis* (Manning and Horton, 1969).

Injections of antigens mixed with complete

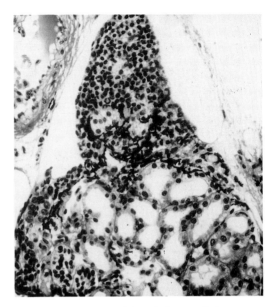

Figure 3.25 Presence of lymphohemopoietic aggregates between the renal tubules of an adult *Pleurodeles waltlii* ($\times$ 80).

Freund's adjuvant into *Bufo marinus* induce a considerable immune response in the lymphohemopoietic tissue of the kidney (Evans *et al.*, 1966; Cowden *et al.*, 1968a, b; Cowden and Dyer, 1971), but similar responses were not observed in *Rana pipiens* immunized with *Aeromonas hydrophila* (Cowden and Dyer, 1971). To localize the antigen, carbon particles and various antigenic materials have been traced to intertubular lymphohemopoietic areas where they appear in association with scattered or small groups of cells (Diener and Nossal, 1966; Turner, 1969, 1970). Turner (1973) explains the route in the following way: antigen may reach the kidney by the circulation or by means of entrapment in mobile macrophages; it is then phagocytosed by the renal tubular cells (Turner, 1969).

Pronephros and mesonephros later become loci for granulopoiesis (perhaps also for lymphopoiesis) in embryonic *Rana pipiens* (Carpenter and Turpen, 1979). Hemopoietic precursors form the lateral plate mesoderm migrate interstitially to those organs, and differentiate into blood cells under the possible influence of local cell microenvironments (Turpen and Knudson, 1980). Moreover, B-cell generation seems to occur within larval kidneys of *Rana pipiens* during premetamorphic stages (Zettergren *et al.*, 1980). During that phase and later during stage II, sIgM⁻ cIgM⁺ cells occur in the pronephros and mesonephros. During premetamorphosis, these cells are more abundant in the kidney than in any other sites. The pre-B-cells develop also sIgM⁺ lymphocytes by the time young *Rana pipiens* begin to feed. sIgM⁺ lymphocytes seem to be precursors for sIgM⁺ sIgG⁺ B-lymphocytes. Finally, sIgM⁻ cIgG⁺ B-lymphocytes appear to be more prominent in ontogeny than during later stages.

FINAL COMMENT

Almost all terrestrial vertebrates possess hemopoietic bone marrow. Beginning with amphibians, this specialized site of hemocytopoiesis becomes more and more differentiated during evolution. The obvious questions that arise are: why only terrestrial vertebrates? why inside bone marrow compartments? One simplistic interpretation is related to the tetrapod condition and the development of long, hollow bones. However, this does not explain the presence of bone marrow or its equivalents in sites other than these long bones. There is also no explanation for the absence of marrow in fish and other lower forms where abundant osteological organization occurs. Hemopoietic bone marrow-like microenvironments are well developed in Osteichthyes, Chondrichthyes and Cyclostomata, located in organs such as the esophageal wall, kidneys, supraneural organs, spleen, Leydig organ and liver. However, adult amphibians and all higher forms show a shift in such hemopoietic sites with increased development of bone marrow. Whatever the condition, probably due to the external and internal environments, all vertebrates possess sites where stem cells and blood cells, including immunocompetent cells, are generated. These immunocytes circulate freely within the blood and lymph, gaining access to tissue spaces and organs of the immune system where they can generate immune responses after specific stimulation via antigen − receptor interactions.

REFERENCES

Al-Adhami MA and Kunz YW (1976). Haemopoietic centres in the developing angelfish *Pterophyllum scalare* (Curier and Valenciennes). *Wilheim Roux's Arch* **179**: 393−401.

Anderson DP (1978). Passive hemolytic plaque assay as a means for detecting antibody producing cells in rainbow trout immunized with the O-antigen of enteric redmouth bacteria. Doctoral thesis, University of Maryland.

Ardavin CF and Zapata A (1987). Ultrastructure and changes during metamorphosis of the lympho-hemopoietic tissue of the larval anadromous sea lamprey *Petromyzon marinus*. *Dev Comp Immunol* **11**: 79−93.

Ardavin CF and Zapata A (1988). Lymphoid components in the branchial cavernous body of the ammocoete of *Petromyzon marinus*. *Acta Zool Stockh* **69**: 23−28.

Ardavin CF, Gomariz RP, Barrutia MG, Fonfria J and Zapata A (1984). The lympho-hemopoietic organs of the anadromous sea lamprey *Petromyzon marinus*. A comparative study throughout its life span. *Acta Zool Stockh* **65**: 1−15.

Biermann A and Graf von Keyserlingk D (1978). Ultrastructure of reticulum cells in the bone marrow. *Acta Anat* **110**: 34−43.

Campbell F (1967). Fine structure of the bone marrow of the chicken and pigeon. *J Morph* **123**: 405−440.

Campbell F (1970). Ultrastructure of the bone marrow of the frog. *Am J Anat* **129**: 329−356.

Campbell F (1972). Ultrastructural analysis of transmural migration of blood cells in the bone marrow of rats, mice, and guinea pigs. *Am J Anat* **135**: 521−536.

Carpenter KL and Turner JB (1979). Experimental studies on hemopoiesis in the pronephros of *Rana pipiens*. *Differentiation* **14**: 167−174.

Caspi RR and Avtalion RR (1984). Evidence for the existence of an Il-2 like lymphocyte growth promoting factor in a bony fish *Cyprinus carpio*. *Dev Comp Immunol* **8**: 51−60.

Chen LT and Weiss L (1975). The development of vertebral bone marrow of human fetuses. *Blood* **46**: 389−408.

Chiller JM, Hodgins HO and Weiser RS (1969). Antibody response in rainbow trout *Salmo gairdneri*. II. Studies of the kinetics of development of antibody-producing cells and on complement and natural hemolysin. *J Immunol* **102**: 1202−1207.

Citterio V (1931). Capacita eritropoietica dell'endotelio cardiaco nella larva di *Chimaera monstrosa*. *Monit Zool Ital* **42**: 184−289.

Claridge PN and Potter IC (1974)). Heart ratios at different stages in the life cycle of lampreys. *Acta Zool Stockh* **55**: 61−69.

Cohen N (1971). Amphibian transplantation reactions: a review. *Am Zool* **11**: 193−205.

Cooper EL (1976). Immunity mechanisms. In Lofts B (Ed), *Physiology of the Amphibia*. Vol III. Academic Press: New York. pp 163−272.

Cooper EL and Schaefer DW (1970). Bone marrow restoration of transplantation immunity in the leopard frog *Rana pipiens. Proc Soc Exp Biol Med* **135**: 406−411.

Cowden RR and Dyer RF (1971). Lymphopoietic tissue and plasma cells in amphibians. *Am Zool* **11**: 183−192.

Cowden RR, Dyer RF, Gebhardt BM and Volpe EP (1968a). Amphibian plasma cells. *J Immunol* **100**: 1293−1295.

Cowden RR, Gebhardt BM and Volpe EP (1968b). The histophysiology of antibody forming sites in the marine toad. *Z Zellforsch* **85**: 196−205.

Cuchens MA and Clem LW (1977). Phylogeny of lymphocyte heterogeneity. II. Differential effects of temperature on fish T-like and B-like cells. *Cell Immunol* **34**: 219−227.

Cuchens M, McLean E and Clem LW (1976). Lymphocyte heterogeneity in fish and reptiles. In Wright RK and Cooper EL (Eds), *Phylogeny of Thymus and Bone Marrow—Bursa Cells*. Elsevier/North-Holland Biomedical Press: Amsterdam. pp 205−213.

Curtis SK, Cowden RR and Knagel JW (1979). Ultrastructure of the bone marrow of the salamander *Plethodon glutinosus* (Caudata: Plethodontidae). *J Morph* **123**: 405−440.

DeBruyn PP, Michelson S and Thomas TB (1971). The migration of blood cells of the bone marrow through the sinusoidal wall. *J Morph* **133**: 417−437.

Dexter TM (1981). Self-renewing haemopoietic progenitor cells and the factors controlling proliferation and differentiation. In *Microenvironments in Haemopoietic and Lymphoid Differentiation, Ciba Foundation Symposium 84*. Pitman: London. pp 22−37.

Diener E and Nossal GJ (1966). Phylogenetic studies on the immune response in the toad *Bufo marinus. Immunology* **10**: 535−541.

Du Pasquier L (1968). Les proteines seriques et le complex lymphomyeloide chez le tetard d'*Alytes obstetricans* normal et thymectomise. *Ann Inst Pasteur* **114**: 490−502.

Eipert EF, Wright RK and Cooper EL (1977). Comparison of spleen and bone marrow mitogen responses in *Rana catesbeiana* (Abstract). *Am Zool* **17**: 892.

Eipert EF, Klempau AE, Lallone RL and Cooper EL (1979). Bone marrow antibody synthesis in *Rana. Cell Immunol* **46**: 275−280.

Ellis AE (1977). Ontogeny of the immune response in *Salmo salar*. Histogenesis of the lymphoid organs and appearance of membrane immunoglobulin and mixed leukocyte reactivity. In Solomon JB and Hortons JD (Eds), *Developmental Immunobiology*. Elsevier/North Holland Biomedical Press: Amsterdam. pp 225−231.

Ellis AE (1980). Antigen trapping in the spleen and kidney of the plaice *Pleuronectes platessa. J Fish Dis* **3**: 413−426.

Ellis AE and de Sousa M (1974). Phylogeny of the lymphoid system. I. A study of the fate of circulating lymphocytes in plaice. *Eur J Immunol* **4**: 338−343.

Ellis AE, Monroe ALS and Roberts RJ (1976). Defense mechanisms in fish. I. A study of the phagocytic system and the fate of intraperitoneally injected particulate material in the plaice *Pleuronectes platessa. J Fish Biol* **8**: 67−78.

Etlinger HM, Hodgins HO and Chiller JM (1976). Evolution of the lymphoid system. I. Evidence for lymphocyte heterogeneity in rainbow trout revealed by the organ distribution of mitogenic responses. *J Immunol* **116**: 1547−1553.

Etlinger HM, Hodgins HO and Chiller JM (1977). Evolution of the lymphoid system. II. Evidence for immunoglobulin determinants on all rainbow trout lymphocytes and demonstration of mixed leukocyte reaction. *Eur J Immunol* **7**: 881−887.

Evans DL, Graves SS, Cobb D and Dawe DL (1984). Nonspecific cytotoxic cells in fish *Ictalurus punctatus*. II. Parameters of target cell lysis and specificity. *Dev Comp Immunol* **8**: 303−312.

Evans EE, Kent SP, Bryant RE and Moyer M (1966). Antibody formation and immunological memory in the marine toad. In Smith R, Miescher P and Good RA (Eds), *Phylogeny of Immunity*. University of Florida Press: Gainesville. pp 218−226.

Fahrenholz C (1929). Eine rachendach hypophyse bei *Chimaera monstrosa. Anat Anz* **66**: 342−348.

Fange R (1963). Structure and function of the excretory organs of myxinoids. In Brodal A and Fange R (Eds), *The Biology of Myxine*. Universtetsforlaget: Oslo. pp 516−529.

Fange R (1966). Comparative aspects of excretory and lymphoid tissue. In Smith RT, Miescher PA and Good RA (Eds), *Phylogeny of Immunity*. University of Florida Press: Gainesville. pp 140−145.

Fange R (1982). A comparative study of lymphomyeloid tissue in fish. *Dev Comp Immunol* Suppl **2**: 22−33.

Fange R and Johansson-Sjobek M-L (1975). The effect of splenectomy on the haematology and on the activity of 6-amino-levulinic acid dehydratase (ALA-D) in hemopoietic tissues of the dogfish *Scyliorhinus canicula* (Elasmobranchii). *Comp Biochem Physiol* **52A**: 577−580.

Fange R and Mattisson A (1981). The lymphomyeloid (hemopoietic) system of the Atlantic nurse shark *Ginglymostoma cirratum. Biol Bull* **160**: 240−249.

Fange R and Pulsford A (1983). Structural studies on lymphomyeloid tissues in the dogfish *Scyliorhinus canicula* L. *Cell Tissue Res* **230**: 337−351.

Fange R and Sundell G (1969). Lymphomyeloid tissues, blood cells and plasma proteins in *Chimaera monstrosa* (Pisces, Holocephali). *Acta Zool* **50**: 155−168.

Finstad J and Good RA (1964). Evolution of the immune response. III. Immunologic responses in the lamprey. *J Exp Med* **120**: 1151−1168.

Finstad J, Papermaster B and Good RA (1964). Evolution of the immune responses. II. Morphologic studies on the origin of the thymus and organized lymphoid tissue. *Lab Invest* **13**: 490−512.

Fujii T (1981). Antibody-enhanced phagocytosis of lamprey polymorphonuclear leucocytes against sheep erythrocytes. *Cell Tissue Res* **219**: 41−51.

Fujii T (1982). Electron microscopy of the leucocytes of the typhlosole in ammocoetes with special attention to the antibody producing cells. *J Morph* **173**: 87−100.

Fujii T, Nakagawa H and Murakawa S (1979). Immunity in lamprey. II. Antigen-binding responses to sheep erythrocytes and hapten in the ammocoete. *Dev Comp Immunol* **3**: 609−620.

Fujita T (1963). Uber das zwischenhirn-hypophysensystem von *Chimaera monstrosa*. *Zeitschr F Zellforsch* **60**: 147−162.

Good RA, Finstad J, Pollara B and Gabrielsen AE (1966). Morphological studies on the evolution of the lymphoid tissues among the lower vertebrates. In Smith RT, Miescher PA and Good RA (Eds), *Phylogeny of Immunity*. University of Florida Press: Gainesville. pp 149−167.

Grace MF and Manning MJ (1980). Histogenesis of the lymphoid organs in rainbow trout *Salmo gairdneri* Rich. 1836. *Dev Comp Immunol* **4**: 255−264.

Graves SS, Evans DL, Cobb D and Dawe DL (1984). Non-specific cytotoxic cells in fish *Ictalurus punctatus*. I. Optimum requirements for target cell lysis. *Dev Comp Immunol* **8**: 293−302.

Green N and Cohen N (1979). Phylogeny of immunocompetent cells. III. Mitogen response characteristics of lymphocyte subpopulations from normal and thymectomized frogs *Xenopus laevis*. *Cell Immunol* **48**: 59−70.

Grodzinski Z (1926). Uber das blutgefass-system von *Myxine glutinosa* L. *Bull Acad Pol Sci Cl Sci Math Nat Ser B*. 123−125.

Hadji-Azimi I and Fischberg M (1967). Hematopoiese perihepatique chez le batracien anoure *Xenopus laevis*. Comparaison entre les individus normaux et les porteurs de tumeurs lymphoides. *Rev Suisse Zool* **74**: 642−647.

Hadji-Azimi I, Schwager J, Thiebard CH and Perrenot N (1982). B-Lymphocyte differentiation in *Xenopus laevis* larvae. *Dev Biol* **90**: 253−258.

Hagen M, Filosa MF and Youson JH (1983). Immunocytochemical localization of antibody-producing cells in adult lamprey. *Immunol Letters* **6**: 87−92.

Hardisty MW and Potter IC (1971a). The behavior, ecology and growth of larval lampreys. In Hardisty MW and Potter IC (Eds), *The Biology of Lampreys*. Vol I. Academic Press: London. pp 85−125.

Hardisty MW and Potter IC (1971b). The general biology of adult lampreys. In Hardisty MW and Potter IC (Eds), *The Biology of Lampreys*. Vol I. Academic Press: London. pp 127−206.

Henry M and Charlemagne J (1977). Plasmacytic series in the perihepatic layer of the urodele amphibian *Pleurodeles walthi* Michah (Salamandridae). *Dev Comp Immunol* **1**: 23−32.

Holmgren N (1942). Studies on the head of fishes. An embryological, morphological and phylogenetical study. *Acta Zool Stockh* **23**: 129−261.

Holmgren N (1950). On the pronephros and the blood in *Myxine glutinosa*. *Acta Zool Stockh* **31**: 233−348.

Horton JD (1971). Ontogeny of the immune system in amphibians. *Am Zool* **11**: 219−228.

Hoshi H and Weiss L (1978). Rabbit bone marrow after administration of saponin. An electron microscopic study. *Lab Invest* **38**: 67−80.

Idler DR and Burton MP (1976). The pronephros as the site of presumptive interrenal cells in the hagfish *Myxine glutinosa* L. *Comp Biochem Physiol* **53A**: 73−77.

Jacobshagen E (1915). Zur morphologie des spiraldarms. *Anat Anz* **498**: 220−235.

Jordan HE (1938). Comparative hematology. In Downey H (Ed), *Handbook of Hematology*. Vol II. Paul B Hocker: New York. pp 700−862.

Jordan HE and Speidel CC (1930). Blood formation in cyclostomes. *Am J Anat* **46**: 355−391.

Jordan HE and Speidel CC (1931). Blood formation on the African lungfish, under normal conditions and under conditions of prolonged estivation and recovery. *J Morphol Physiol* **51**: 319−371.

Kilarski W and Plytycz B (1981). The presence of plasma cells in the lamprey (Agnatha). *Dev Comp Immunol* **5**: 361−366.

Kolmer W (1923). Uber das vorkommen eines knochenmarkahnlichen gewebes bei einem selachier (Knorpelmark bei *Chimaera monstrosa*). *Anat Anaz* **56**: 529−534.

Leach WJ (1951). The hypophysis of lampreys in relation to the nasal apparatus. *J Morphol* **189**: 217−246.

Le Douarin N (1966). L'hematopoiese dans les formes embryonnaires et jeunes des vertebres. *L'Annee Biol* **5**: 105−171.

Leydig F (1851). Zur anatomie und histologie der *Chimaera monstrosa*. *Mullers Arch Anat Physiol* **10**: 241−272.

Leydig F (1857). Von blut und der lymphe der wirbelthiere. In *Jahrbuch der Histologie des Menschen und der Thiere*. Meidinger Sohn: Frankfurt am Main. pp 448−450.

Lucas AM and Jamroz C (1961). Atlas of avian hematology. Agri. Monograph No. 25. US Dept Agriculture: Washington.

Manning MJ (1981). The evolution of vertebrate lymphoid organs. In Solomon JB (Ed), *Aspects of Developmental and Comparative Immunology I*. Pergamon Press: Oxford. pp 67−72.

Manning MJ (1984). Phylogenetic origins and ontogenetic development of immonocompetent cells in fish. In Cooper EL and Wright RK (Eds), *Aspects of Developmental and Comparative Immunology II. Dev Comp Immunol* Suppl **3**: 61−68.

Manning MJ and Horton JD (1969). Histogenesis of lymphoid organs in larvae of the South African clawed toad, *Xenopus laevis* (Daudin). *J Embryol Exp Morphol* **22**: 265−277.

Matthews LH (1950). Reproduction in the basking shark *Cetorhinus maximus*. *Phil Trans R Soc London (B)* **234**: 247−315.

Mattisson A and Fange R (1982). The cellular structure of

the Leydig organ in the shark *Etmopterus spinax* L. *Biol Bull* **162**: 182−194.

Maximow A (1910). Untersuchungen uber blut und bindegewebe III. Die embryonale histogenese des knochenmarks der sauge tiere. *Arch Mikr Anat Entwgesch Bd* **76**: S 1−113.

McKinney EC, Ortiz G, Lee JC, Sigel MM, Lopez DM, Epstein RS and McLeod TF (1976). Lymphocytes of fish: multipotential or specialized?. In Wright RK and Cooper EL (Eds), *Phylogeny of Thymus and Bone Marrow— Bursa cells*. Elsevier/North-Holland Biomedical Press: Amsterdam. pp 73−82.

Mimura OM and Mimura I (1977). Timo de *Lepidosiren paradoxa* (Fitz, 1836). Peize dipnoico. *Bol Fisiol Anim Univ S Paulo* **1**: 29−38.

Minigawa Y, Ohnishi K and Murakawa A (1975). Structure and immunological function of lymphomyeloid organs in the bullfrog *Rana catesbeiana*. In Hildemann WH and Benedict AA (Eds), *Immunological Phylogeny*. Plenum Press: London. pp 257−266.

Neale NL and Chavin W (1971). Lymphocytic tissue alterations during the primary immune response of the goldfish *Carassius auratus*. *Mich Acad* **3**: 21−30.

Ooi EC and Youson JH (1979). Regression of the larval opisthonephros during metamorphosis of the sea lamprey *Petromyzon marinus* L. *Am J Anat* **154**: 57−59.

Page M and Rowley AF (1984). The reticulo-endothelial system of the adult river lamprey, *Lampetra fluviatilis* L.: the fate of intravascularly injected colloidal carbon. *J Fish Dis* **7**: 339−353.

Percy Lord R and Potter IC (1976). Blood cell formation in the river lamprey *Lampetra fluviatilis*. *J Zool Lond* **178**: 319−340.

Percy Lord R and Potter IC (1977). Changes in haemopoietic sites during metamorphosis of the lampreys *Lampetra fluviatilis* and *Lampetra plameri*. *J Zool Lond* **183**: 111−123.

Percy Lord R and Potter IC (1979). The intestinal blood circulation in the river lamprey *Lampetra fluviatilis*. *J Zool Lond* **187**: 415−431.

Pontius H and Ambrosius H (1971). Lymphozytares system und immunantwort bei niederen wirbeltieren. *Folia Haematol* **96**: 333−341.

Potter IC and Huggins RJ (1973). Observations on the morphology, behavior and salinity tolerance of downstream migrating river lampreys (*Lampetra fluviatilis*). *J Zool Lond* **169**: 365−379.

Price GC (1910). The structure and function of the adult head kidney of *Bdellostoma stouti*. *J Exp Zool* **9**: 848−864.

Raison RL and Hildemann WH (1984). The unique structure and cell surface expression of immunoglobulin in the Pacific hagfish. In Cooper EL and Wright RK (Eds), *Aspects of Developmental and Comparative Immunology II*. *Dev Comp Immunol* Suppl 3: 157 (Abstract).

Raison RL, Hull CJ and Hildemann WH (1978). Production and specificity of antibodies to streptococci in the Pacific lagfish *Eptatretus stoutii*. *Dev Comp Immunol* **2**: 253−262.

Romer AS (1971). *The Vertebrate Body*. Saunders: Philadelphia.

Ruben LN, van der Hoven A and Dutton RW (1973). Cellular cooperation in hapten-carrier responses in the newt *Triturus viridescens*. *Cell Immunol* **6**: 300−314.

Ruben LN, Warr GW, Decker JM and Marchalonis JJ (1977). Phylogenetic origins of immune recognition: Lymphoid heterogeneity and the hapten/carrier effect in goldfish *Carassius auratus*. *Cell Immunol* **31**: 266−283.

Saliendri K and Muthukkaruppan VR (1975a). Morphology of lymphoid organs in a cichlid teleost *Tilapia mossambica* (Peters). *J Morphol* **147**: 109−122.

Sailendri K and Muthukkruppan VR (1975b). The immune response of the teleost *Tilapia mossambica* to soluble and cellular antigens. *J Exp Zool* **191**: 79−92.

Secombes CJ and Manning MJ (1980). Comparative studies on the immune system of fishes and amphibians: antigen localization in the carp *Cyprinus carpio* L. *J Fish Dis* **3**: 399−412.

Secombes CJ and Manning MJ (1982). Histological changes in lymphoid organs of carp following injection of soluble or particulate antigens. *Dev Comp Immunol* Suppl **2**: 53−58.

Secombes CJ, Manning MJ and Ellis AE (1981). Antigen trapping in the carp *Cyprinus carpio*. In Solomon JB (Ed), *Aspects of Developmental and Comparative Immunology I*. Pergamon Press, Oxford. pp 465−466.

Smith AM, Potter M and Merchant EB (1967). Antibody-forming cells in the pronephros of the teleost *Lepomis macrochirus*. *J Immunol* **99**: 876−882.

Smith AM, Wivel NA and Potter M (1970). Plasmacytosis in the pronephros of the carp *Cyprinus carpio*. *Anat Rec* **167**: 351−370.

Stanley HP (1963). Urogenital morphology in the chimaeroid fish *Hydrolagus colliei* (Lay and Bennett). *J Morphol* **112**: 99−128.

Sterba G (1962). Die neunagen (Petromyzontidae). *Handb Binnenfish Mitteleur* **3B**: 263−352.

Tahan AM and Jurd RD (1981). Antigen trapping in *Ambystoma mexicanum*: role of secondary lymphoid organs. *Dev Comp Immunol* **5**: 219−300.

Taliaferro WH and Taliaferro LG (1955). Reactions of the connective tissue in chickens to *Plasmodium gallinaceum* and *Plasmodium lophurae*. I. Histopathology during initial infections and superinfections. *J Infect Dis* **97**: 99−136.

Tam MR, Reddy AL, Karp RD and Hildemann WH (1977). Phylogeny of cellular immunity among vertebrates. In Marchalonis JJ (Ed), *Comparative Immunology*. Blackwell, Oxford. pp 98−119.

Tanaka Y (1976). Architecture of the marrow vasculature in three amphibian species and its significance in hematopoietic development. *Am J Anat* **145**: 485−498.

Tanaka Y, Saito Y and Gotoh H (1981). Vascular architecture and intestinal hematopoietic nests of two cyclostomes, *Eptatretus burgeri* and ammocoetes of

Entosphenus reissneri: A comparative morphological study. *J Morph* **170**: 71−93.

Tavassoli M (1977). Adaptation of marrow sinus wall to fluctuation in the rate of cell delivery: studies in rabbits after blood letting. *Br J Haematol* **35**: 25−32.

Tavassoli M and Shaklai M (1979). Absence of tight junction in endothelium of marrow sinuses: possible significance for marrow cell egress. *Br J Haematol* **41**: 303−307.

Thoenes GH and Hildemann WH (1969). Immunological responses of Pacific hagfish. II. Serum antibody production to soluble antigen. In Sterzl J and Riha J (Eds), *Developmental Aspects of Antibody Formation and Structure*. Czechoslovakian Academy of Sciences: Prague. pp 711−722.

Thompson A (1971). Quantitative and cytological studies on the adenohypophysis of *Lampetra planeri* and *Lampetra fluviatilis* with special reference to metamorphosis. MSc Thesis. Bath University.

Tomonaga S, Hirokane T, Shinohara H and Awaya K (1973). The primitive spleen of the hagfish. *Zool Mag* **82**: 215−217.

Tomonaga S, Kobayashi K, Kajii T and Awaya K (1984). Two populations of immunoglobulin-forming cells in the skate *Raja kenojei*: their distribution and characterization. *Dev Comp Immunol* **8**: 803−812.

Turner RJ (1969). The functional development of the reticulo-endothelial system in the toad *Xenopus laevis* (Daudin). *J Exp Zool* **170**: 467−480.

Turner RJ (1970). The influence of colloidal carbon on hemagglutinin production in the toad *Xenopus laevis*. *J Ret Soc* **8**: 434−445.

Turner RJ (1973). Response of the toad *Xenopus laevis* to circulating antigens. I. Responses after splenectomy. *J Exp Zool* **183**: 35−46.

Turpen JB and Knudson CM (1982). Ontogeny of hemopoietic cells in *Rana pipiens*: Precursor cell migration during embryogenesis. *Dev Biol* **89**: 138−151.

Warr GW and Marchalonis JJ (1977). Lymphocyte surface immunoglobulin of the goldfish differs from its serum counterpart. *Dev Comp Immunol* **1**: 15−22.

Weiss L (1965). The structure of bone marrow. Functional interrelationships of vascular and hematopoietic compartments in experimental hemolytic anemia: An electron microscopic study. *J Morph* **117**: 467−537.

Weiss L (1981). Haemopoiesis in mammalian bone marrow. In *Microenvironments in Haematopoietic and Lymphoid Differentiation*. Ciba Foundation Symposium 84. Pitman: London. pp 5−21.

Weiss L and Greep RD (1977). *Histology*. McGraw-Hill: New York.

Westen H and Bainton DF (1979). Association of alkaline-phosphatase-positive reticulum cells in bone marrow with granulocytic precursors. *J Exp Med* **150**: 919−937.

Willmer EN (1960). *Cytology and Evolution*. Academic Press: New York.

Wright GM and Youson JH (1976). Transformation of the endostyle of the anadromous sea lamprey *Petromyzon marinus* L. during metamorphosis. I. Light microscopy and autoradiography with ^{125}I. *Gen Comp Endocrinol* **30**: 243−257.

Youson JH (1980). Morphology and physiology of lamprey metamorphosis. *Can J Fish Aquat Sci* **37**: 1687−1710.

Youson JH and Connely KL (1978). Development of longitudinal mucosal folds in the intestine of the anadromous sea lamprey *Petromyzon marinus* L. during metamorphosis. *Can J Zool* **56**: 2364−2371.

Youson JH and Horbert WR (1982). Transformation of the intestinal epithelium of the larval anadromous sea lamprey *Petromyzon marinus* during metamorphosis. *J Morphol* **171**: 89−117.

Youson JH and Ooi EC (1979). Development of the renal corpuscle during metamorphosis in the lamprey. *Am J Anat* **155**: 201−222.

Youson JH and Potter IC (1979). A description of the stages in the metamorphosis of the anadromous sea lamprey *Petromyzon marinus* L. *Can J Zool* **57**: 1808−1817.

Zapata A (1979). Ultrastructural study of the teleost fish kidney. *Dev Comp Immunol* **3**: 55−65.

Zapata A (1981a). Ultrastructure of elasmobranch lymphoid tissue. II. Leydig's and epigonal organs. *Dev Comp Immunol* **5**: 43−52.

Zapata A (1981b). Lymphoid organs of teleost fish. II. Ultrastructure of renal lymphoid tissue of *Rutilus rutilus* and *Gobio gobio*. *Dev Comp Immunol* **5**: 685−690.

Zapata A, Villena A and san Miguel R (1979). Estudio ultra-structural de los microambientes hematopoieticos de *Pleurodeles waltlii*. *Morf Norm Pathol Sec A* **31**: 445−456.

Zapata A, Leceta J and Villena A (1981a). Ultrastructure of reptilian bone marrow: A study in the Spanish lizard *Lacerta hispanica*. *J Morph* **168**: 137−149.

Zapata A, Ardavin CF, Gomariz RP and Leceta J (1981b). Plasma cells in the ammocoete of *Petromyzon marinus*. *Cell Tissue Res* **221**: 203−208.

Zapata A, Fange A, Mattisson A and Villena A (1984). Plasma cells in adult Atlantic hagfish *Myxine glutinosa*. *Cell Tissue Res* **235**: 691−693.

Zettergren LD, Kubagawa H and Cooper MD (1980). Development of B cells in *Rana pipiens*. In Manning MJ (Ed), *Phylogeny of Immunological Memory*. Elsevier/North-Holland Biomedical Press: Amsterdam. pp 117−186.

4

The Bursa of Fabricius

INTRODUCTION

The bursa of Fabricius, a lymphoepithelial organ unique in birds, located in the distal side of the cloaca, was first described by Leydig in 1857. Its immunological role was firmly established after Glick and his coworkers demonstrated a deficiency in antibody formation in chickens whose bursa had been removed at or prior to hatching (Chang et al., 1955; Glick et al., 1956). More recent discussions have, however, assigned the bursa's role in initiating B-cell development. Actually the bursa seems to function as a central or peripheral lymphoid organ during distinct life stages. During embryonic periods and the first few weeks post-hatching, the bursa is a central organ involved in the generation of immunological diversity (Toivanen et al., 1987; Weill and Reynaud, 1987). After seeding immunocompetent cells to peripheral lymphoid organs, i.e spleen, primitive lymph nodes, cecal tonsils, Harderian glands, etc., the bursa functions as a peripheral lymphoid organ for local antibody production (Kincade and Cooper, 1971; Toivanen et al., 1972a, b, c; van Alten and Meuwissen, 1972; Waltenbaugh and van Alten, 1974; Sorvari and Sorvari, 1977). In perianum-stimulated chickens the major immune response is elicited in the bursa, whereas the spleen is the main site where responses to intravenously administered antigens occur (Naukkarinen, 1982). On the dorsal surface of the bursa near its duct, there is a diffusely infiltrated area, the so-called DIA (Odend'hal and Breazile, 1979a, b), which is filled with lymphocytes. Most lymphocytes are probably T-derived cells which do not actually appear until immediately after hatching (Odend'hal and Breazile, 1980). After this productive period, the bursa finally undergoes involution (Glick, 1977), gradually losing its lymphoid structure at 15–24 weeks (Naukkarinen and Sorvari, 1984) and disappearing completely in chickens at 6–12 months of age (Glick, 1960). In addition to morphology, histology and functional development of B-cells, a good deal of this chapter will focus on developmental changes. In fact, without this discovery all of immunology, not just comparative immunology, might have been detained and not developed as one of the pre-eminent fields it is today.

ANATOMY

The bursa of most birds is an appendix of the proctodeum which lies dorsally to the urodeum. It is connected to the cloacal proctodeum by a short stalk (Figure 4.1(a)) which may be lacking in some species, e.g. the ostrich (Grimpe, 1930). Although structural and functional immunological studies on the bursa have been mainly performed in *Gallus domesticus* (see review by Glick, 1982), it has been analyzed both anatomically and histologically in several groups of birds: Struthioniformes (Forbes, 1877; von Rautenfeld and Budras, 1982); Rheiformes and Cavaniformes (von Rautenfeld and Budras, 1982); Tinamiformes (Forbes, 1877); Pelecaniformes

(Ackerman and Knouff, 1964); Ciconiiformes and Coraciiformes (Dominic, 1962); Anseriformes (Ward and Middleton, 1971; Sugimura *et al.*, 1975); Falconiformes and Strigiformes (Wemckebach, 1888; Jolly, 1915; Mathis, 1938); Caprimulgiformes (Jolly, 1915); and Passeriformes (Glick and Olah, 1982; Fonfria, 1988).

(a)

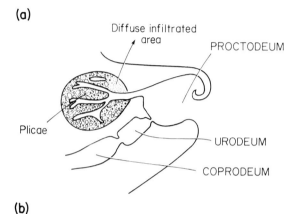

(b)

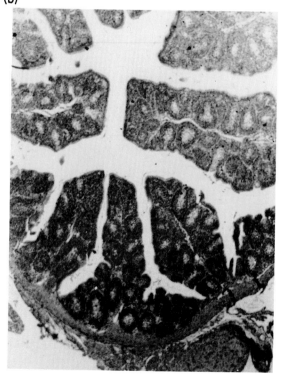

Figure 4.1 (a) Anatomical location of the bursa of Fabricius in the avian cloaca. Note the presence of a diffusely infiltrated lymphoid area in the bursal duct. (b) Histological organization of the bursa in an adult chicken (× 30).

At hatching and during early development, the bursa consists of 12 − 15 internal plicae found in the bursal lumen (Glick, 1979). Within the plicae, there are several lymphoid elements organized into follicles (Figure 4.1(b)). Externally, the bursa is enveloped by a connective tissue framework (Figure 4.2). In a 4-week-old chicken, there is an average of 820 lymphoid follicles in each fold (Olah and Glick, 1978a; Romppanen, 1982). Contrary to the morphology in the majority of avian species, the so-called lobuli bursales in Struthioniformes, including the ostrich, *Struthio camelus australis*, emu, *Dromaius novaehollancliae*, and rhea, *Rhea americana*, are not invaginated into the mucosa but project into the lumen (von Rautenfeld and Budras, 1982). Projecting follicles might represent a primitive condition that has been retained (von Rautenfeld and Budras, 1982) since they have been observed during bursal ontogenesis in *Gallus* (Holbrook *et al.*, 1974; Glick *et al.*, 1977) and *Anas* (Mark, 1944), disappearing in late embryonic development.

Major blood vessels which nourish the bursa are the pudendal arteries and veins and posterior mesenteric vein (Pintea *et al.*, 1967). Lymphatics drain the bursal area (Uyematsu, 1940; Dransfield, 1945; Ekino *et al.*, 1979) although the lymph vessels apparently never enter lymphoid follicles but commence in their immediate exterior (Ekino *et al.*, 1979). The chicken bursa receives its innervation from sympathetic fibers, the pelvic nerve and intestinal nerves that enter the first bursal cloacal ganglion at its anterior pole (Pintea *et al.*, 1967; Cordier, 1969).

HISTOLOGICAL ORGANIZATION

The bursal plicae are covered by a pseudostratified columnar epithelium where two histologically distinguishable regions are differentiated, namely mucus-secreting interfollicular epithelial cells and lymphoid follicle-associated epithelial cells which possess endocytic capabilities. The follicle-associated epithelium passes in towards the inner part of the plicae where they are accompanied by its basement membrane (Figure 4.2). This basement membrane, easily demonstrable by silver impregnation (Figure 4.3) divides the lymphoid follicle into a lightly staining follicular medulla and a dense follicular cortex (Figure 4.2).

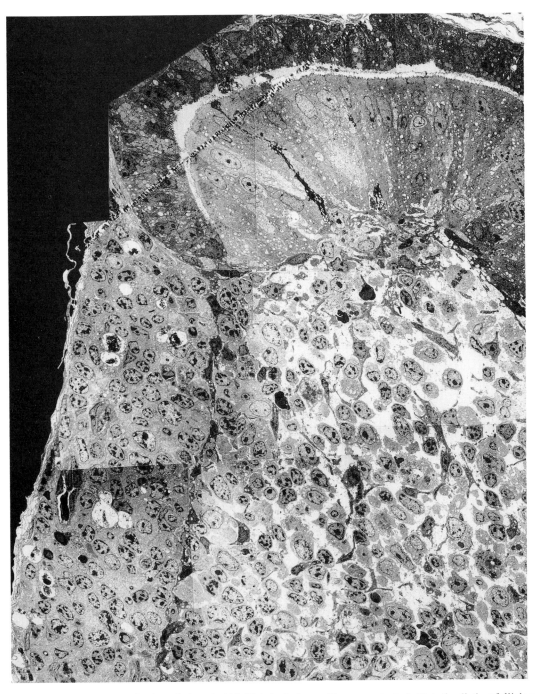

Figure 4.2 Ultrastructural organization of a lymphoid follicle in the bursa (*Sturnus unicolor*). Note the distinct follicle associated epithelium and the epithelial separation between the cortex and medulla (× 1162).

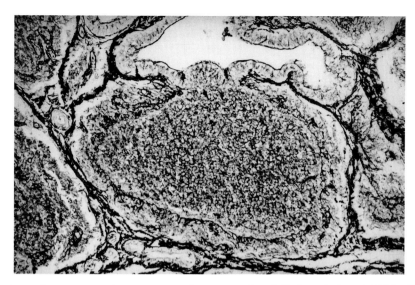

Figure 4.3 A continuous basement membrane separates the cortex and medulla from the bursal follicle (*Sturnus unicolor*). Gomori's silver impregnation (× 190).

The Follicle-associated Epithelium

The follicular epithelium consists of tall, medium to high electron-dense cells with pale, euchromatic nuclei and short microvilli at the apical border (Figure 4.3). They are joined together laterally by desmosomes between them and to the cells of the nearby lining epithelium. In this way, the follicle-associated epithelial cells constitute a continuation of the surface epithelium. Surrounding epithelial cells are in any case clearly distinguishable because they contain light, flocculent material in the apical cytoplasm but pinocytotic capabilities are lacking. In contrast, a myriad of electron-lucent vesicles and vacuoles arranged apically supports the endocytic capacity of the follicle-associated epithelial components (Figure 4.2). In *Sturnus unicolor*, unlike in the chicken, there are numerous tingible body macrophages associated with the follicular epithelium (Figure 4.2). Glick and Olah (1982) reported a similar condition in the bursa of *Sturnus vulgaris*.

The follicle-associated epithelial cells have no basal lamina and are inserted in the discontinuity of the epithelium along the surface of the plicae. Thus, they make contacts at their basal surface with the reticuloepithelial cells which form the supporting network of the follicular medulla (Figure 4.4). Classical reports have maintained that the follicle-associated epithelial components are epithelial in origin, but other data, mainly from Lupetti and coworkers, supported a mesenchymal nature. They have certain characteristics in common with mesenchymal cells which support indirectly the hypothesis that they would be mesenchymal cells with epithelioid features: (1) they appear in the lining epithelium after migration of colony-forming units (Glick, 1977; Naukkarinen *et al.*, 1978); (2) they have no basement membrane (Figure 4.2) (Ackerman and Knouff, 1959; Hodges, 1974); (3) they show high esterase (Schaffner *et al.*, 1974; Ruuskanen *et al.*, 1977) and micropinocytotic activity (Bockman and Cooper, 1973, 1975; Schaffner *et al.*, 1974; Gilmore and Bridges, 1977; Naukkarinen *et al.*, 1978; Lupetti and Dolfi, 1980); (4) like macrophages, the follicle-associated epithelial cells, but not the surrounding epithelial cells, are sensitive to carragenan (Dolfi *et al.*, 1981) and silica (Lupetti *et al.*, 1983); (5) they are in morphological continuity with cells of the centromedullary zone (Figure 4.2) which are mesenchymal in origin (Lupetti and Dolfi, 1982); and finally (6) they show a marked ability to trap India ink (Bockman and Cooper, 1973; Schaffer *et al.*, 1974), ferritin (Bockman and Cooper, 1973), latex particles, thorotrast (Schaffner *et al.*, 1974), horseradish perox-

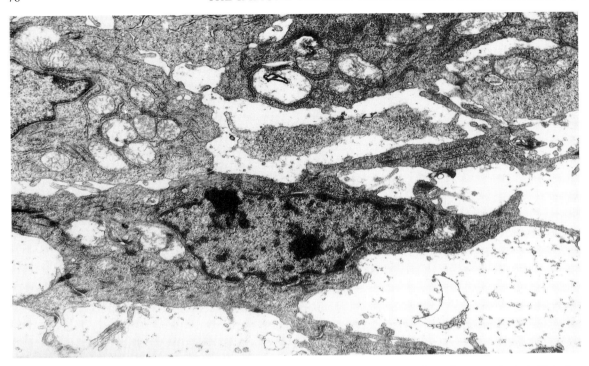

Figure 4.4 Absence of basement membrane at the base of the follicle-associated epithelium (*Sturnus unicolor*). Note the desmosomal junctions between follicle-associated epithelial cells and the medullary reticular epithelial cells (× 13300).

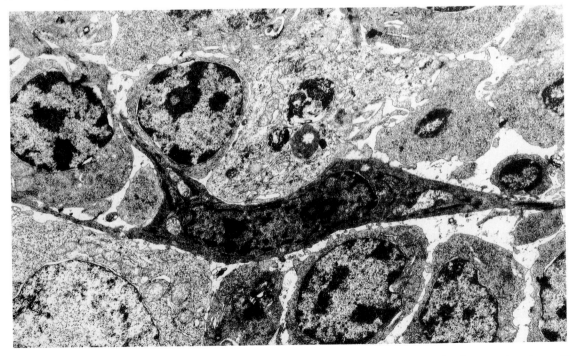

Figure 4.5 Electron-dense reticular epithelial cells in the bursal medulla (*Sturnus unicolor*). Abundant cytoplasmic tonofilaments and desmosomes characterize this cell type (× 5250).

idase (Bockman and Stevens, 1977; Lupetti and Dolfi, 1980; Naukkarinen, 1982).

How the follicle-associated epithelium in the bursa functions seems to be related to its endocytotic capacity, which has been just mentioned. Some comparative immunologists have claimed that the presence of an actively endocytosing follicle-associated epithelium is essential to the peripheral immune system residing in the bursa (Schaffner *et al.*, 1974; Sorvari *et al.*, 1975) and even to the central one as well (Ekino *et al.*, 1980). The functional activity of the adult bursa as a peripheral lymphoid organ is due to the capability of chickens to suck in suspensions from the anal lips to the bursal lumen, where they can be transported further to lymphoid follicles by the follicle-associated epithelium. Naukkarinen (1982) studied this phenomenon extensively, reporting its distinct physiological significance during embryonic and post-hatching life. The anal, sucking-like movements are observed in chick embryos from the 15th day of incubation onwards, but apparently they have no biological importance during the embryonic period because: (a) the sucking movements do not occur spontaneously; (b) the embryo within the eggshell has not actually been exposed to environmental antigens; and (c) the follicle-associated epithelium is not mature to accept the material possibly present in the bursal lumen until some few days before hatching (Naukkarinen, 1982). Effectively, active endocytosis in the follicle-associated epithelium probably does not begin until the end of the fetal period. In the developing follicle-associated epithelium, small apically located vacuoles appear on day 15 and invaginations of the apical plasma membrane 2 days later. Both are signs of endocytic function. Colloidal carbon introduced into the bursal lumen was not endocytosed by the follicle-associated epithelium at 15 or 17 days, and in only four out of ten 19-day-old embryos endocytosis of colloidal carbon by the follicle-associated epithelium was found (Bockman and Cooper, 1973).

In newly hatched chickens, the sucking movements are spontaneous, even faster than the respiratory movements, and they transport into the bursa most of the material applied on the anal lips (Naukkarinen, 1982). Nevertheless, even after hatching, the endocytic capacity of bursal follicle-associated epithelium reaches its highest activity in 10-week-old chickens (Waltenbaugh and van Alten, 1974; Sorvari and Sorvari, 1977). Naukkarinen (1982) concluded that in

chickens the function of the anal sucking-like movements is to transport environmental antigens from the anal lips to the bursal lumen. After involution of the bursa, these movements direct material to the cecal tonsils.

The need for antigenic transport through the follicle-associated epithelium to induce bursal lymphopoiesis and B-cell differentiation is a matter of discussion. One research group (Beezhold *et al.*, 1983) has proposed that embryonic transport of lumenal contents may influence B-cell differentiation and in combination with follicular medullary macrophages, which trap the antigenic and non-antigenic materials after the follicle-associated epithelium (Sorvari and Sorvari, 1977; Naukkarinen, 1982; Naukkarinen and Sorvari, 1982a), may affect the expansion of B-cell populations. In contrast, Lupetti and Dolfi (1980) demonstrated that lymphopoiesis may occur in the bursa without the influence of any factor from the intestinal lumen. Similar conclusions were reached by von Rautenfeld *et al.* (1979), who used the bursa of emus. More recent reports suggest that antigenic stimulation via the bursal route might accelerate rather than induce the development of a lineage of antibody-forming cells (Boyd and Ward, 1984; Ekino *et al.*, 1985). These authors emphasize that this accelerating mechanism might play a major role in a rapid adaptation of the avian immune system to the environment. Other factors which may be responsible for B-cell proliferation in the bursa will be discussed later, along with the rapidly emerging information concerning an active role of the diffusely infiltrated area (DIA) in local antibody production.

The Follicular Medulla and Cortex

The follicular medulla of the adult bursa shows a loose, electron-lucent appearance, especially under the follicle-associated epithelium (Figure 4.2). Its non-lymphoid supporting stroma is formed by long irregular reticular epithelial cells whose processes are apparently joined by desmosomes (Figures 4.2, 4.4–4.6). Between the cytoplasmic extensions of these cells, macrophages, dendritic-like cells, presumptive secretory cells and lymphoid cells of varying size occur (Figure 4.2). Such a histological organization has been reported by numerous workers (Ackerman, 1962; Sherman and Auerbach, 1966; Clawson *et al.*, 1967; Aramaki, 1968; Frazier, 1974;

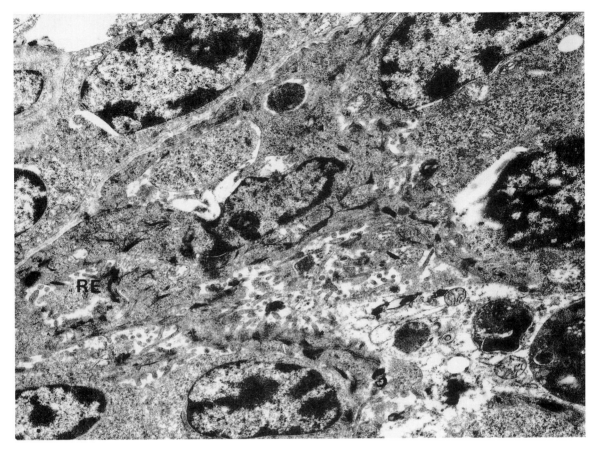

Figure 4.6 Electron-lucent reticular epithelial cells (RE) in the medullary border of a bursal follicle (*Sturnus unicolor*). Together with bundles of cytoplasmic filaments (arrows) and desmosomes which join other stromal components, there are small cavities where these cells project short microvilli (× 6300).

Stinson and Glick, 1978; Naukkarinen and Sorvari, 1982b).

Most reticuloepithelial cells of follicular medulla are very electron-dense, irregularly elongated elements (Figures 4.4, 4.5) resembling those which line the follicular cortex and medulla (Figures 4.2, 4.10). They show an elongated nucleus with a prominent nucleolus and condensed chromatin arranged peripherally (Figure 4.5). In the cytoplasm, bundles of microfilaments abound, basically in the long cell extensions which are joined together by surface desmosomes (Figures 4.4, 4.5). Occasionally, pale reticuloepithelial cells occur in the bursal medulla (Figure 4.6). They are mainly prominent in the limits between follicular cortex and medulla beneath the continuous basement membrane which separates both bursal regions (Figure 4.6). These pale reticuloepithelial cells also show abundant cytoplasmic filaments, desmosomes and remarkably empty cavities into which short microvilli seem to be projected (Figure 4.6). Frazier (1974) also reported on two types, pale and dark, of medullary reticuloepithelial cells. On the other hand, morphologically similar cells have been described by other authors who used a different nomenclature (Ackerman, 1962, endodermal epithelial cells; Naukkarinen and Sorvari, 1982b, dendritic reticulum cells). Recently, keratin-positive reticuloepithelial cells of the bursal medulla have been demonstrated to be positive for B-l antigens (Hoshi *et al.*, 1988).

Free macrophages are a common feature both in the bursal medulla and cortex (Figure 4.7). They are sometimes voluminous cells which contain numerous, engulfed cell debris, more or less degraded in their cytoplasm (Figure 4.7). Some authors have pointed out that macrophages in the follicular medulla are quite similar, if not identical, to the tingible body macrophages of germinal centers (Naukkarinen, 1982). Naukkarinen and Sorvari (1980) studied the role of medullary macrophages in the trapping of per anum injected materials. As early as 15 minutes after this application of colloidal carbon, when it has already been endocytosed by the follicle-associated epithelium, it appears in the stromal intercellular spaces of the bursal medulla. Here, carbon appears in the cytoplasm of macrophages, some of them apparently migrate to the interfollicular surface epithelium. Thus, the number of carbon-containing medullary macrophages gradually decreases. In these conditions, macrophages have never been found in the follicle-associated epithelium in chicken bursa (Naukkarinen

and Sorvari, 1980). Niedorf and Wolters (1974) reported that bursal macrophages in embryos and young chickens migrated from the cortical to the medullary zone and reached the bursal lumen through the follicle-associated epithelium. In this regard, the presence of macrophages in the follicle-associated epithelium is a common feature in the bursa of *Sturnus unicolor* (Figure 4.2).

Cells which resemble dendritic types also occur in the bursal medulla (Figure 4.8). They are electron lucent, and bear numerous cell extensions which project and make contact on the surfaces of neighboring lymphoblasts and lymphocytes (Figure 4.8). In the cytoplasm there are numerous membranous organelles, including pale mitochondria, abundant profiles of rough endoplasmic reticulum, small vesicles and electron-dense granules. Whether these cells represent antigen-presenting Ia-positive cells or monocytic-like cells, precursors of macrophages, is difficult to ascertain from mere morphological analyses. Recently, Houssaint (1987) has reported that the first cells which

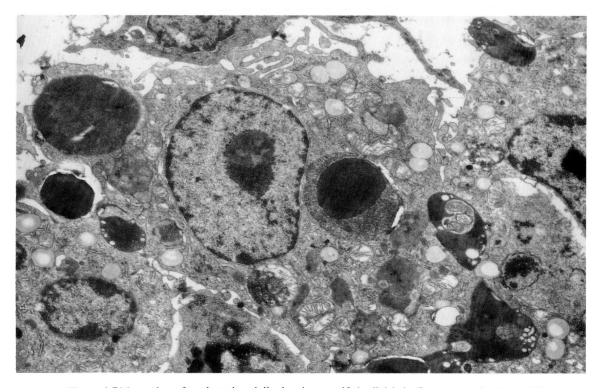

Figure 4.7 Macrophage from bursal medulla showing engulfed cell debris (*Sturnus unicolor*) (× 11 495).

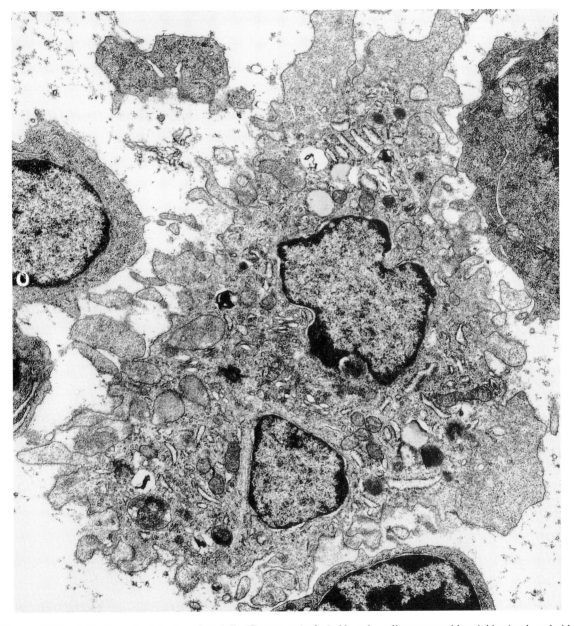

Figure 4.8 Dendritic-like cell of the bursal medulla (*Sturnus unicolor*). Note the cell contacts with neighboring lymphoid cells (× 13 600).

colonize the bursal epithelium are dendritic in morphology and express Ia like antigens at a high level. Glick and Olah have repeatedly described the existence of a secretory-like cell in the medulla of bursal follicles. They have been localized in the medullary area, usually parallel to the corticomedullary border (Olah and Glick, 1978b). In addition, they increase in number and apparently engage in secretory activity after cyclophosphamide treatment (Olah et al., 1979).

From morphological evidence, Olah and Glick (1981) have suggested that small lymphocyte-like cells which belong to the null cell population of the bursa are precursors of these secretory cells. More recently, Olah and Glick found, however, that dark mesenchymal cells which are present in the bursal anlage during early embryonic periods are precursor secretory cells (Glick and Olah, 1987). Furthermore, there is an apparent relationship between these bursal cells and ellipsoid-associated reticulum cells which are involved in antigen trapping and processing in chicken spleens (Glick and Olah, 1984) (see also Chapter 6). Unfortunately other workers have been unable to demonstrate these secretory-like cells in the avian bursa. Von Rautenfeld and Budras (1980) detected such secretory cells in germinal centers of the intestinal tonsils of *Gallus* and various other birds, but not in the bursa species of Struthioniformes.

In histological sections, a monoclonal antibody (CVI-ChNL-68.2) specific for splenic ellipsoid-associated reticulum cells stains positive cells in the surrounding mesenchyme of chicken bursa but never in the follicular medulla (Teurissen, personal communication). In the bursal medulla of *Sturnus unicolor* there are a few cells with certain structural features that resemble those of the secretory cells described by Olah and Glick (Figure 4.9). These cells exhibit some secre-

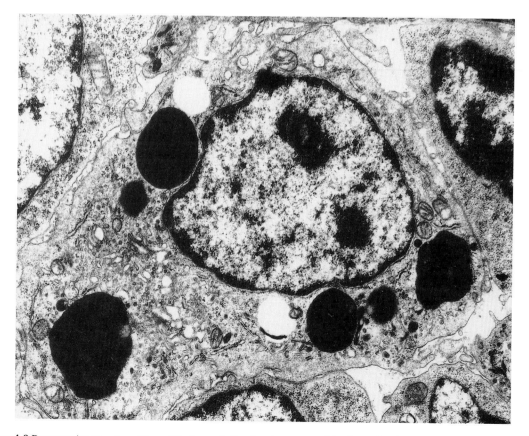

Figure 4.9 Presumptive secretory-like cell in the medulla often in contact with other cells (*Sturnus unicolor*). Note the rough endoplasmic reticulum and the small vesicles and granules (× 22 500).

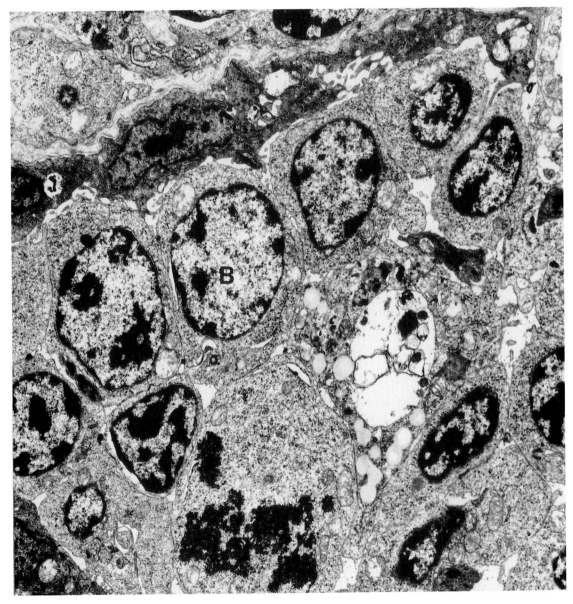

Figure 4.10 A continuous layer of electron-dense epithelial cell (EC) delimits the bursal medulla and cortex (*Sturnus unicolor*). Note the cluster of medullary medium and large lymphocytes as well as lymphoblasts (LB), some in mitosis (arrow), just under this epithelial layer (× 11 875).

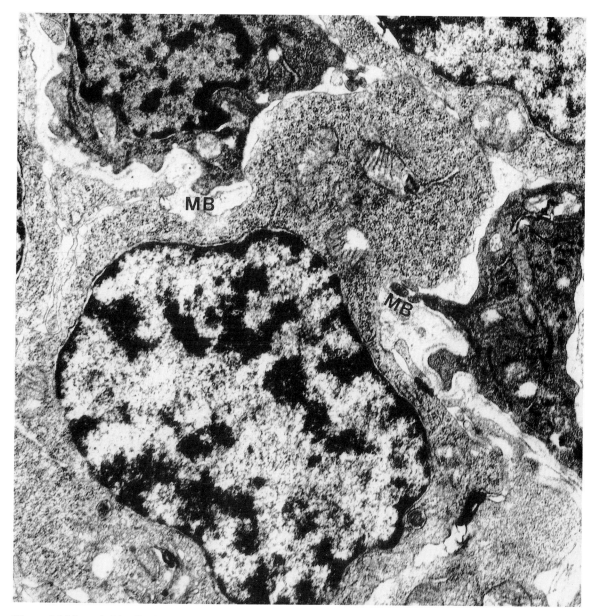

Figure 4.11 Lymphoid cell migrating through the epithelial layer which separates the bursal cortex and medulla (*Sturnus unicolor*) (× 20 900).

tory capacity as evidenced by the existence of a well-developed rough endoplasmic reticulum, Golgi complex, numerous small vesicles and granules (Figure 4.9). Several electron-dense granules of varying sizes occur, some of which contain inside other, smaller electron-dense, granular inclusions. They are often found in contact with other cells; we cannot, in any case, be sure about the true nature of this cell type.

Medium and large lymphocytes are the predominant lymphoid components found mainly in the periphery of the bursal medulla (Figure 4.10). They exhibit the classical characteristics which are a high nucleus: cytoplasm ratio and electron density, abundant condensed chromatin, scarcity of cytoplasmic membranous organelles and numerous polyribosomes (Figures 4.10, 4.11). Frequently, lymphoid cells have been observed to cross the epithelial limits between medulla and cortex. Then the continuous layer of electron-dense epithelial cells is apparently no longer present (Figure 4.11). These epithelial cells resemble morphologically the medullary reticuloepithelial

elements (Figures 4.2, 4.11), and Frazier (1974) has considered them to be identical. Other data, however, suggest that although both cell types are probably of the same epithelial origin they eventually mature into bursal cells with different functions (Eerola, 1980; Naukkarinen and Sorvari, 1982).

Lymphoid migrations between bursal medulla and cortex like those described in Figure 4.10 have been observed extensively, but the usual route for the release of B-lymphocytes from the bursa is a matter of discussion. Ekino *et al.* (1979) reported that the bursal cells are seeded to peripheral lymphoid tissue via lymph vessels. Other workers, however, have pointed out that for this process to occur it must be via the subepithelial system of blood capillaries (Clawson *et al.*, 1967; Holbrook *et al.*, 1974). Finally, according to the interpretation of von Rautenfeld and Budras (1982), B-lymphocytes are probably released via postcapillary venules. These authors have also suggested that hormonal bursectomy in species of Struthioniformes involves an increase in lymphocytes

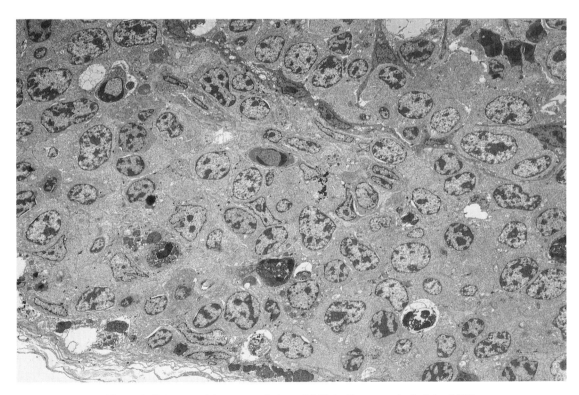

Figure 4.12 Survey of the cortex of a bursal follicle (*Sturnus unicolor*) ($\times$ 2450).

in thin-walled postcapillary venules without exerting a remarkable influence on lymphocyte populations in the peripheral venous blood (von Rautenfeld *et al.*, 1979). Most medullary lymphocytes show an ANAE pattern of staining which suggests that they are B-cells (Naukkarinen and Sorvari, 1982b). However, a few lymphocytes with focal cytoplasmic ANAE activity appear in the follicular medulla. The presence of T-derived lymphocytes in the avian bursa will be commented upon later.

IgM and IgG expression by bursal lymphocytes was first reported only in medullary lymphocytes (Thorbecke *et al.*, 1968; Kincade and Cooper, 1971). Grossi and his coworkers have observed, however, that cells showing diffuse cytoplasmic IgM appear in the follicular cortex, whereas cells with dispersed IgM-containing vesicles are present in the medulla of mature follicles (Grossi *et al.*, 1977a, b). The phenotypic characterization of bursal lymphocytes has also been studied by analyzing mainly the expression of two cell markers, B-L (Ewert *et al.*, 1984) and Bu-l (Gilmour *et al.*, 1976). In addition to surface Ig, they are the most prominent B-cell antigens in chickens and both B-L[+] B-cells (Ewert and Cooper, 1978, 1979; Eerola *et al.*, 1983b) and Bu-l[+] B-cells (Brand *et al.*, 1976, 1983; Audhya *et al.*, 1986) are considered to be bursa dependent. At 8 weeks of age, B-L antigen expression ranged from negative to highly positive, which indicates differences in expression during maturation. In contrast, all the Bu-l[+] bursal cells expressed the antigen but with uniform intensity (Veromaa, 1988). This may indicate that during

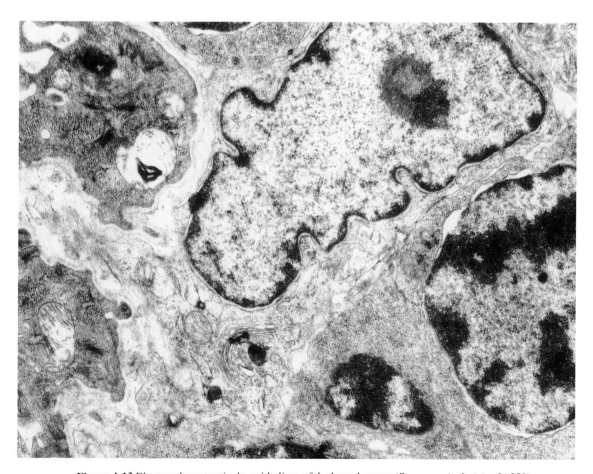

Figure 4.13 Electron-lucent reticulo-epithelium of the bursal cortex (*Sturnus unicolor*) (× 21 350).

ontogeny the level of expression of Bu-l antigen is kept constant but the expression of B-L antigen is increased during the bursal phase of B-cell differentiation.

The follicular cortex develops later than the bursal medulla, which is poorly organized in 1-day-old chickens (Frazier, 1974). In this region, electron-dense small lymphocytes predominate, but macrophages are fairly frequent (Figure 4.12). The cortical stroma has also an epithelial origin but cortical reticuloepithelial cells show less electron density than those of the medulla (Figure 4.13). They show, nevertheless, cytoplasmic fragments as well as a well-developed Golgi complex and possess contacts by desmosomes on their surfaces with other epithelial components of the bursal cortex (Figure 4.13).

Finally, mature granulocytes and plasma cells which are arranged among collections of fibroblasts and collagenous fibers are the main components of the interfollicular stroma (Figure 4.14).

In recent years, heteroantisera and monoclonal antibodies have been produced against distinct bursal cells in order to characterize the main components of the non-lymphoid stroma. Using heteroantisera, antigenic specificity of the cortical reticular fibers (Boyd et al., 1976) and medullary reticuloepithelial cells (Barr et al., 1982) have been observed. More recently, Boyd and coworkers have used a set of monoclonal antibodies to reveal antigenically distinct elements in the chicken bursa such as plicae surface epithelium, follicle-associated epithelium, basement membrane-

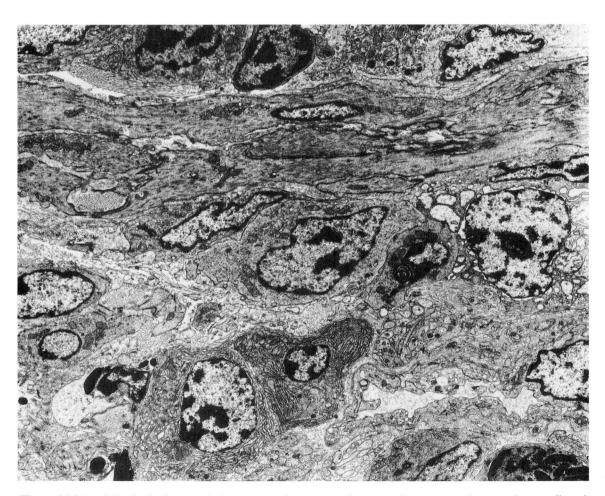

Figure 4.14 Interfollicular lamina propria in the bursa (*Sturnus unicolor*). Note the presence of mature plasma cells and granulocytes among a fibroblastic supporting meshwork under the interfollicular epithelium ($\times$ 6600).

associated epithelium, outer medullary epithelium, medullary reticuloepithelial meshwork, isolated medullary secretory cells, stellate cortical cells, macrophages in the interstitium between follicles and macrophages present in both the cortex and medulla (Boyd *et al.*, 1987a). They also reported that a monoclonal antibody (MUI69) detected an apparently secreted product on the medulla and stained discrete follicles to a different extent, which indicates their heterogeneous nature.

According to these results, which are analogous to those in the thymus, the bursal cortex and medulla seem to be distinguishable by a number of cell determinants, although the role of these regions, if any, in various aspects of B-cell differentiation is unclear. Moreover, evidence for specific bursal hormones, homologous to those of the thymus, is currently somewhat inconclusive.

Involution

Histological changes in the avian bursa of Fabricius, during its natural regression, have been described by numerous authors (Wolfe *et al.*, 1962; Hoffmann-Fezer and lade, 1972; Yamada *et al.*, 1973; Glick, 1977; Naukkarinen and Sorvari, 1984). Naukkarinen and Sorvari (1984), whose results agree with those of others, have found the following morphological changes in the involuting chicken bursa: (a) Bursal weight begins to decrease after 12 weeks. (b) Histological involution occurs between 10 and 23.5 weeks. The earliest histological change in the senescent bursa occurs as a folding of the interfollicular surface epithelium. At that time, the bursa undergoes mucoid involution, i.e. the degenerated lymphoid tissue is then replaced by fibrotic tissue, the amount of which begins to increase in subepithelial regions. Finally, at the age of about 6 months, the bursa appears as a fibrotic residue devoid of its lumen and intact lymphoepithelial structures. (c) The follicle-associated epithelium is capable of endocytosing carbon until week 16. The endocytic function is regressive and practically ends during week 19. (d) A highly significant decline in the number of mitoses per follicle is observed between 10 and 16 weeks. Another significant decline occurs between 20.5 and 23.5 weeks which coincides with the strong deterioration of lymphoid follicles. The number of mitoses was, in any case, twice as high in the follicular cortex as in the medulla at all age groups, a finding which agrees with that of Betti and Borella (1979).

Although the development and involution of the bursa varies prominently in different chicken strains (Wolfe *et al.*, 1962; Hoffmann-Fezer and Lade, 1972; Giurgea, 1977; Glick, 1977; Romppanen, 1982) it is a step-by-step phenomenon in all of them. In contrast, the bursa of Struthioniformes seems to undergo metaplasia rather then involution (von Rautenfeld and Budrus, 1982). As a consequence, the bursa changes from a modified proctodeal mucosa in juveniles to a cutaneous-like mucosa in adults.

The Diffusely Infiltrated Lymphoid Area

Basically in chickens but also in ducks and spotless starlings (*Sturnus unicolor*), a non-follicular region of diffusely infiltrated lymphoid cells, both histologically and probably functionally different from the bursal follicles, occurs around the bursal duct (Diagram 4.l) (Fonfria, 1990). A non-follicular organization is observed in the diffusely infiltrated area (DIA) of *Sturnus unicolor* (Figure 4.15). In a reticular stroma, lymphoid cells of varying sizes, mature, developing plasma cells and macrophages have been observed (Figure 4.15). Moreover, postcapillary venules and interdigitating cells, two typical features of the T-dependent areas of mammalian peripheral lymphoid organs, appear in these regions (Figure 4.15).

This area, which does not appear until after hatching (Odend'hal and Breazile, 1980), was first described by Odend'hal and coworkers (Odend'hal and Breazile, 1979a, b, 1980; Odend'hal and Player, 1979) and later they suggested that it is a T-dependent region of the avian bursa of Fabricius. Previously, reports of T-cells in bursal cell suspensions found important differences (0−20%) (Potworowski, 1972; Hudson and Roitt, 1973; Albini and Wick, 1974; Donnelly *et al.*, 1975; Payne and Rennie, 1976).

Evidence for a probable thymic origin of lymphocytes in the diffusely infiltrated area of the bursa has been explained. First there is the presence of postcapillary venules (high endothelial venules) (Odend'hal and Breazile, 1979a, b, 1980 (Figure 4.15); Odend'hal and Player, 1979; Syrjanen and Naukkarinen, 1982)—the site of preferential recirculation of lymphocytes in mammalian secondary lym-

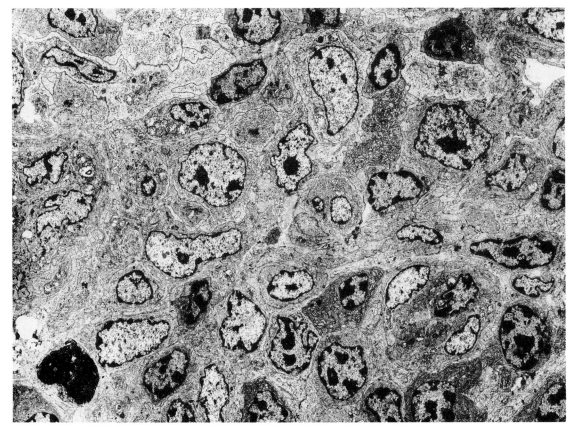

Figure 4.15 Survey of the diffusely infiltrated lymphoid area of the bursa (*Sturnus unicolor*). Together with lymphoid cells of varying sizes, postcapillary venules and interdigitating cells are characteristics of these areas (× 2845).

phoid organs. Second, there is an increased migration of lymphocytes through postcapillary venules in the diffusely infiltrated area after per anum immunization with SRBC (Syrjanen and Naukkarinen, 1982). The highly developed reticular fiber component has been observed in this bursal region (Figure 4.16). Finally, the homing of tritiated uridine-labeled thymocytes to the diffusely infiltrated lymphoid area 6−24 hours after intravenous injection has been determined by autoradiography (Odend'hal and Breazile, 1980).

Unfortunately, results after neonatal thymectomy have been equivocal (Odend'hal and Breazile, 1980), although previously Jankovic and Isakovic (1966) have reported lymphocyte depletion in the bursa after thymectomy. Local treatment with anti-T-lymphocyte serum preceding SRBC stimulation causes prominent changes in the DIA (Naukkarinen and Syrjanen, 1984) which include a decrease in diameter and lumen of postcapillary venules and in the numbers of lymphocytes. Observations have revealed the T-cell staining patterns following histochemical studies of the area using the acid alpha-naphthyl acetate esterase technique, fluorescence antibody assays and resistance to cyclophosphamide treatment (Murthy *et al.*, 1984).

The diffusely infiltrated area has been suggested as a major source of luminal lymphocytes found free in the lumen (Oden'hal and Breazile, 1979b) as well as the site of developing bursal follicles. In contrast, the diffusely infiltrated area is strategically located to ensure intimate contact with environmental antigens although its true role in the above-mentioned local antibody production in the bursa is unclear.

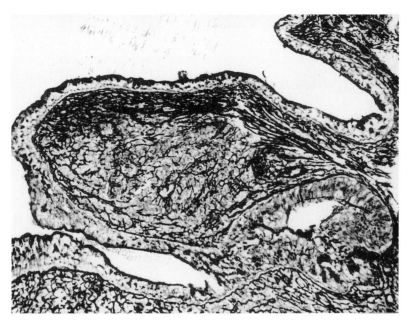

Figure 4.16 Distribution patterns of reticular fibers after silver impregnation in the diffusely infiltrated area of the bursa (*Sturnus unicolor*). Compare this pattern with that of the bursal follicles shown in Figure 4.3 ($\times$ 250).

ONTOGENY

Anatomy and Histology of Bursal Embryonic Development

The development of the bursa of Fabricius has been viewed as occurring in three stages: formation of the anlage; lymphoid follicle formation; and maturation of the follicles. The bursa arises in chick embryos as a dorsocaudal outgrowth of the cloaca at 5−6 days of incubation, and appears initially in the form of a median lamina of endodermal epithelium permeated with varying sizes of spherical vacuoles (Hamilton, 1952; Romanoff, 1960). These vacuoles eventually coalesce and the cavity which is formed communicates with the cloacal lumen (Hamilton, 1952). The bursa undergoes marked growth during development as its shape changes from round to oval. Hypertrophy of the mesoderm which surrounds the bursal epithelium produces longitudinal plicae that project into the bursal lumen. These plicae ultimately house lymphoid follicles (Ackerman and Knouff, 1959; Romanoff, 1960; Ackerman, 1962). During a period up to and including

the 10th day of incubation, 11 or 12 longitudinal plicae which protrude inside the bursal lumen are formed on the 13th or 14th days of development. Numerous button-like epithelial formations proliferate from the epithelial lining of the plicae and penetrate the tunica propria. lymphopoiesis begins inside these 'epithelial buds' and the bursal medulla of the follicle develops thereafter (Jolly, 1915; Ackerman and Knouff, 1959; Ackerman, 1962).

On day 11 of incubation, well-developed bursal plicae are surrounded by a multilayered epithelium and a discontinuous basement membrane. At that time, large basophilic cells are present in the plical mesenchyme. Among them, Glick and Olah (1987) have recognized two populations of mesenchymal cells: one pale and the other darkly stained. These workers suggest, also, the existence of intermediate forms. By day 12, dark mesenchymal cells cluster beneath the epithelium, whereas the light mesenchymal cells remain spherical and show no evidence of migration. Then, bud formation will be observed in those epithelial locations invaded by dark mesenchymal cells, which have previously developed cytoplasmic granules (Glick and Olah, 1987). These two cell types can be identified ultrastructurally by their different electron density. The more electron-lucent cells are the most primitive mesenchymal cells, whereas the dark cells seem to undergo a gradual process of transformation towards a fibroblastic state (Figure 4.17).

Other workers (Lupetti *et al.*, 1986) have suggested, however, that the mesenchymal cells approach the epithelium without penetrating it. They then remain in the lamina propria, separated from the epithelium by the basement membrane, where they form a cell mass which becomes progressively more highly packed, apparently pushing themselves towards the bursal lumen. The lining epithelium in this mesenchymal mass becomes flattened and necrotized so that the uppermost cells of the mesenchymal mass face the bursal lumen. There is currently insufficient evidence

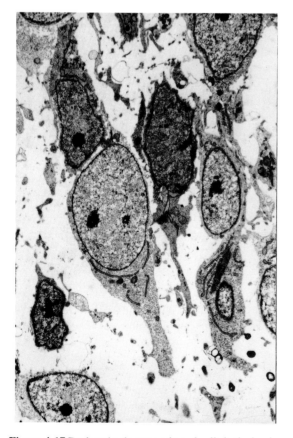

Figure 4.17 Dark and pale mesenchymal cells in the lamina propria of a 11-day-old chicken embryo (× 9120).

to support the precise manner by which the bursal follicles appear. However, as commented upon earlier, certain properties of the follicle-associated epithelium suggest a mesenchymal rather than an epithelial origin for the bursal follicles.

In 13-day-old embryos, lymphoid follicles appear for the first time (Figure 4.18). At this stage, the follicles, showing a variable degree of development, have been observed in the epithelial layer and their basement membranes are easily identified by silver impregnation (Figure 4.19). The follicle-associated epithelial cells are already distinguishable ultrastructurally from those of the interfollicular epithelium. They are pale, electron-lucent with scant condensed chromatin, patent nucleoli, groups of cytoplasmic polyribosomes, profiles of rough endoplasmic reticulum, small, round mitochondria, a well-developed Golgi complex, and short apical microvilli (Figure 4.18). Although at this stage follicles are basically epithelial, lymphoid elements do occur in the most developed ones. Moreover, blast cells apparently migrate through the basement membrane and the epithelial cell processes into the bursal follicles. In the lamina propria, there are accumulations of granulocytes, macrophages and monocytic-like cells. During embryonic life, active granulopoiesis is restricted to the mesenchymal component beginning from day 9 of incubation and disappearing at hatching (Houssaint *et al.*, 1976). Even discrete erythropoiesis has been observed in the bursal mesenchyme *in ovo* (Houssaint, 1987).

On day 15 of incubation there is a notable increase in number, size and organization of the bursal follicles (Figure 4.20). These latter are not more circumscribed to the epithelium but clearly included in the bursal stromal. At the ultrastructural level, the most remarkable changes occur: the appearance of two types of reticuloepithelial cells which form the supporting stroma of the bursal follicles; appearance of macrophages or their precursors inside the follicle; migration of lymphoid cells through the surrounding basement membrane on both sides; and accumulation of lymphoid elements in the mesenchyme which surrounds the bursal follicles.

With various degrees of development, the bursal follicles of 17-day-old embryos increase in number and size with respect to the above stages (Figure 4.21). In the most developed follicles, the cortex begins to be apparent. Moreover, the follicle-associated epithelial

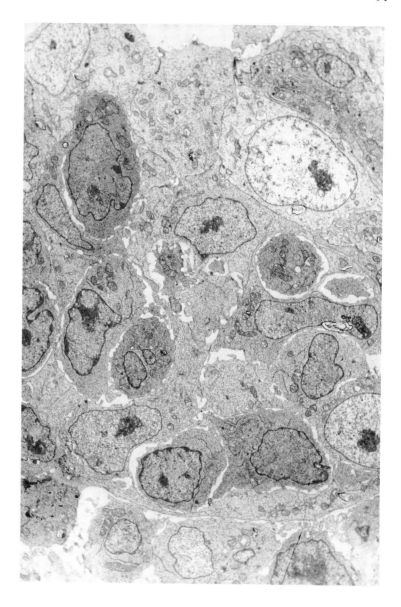

Figure 4.18 Thirteen-day-old bursal follicle (× 4000).

cells develop a canalicular membranous system in the apical border which consists of invaginations of the surface membrane and of the electron-lucent vesicles. In bursas of 19-day-old embryos, the lymphoid follicles have increased considerably in size and number, thus they occupy almost all of the bursal stroma. The cortex – medulla differentiation is more evident and granulocytes cluster in the base of lymphoid follicles (Figure 4.22).

The pattern of vascularization in the embryonic bursa of Fabricius, probably important for the growth and specialization of bursal follicles, has been analyzed extensively by Schoenwolf et al. (1981). In the early stages of development, the bursal blood vessels form a superficial, somewhat hexagonal plexus. As longitudinal plicae form and grow inward, some of the superficial vessels are apparently pulled internally, where they establish the middle plical

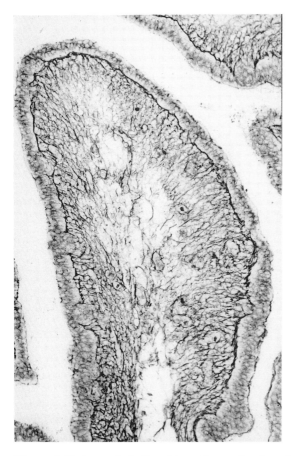

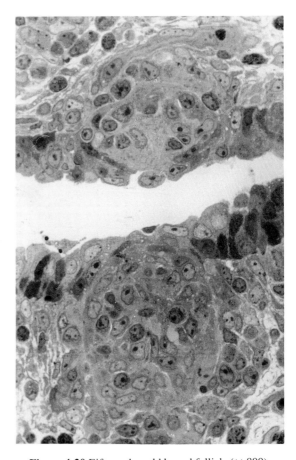

Figure 4.19 Anatomical disposition of emerging bursal follicles in a 13-day-old embryo. The basement membrane stained by silver impregnation indicates the position of the follicles in the bursal stroma ($\times$ 380).

Figure 4.20 Fifteen-day-old bursal follicle ($\times$ 800).

vessels. As the plicae form, hexagonally arranged vessels are progressively recruited as middle plicae and cross-connecting vessels. Thus, the superficial plexus no longer exists at the end of incubation.

The epithelial buds are always closely associated with small vascular sprouts from the middle capillary bed. The capillaries which supply each follicle form complex, net-like configurations concomitant with the differentiation of developing lymphatic follicles into clearly recognizable cortical and medullary regions. Progressively more blood is needed as the bursa continues to grow. During post-hatching, the extrinsic bursal vessels continue to increase gradually in

diameter, whereas the diameters of the middle plical vessels as well as those of all other intrinsic bursal vessels no longer increase, but actually decrease from late pre-hatching stages. The physiological significance, if any, of this decrease in diameter of intrinsic bursal vessels is unknown.

In contrast to these morphological observations, the ontogenetic analysis using monoclonal antibodies shows a sequential development of stromal antigens in the bursa (Boyd *et al.*, 1987b). Those monoclonal antibodies which react with the adult bursal surface epithelium are positive as early as day 10 of embryogenesis. Most of the monoclonal antibodies specific

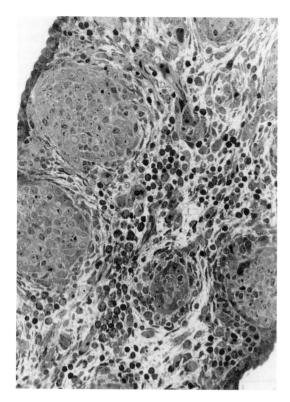

Figure 4.21 Seventeen-day-old bursal follicle ($\times$ 330).

for the adult bursal cortex stain exclusively the embryonic lamina propria during development, beginning at about day 12. Certain of these antibodies which are reactive for the adult medulla only stain this region throughout development (beginning around day 15), while most of the anti-medulla monoclonal antibodies react with the surface epithelium in embryos. Various relationships between the distinct origin of bursal components deserve special attention (Boyd *et al.*, 1987b). The finding that many monoclonal antibodies reacting with the adult medulla initially stain the embryonic surface epithelium is further evidence for developmental relationships between these areas (Le Douarin *et al.*, 1975; Houssaint *et al.*, 1976). The restriction of staining by monoclonal antibodies reactive with the adult cortex to the embryonic lamina propria also reflects this developmental relationship (Le Douarin *et al.*, 1975).

Bursal Precursor Cells and B-cell Maturation

Hemopoietic differentiation in the bursa depends upon migration of blood-derived stem cells (Moore and Owen, 1966, 1967; Le Douarin and Houssaint, 1974; Dieterlen-Lievre, 1975; Houssaint *et al.*, 1976; Lassila *et al.*, 1978). From about day 8 to day 15 of the chicken's embryonic life, precursor cells migrate from extrabursal mesenchyme into the developing organ, where they proliferate in bursal follicles. Houssaint has proposed that colonization of the bursal epithelium by hemopoietic precursors, defined by specific monoclonal antibodies (CL-1, L-232), is a two-step process (Houssaint, 1987; Houssaint *et al.*, 1987). According to her observations, the first cells (CL-1$^+$, L-22$^-$) which represent the macrophage/dendritic cell lineage are responsible for forming the epithelial buds which during subsequent phases are colonized by lymphoid precursors (C-L$^+$, L-22$^+$). From this interpretation, there is no clearly defined pre-B phase in the development of avian B-cells.

To extend these observations, Cooper (1986) recently summarized development using molecular markers which are expressed on bursal cells: (a) lymphoid precursor cells that enter the bursal epithelium appear to express Ia antigen (Ewert *et al.*, 1984) and a common leukocyte antigen which is shared with other hemopoietic progenitors and retained on mature T-cells (Chen and Cooper, 1987); (b) the CB-1 homodimer is expressed exclusively on intrabursal B-cells but is lost when B-cells migrate to peripheral regions; (c) two other antigenic molecules, CB-2 and HNK-1, which are present on bursal B-cells but not on peripheral B-cells also appear on cells of other lineages. The molecule detected by antibody HNK-1, is similar in molecular weight ($\sim$ 100 000) to the HNR-1$^+$ myelin-associated glycoprotein; (d) Bu-1, CB-3, CB-4 and CB-5 are similar to surface IgM in that they are expressed on B-cells throughout the body; CB-5 expression continues through to the appearance of the plasma cell stage. Using other markers, MUI 36 positive cells which express a non-Ig, non-BL B-lymphocyte determinant, similar to L-22 or Bu-1a, are first detected in the lamina propria of 10-day embryos and are localized by day 12 in both the lamina propria and developing epithelial buds (Boyd *et al.*, 1987b).

From another viewpoint, it has been suggested that precursors of chicken B-lymphocytes are different

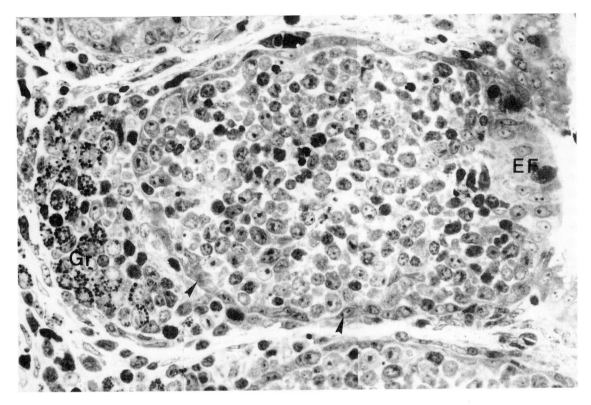

Figure 4.22 Bursal follicle of a 19-day-old chicken embryo. Note the incipient development of the bursal cortex and the cluster of granulocytes (Gr) which surround the bursal follicle (EF) (× 666).

from those of T-lymphocytes (at least for the majority of them) (Houssaint, 1987; Houssaint *et al.*, 1987; Veromaa, 1988). Weber had already shown that 14-day embryonic bone marrow contains cells which are capable of repopulating both thymus and bursa of irradiated embryonic recipients, whereas 1-day post-hatching chick bone marrow no longer contained the bursal-homing precursor cells (Weber and Mausner, 1977; Weber and Alexander, 1978). Furthermore, the capacity of hemopoietic precursors to home to embryonic bursal and thymic rudiments has been investigated in embryonic and newly hatched chick recipients (Houssaint *et al.*, 1983). Whereas thymic grafts developed normal lymphopoiesis in both recipients, the bursal rudiment was colonized in embryonic but not in post-hatching recipients. According to one conclusion, there was a selective disappearance of B-cell precursors around hatching time. Other data using the now classic quail chicken

chimeras suggest, however, that the bursal-colonizing hemopoietic cells might be multipotential because at least some cells from an 11-day quail bursa can migrate into a chicken thymus in an organ culture system (Jotereau *et al.*, 1980).

The number of lymphoid stem cells populating a bursal follicle is, in any case, small, i.e. less than ten (Pink *et al.*, 1985) and little is known about their phenotype. They probably do not express Ig (Szenberg, 1976; Ewert and Cooper, 1978) and might even contain unrearranged Ig genes. Ratcliffe *et al.* (1978) propose that these lymphoid precursor cells rapidly become committed to the expression of particular V region genes, probably as a consequence of productive V region recombination. This recombination is restricted to the embryo and may not require the bursal microenvironment for its induction. The available germ-line repertoire of heavy and light chain V regions in the chicken is very limited and little diversity can be generated from this initial recombination event (Weill *et al.*, 1986).

Apparently B-cell development in chickens develops by a discrete series of ontogenically restricted stages. lymphoid cell proliferation in separate follicles proceeds independently, with very little cell traffic from one follicle to another, since neighboring follicles in chimeric birds often contain cell populations of distinct origins (Pink *et al.*, 1985). Proliferation is rapid, with a population doubling time of about 10 hours in 14−16-day chicken embryos (Lydyard *et al.*, 1976). In addition, cortical and medullary cells in the same follicle are derived from the same precursors, but otherwise the relationships between cells in the two compartments are unclear (Cooper *et al.*, 1972).

As has been mentioned repeatedly, the first antigen to be detected on bursal lymphocytes is the B-L antigen (chicken MHC class II antigen) on day 9 of incubation (Ewert *et al.*, 1984). B-L$^+$ cells increase from about 4% on day 9 to 30% on day 13 and 82% on day 19 of incubation. Moreover, two populations of B-L$^+$ cells have been identified in the bursa. Of the larger bursal cells, 40−60% exhibit brighter immunofluorescence reactivity than the relatively smaller bursal cells (Ewert *et al.*, 1984). Remarkably, there are apparently differences in the proportions of brightly staining B-L$^+$ bursal cells from different MHC homozygous chicken lines. Regulation of this difference has been associated with a non-MHC-linked Bu-1 alloantigen locus (Fredericksen and Gilmour, 1985).

Ig-bearing cells are first visible within the bursa at about day 12 of incubation, and by day 18 about 85% of cells in bursal cell suspensions are Ig$^+$ (Lydyard *et al.*, 1976; Szenberg, 1976; Ewert and Cooper, 1978). From then onward, B-cells are exported from the bursa (Woods and Linna, 1965; Glick, 1977; Ivanyi, 1981). The fraction which is exported is about 1−5% of the cells produced but the rest of the newly produced cells presumably die *in situ* (cited by Pink and Lassila, 1987). At 5−7 weeks after hatching, when the bursa reaches maximum weight, it contains 90% of lymphocytes which carry cell surface IgM (Lydyard *et al.*, 1976). A small percentage (<1%) carry IgG and IgA. Since these cells appear early in ontogeny—IgG on day 14 (Lydyard *et al.*, 1976; Grossi *et al.*, 1977a; Chen, 1978) and IgA on day 16 (Chen, 1978; Lebacq and Ritter, 1979)—it has been proposed that they may be formed in the bursa by intrabursal switching from IgM$^+$ precursors (Pink and Lassila, 1987).

Factors regulating colonization of precursor cells and B-cell maturation in the bursa are poorly understood. Holmes and Haar (1982) demonstrated that embryonic 10-, 11-, 13- and 14-day chicken bursa produce a soluble factor when cultured *in vitro*. It causes a greater than control level migration of age-matched yolk sac cells in a blind well chamber experiment. It is noteworthy that the high migration index which has been observed at day 10 corresponds with the large influx of precursor cells that occurs at this age *in vivo* (Le Douarin *et al.*, 1975). Thus, the *in vivo* function of such a factor could be to increase the invasion of blood-borne stem or progenitor cells into the bursal stroma. In contrast, an *in vivo* function for a migration inhibitory factor, possibly produced by the bursa on day 12, may be to immobilize stem cells once they have been attracted to the bursa. Such a decline of cell movement may permit these cells to associate with epithelial or mesenchymal cells and thereby become susceptible to hemopoietic, microenvironmental influences (Holmes and Haar, 1982).

Bursin, a tripeptide hormone associated with B-cell differentiation, induces Bu-1 alloantigen and B-L antigens on the surface of precursor cells (Brand *et al.*, 1983). The bursal epithelium cultured *in vitro* could therefore induce B-l antigens on the surface of pre-bursal stem cells derived from 7-day-old intra-embryonic mesenchyme (Eerola *et al.*, 1982). The precursor cells cultured with bursal reticular epithelial cells become positive for chicken B-lymphocyte differentiation antigens but negative for fetal-associated antigens after cell to cell contact. However, Ig detected on precursor cells has not been induced successfully (Boyd *et al.*, 1983).

FUNCTION

As mentioned earlier in the introduction to this Chapter, the avian bursa of Fabricius functions as both a central lymphoid organ during ontogeny and an antibody-producing peripheral lymphoid organ after hatching, especially in the *per anum*, antigenic stimulation experiments. Now we will discuss additional evidence for a presumptive role of the bursa in the development of the avian thymus-dependent immune functions which have been proposed by some workers (Fitzsimmons et al., 1973, 1977; Dixon and Fitzsimmons, 1980).

The major function of the bursa is to provide an environment where rapid cell divisions allow the generation of diversity from a limited germ-line repertoire by the accumulation of somatic modifications. On the other hand, a relation of the bursa with T-cell responses has been claimed. It has been suggested to be the source of suppressor T-cells in chickens by various investigators (Droege, 1971, 1976; Moticka, 1977), based on the lack of suppressor T-cell function in bursectomized chickens. Such a possibility is supported by the observation that neonatal bursectomy causes a substantial decrease in a subset of thymocytes in the chicken thymus (Zucker et al., 1973). In contrast, other investigators have demonstrated the presence of suppressor T-cells in chickens which have been bursectomized by a variety of techniques (Blasese et al., 1974; Palladino et al., 1976; Kermani-Arab and Leslie, 1977).

There are reports of cortical atrophy in the thymus in 18-day-old chicken embryos bursectomized at 70 hours of incubation (Fitzsimmons et al., 1973, 1977). Jankovic et al. (1976, 1977) did not, however, find morphological differences in the thymus of bursectomized and cyclophosphamide-treated chickens at 10 weeks of age. In addition, no signs of atrophy or hypoplasia have been observed in the spleen, tonsils, Harderian gland, thymus or bone marrow of bursectomized chickens studied by Granfors et al. (1982) and Jalkanen et al. (1983b). Veromaa (1988) has suggested that these discrepancies could be explained by the fact that Fitzsimmons and coworkers analyzed chicken embryos, and the lymphoid organs of bursectomized birds could develop slower than in normal chickens. In any case, recent results suggest conclusively that the bursa of Fabricius is not necessary for the development of thymus-dependent immune function (Veromaa, 1988).

A systemic antibody response following cloacal antigenic stimulation has been reported by numerous investigators and extensively pointed out in this chapter (Schaffner et al., 1974; Sorvari and Sorvari, 1977; Naukkarinen, 1982). In this respect, Toivanen et al. (1987) recently proposed that the peripheral function of the bursa is to expose the vigorously proliferating stem cells to environmental antigens which could serve to create an antibody repertoire necessary for host survival in a given environment.

The size of the B-cell population in the chicken (Kincade et al., 1973), its clonal diversity (Ivanyi, 1975a, b; Huang and Diener, 1978) and its isotypic heterogeneity (Cooper et al., 1969; Kincade and Cooper, 1973) are dependent on the time allowed for the bursa to function before its elimination. Birds bursectomized at 17 days of incubation fail to develop B-cells and become completely agammaglobulinemic (Cooper et al., 1969), which suggests that normal B-cell differentiation occurs exclusively in the bursa. If, however, the bursal epithelium is experimentally ablated at 60 hours of incubation, the chickens which subsequently develop will show remarkable immune imbalances (Granfors et al., 1982; Eerola et al., 1983a, 1984a, b; Jalkanen et al., 1983a, b, 1984a, b).

Despite the absence of any bursal follicles confirmed histologically, operated birds still have serum Ig of IgM, IgG and IgA classes at 10 weeks of age. Serum IgG levels are decreased but those of IgM and IgA remain normal (Jalkanen et al., 1983a). Furthermore, the number of surface IgG lymphocytes is markedly reduced in the peripheral blood, spleen and thymus of bursectomized birds in comparison with controls. However, these chickens are absolutely unable to produce specific antibodies, even after heavy immunization (Granfors et al., 1982). In addition, bursectomized chickens lack natural antibodies against phosphorylcholine, fecal bacteria, rabbit red blood cells and autoantibodies to the liver, kidney and thyroid as well as the bursa of Fabricius (Jalkanen et al., 1983b). Similar results have been recently observed by Corbel et al. (1987), who used surgical bursectomy at day 5 of incubation. Furthermore, Veromaa (1988) has found B-L[+] and Bu-l[+] cells in bursectomized chickens, although there was a striking decrease in their numbers in the peripheral blood and spleen, but not in the thymus and bone marrow.

lymphoid cells from bursectomized chickens are capable of producing IgM, IgG and IgA in vitro, but no production of specific antibodies has been observed (Eerola et al., 1983a). This inability of pre-immunized bursectomized birds to produce specific antibodies has not been reconstituted by cultured bursal epithelium or in vitro in a bursal epithelium conditioned medium (Eerola et al., 1984a). Moreover, antigen presentation *in vitro* to lymphocytes from bursectomized birds by MHC-compatible normal peripheral blood monocytes does not restore the ability to produce specific antibodies (Eerola *et al.*, 1984b). Jalkanen (1983) transferred bone marrow cells from 2- and 10-week-old bursectomized chickens to newly hatched, cyclophosphamide-treated chickens. These cells could, to some extent, reconstitute serum Ig in recipients, but these cells were totally incapable of homing into the bursa and restoring specific antibody production, which indicates their origin as post-bursal cells (Jalkanen, 1983).

These and related experiments indicate that the bursa is not needed for the induction of B-cell surface antigen, since its specific function is to act as a central lymphoid organ for generating clonal and isotypic diversity and not initiating B-cell development (Toivanen *et al.*, 1987; Weill and Reynard, 1987). These results also imply that Ig gene rearrangement during B-cell development occurs exclusively within the bursa (Cooper, 1986). Although this concept of a self-renewing, bursa-derived B-cell population in adult chickens is currently widely accepted, there is another model which accounts for B-cell development. According to this alternative explanation, adult B-cells are generated from precursors which are not descendants of bursa cells nor are they detectable in transfer experiments (Pink *et al.*, 1987). According to this model, bursectomy induces T-cell-mediated suppression of further B-cell development. This has been substantiated by Blaese *et al.* (1974), who used surgical bursectomy at one day post-hatching in chicks which contained with X-ray irradiation to produce agammaglobulinemic chickens.

The analysis of chicken Ig genes by Weill and colleagues (Dahan *et al.*, 1983; Reynaud *et al.*, 1983, 1985; Weill *et al.*, 1986) has revealed a remarkably different picture from that which has been proposed for mammalian Ig genes. The light chains in chickens are of lambda type, and the lambda locus consists of a single functional V lambda 1, J lambda and C lambda gene lying within 2 kilobases of each other in a germline configuration. Upstream from the V lambda l gene are a dozen or more pseudo V lambda genes. In order to become a B-cell, each bursal precursor appears to undergo a single V lambda l − J lambda rearrangement event. Once this occurs, a somatic mutational mechanism is initiated by bursal B-cells that may involve

donating V lambda pseudogene sequences via a gene-conversion mechanism. less is known about the heavy chain gene locus but available data also suggest the presence of very few V H genes, perhaps no more than three in number. Consequently there may be two ways of generating antibody diversity (Pink and Lassila, 1987); a model in which B-cells are formed during a short period of ontogenesis, and thereafter accumulate somatic mutations in a small number of variable-region genes (functional in chickens and perhaps sheep), and a 'steady-state' model (in mice) in which variability is generated by the continual formation of B-cells with fresh rearrangements of large numbers of Ig variable-region genes.

FINAL COMMENT

The existence of a lymphoid bursa of Fabricius is evidence of a remarkable immunological dissociation in birds (Szenberg and Warner, 1962). This concept proposes that there are two fundamentally distinct populations of immunologically competent cells. The bursal lymphocytes are responsible for Ig synthesis and antibody formation, whereas those that are derived from the thymus are concerned with cell-mediated immune responses.

REFERENCES

Ackerman GA (1962). Electron microscopy of the bursa of Fabricius of the embryonic chick with particular reference to the lympho-epithelial nodules. *J Cell Biol* **13**: 127–146.

Ackerman GA and Knouff RA (1959). Lymphocytopoiesis in the bursa of Fabricius. *Am J Anat* **104**: 163–206.

Ackerman GA and Knouff RA (1964). Lymphocytopoietic activity in the bursa of Fabricius. In Good RA and Gabrielsen AE (Eds), *The Thymus in Immunobiology*. Hoeber Medical Divisions: New York. pp 123–149.

Albini B and Wick G (1974). Delineation of B and T lymphoid cells in the chicken. *J Immunol* **112**: 444–450.

Aramaki T (1968). Morphologic studies of lymphatic tissues (XIII). Light and electron microscope observations on the bursa of Fabricius of the chick and *Coturnix* embryos with special reference to lymphocytopoiesis. *Keio J Med* **17**: 135–155.

Audhya T, Kroon D, Heavner G, Viamontes G and Goldstein G (1986). Tripeptide structure of bursin, a selective B-cell differentiating hormone of the bursa of Fabricius. *Science* **231**: 997–999.

Barr IG, Alderton M, Brumley Rl, Boyd RO, Muller HK and Ward A (1982). Antigens associated with bursal and thymic reticular epithelial cells. *Adv Exp Med* **149**: 711–717.

Beezhold DH, Sachs HG and van Alten PJ (1983). The development of transport ability by embryonic follicle-associated epithelium. *J Ret Soc* **34**: 143–152.

Betti F and Borella MI (1979). Bursa of Fabricius. Mitotic index in the follicles of immunized and non-immunized chicks (*Gallus domesticus*). *Anat Anz* **146**: 439–443.

Blaese RM, Weiden Pl, Koski I and Dooley N (1974). Infectious agammaglobulinemia. Transmission of immunodeficiency with grafts of agammaglobulinemic cells. *J Exp Med* **140**: 1097–1101.

Bockman DE and Cooper MD (1973). Pinocytosis by epithelium associated with lymphoid follicles in the bursa of Fabricius, appendix and Peyer's patches. An electron microscopic study. *Am J Anat* **136**: 455–478.

Bockman DE and Cooper MD (1975). Early lymphoepithelial relationships in human appendix. *Gastroenterology* **68**: 1160–1168.

Bockman DE and Stevens W (1977). Gut-associated lymphoepithelial tissue: Bidirectional transport of tracer by specialized epithelial cells associated with lymphoid follicles. *J Ret Soc* **21**: 245–254.

Boyd RL and Ward HA (1984). Lymphoid antigenic determinants of the chicken: Ontogeny of bursa-dependent lymphoid tissue. *Dev Comp Immunol* **8**: 149–167.

Boyd RL, Ward HA and Muller HK (1976). Antisera specific for the reticulin of the bursa of Fabricius. *Int Arch Allergy Appl Immunol* **50**: 129–132.

Boyd RL, Ward HA and Muller HK (1983). Bursal and thymic reticular cells in the chicken. Induction of B- and T-lymphocyte differentiation by *in vitro* monolayer cultures. *J Ret Soc* **34**: 383–398.

Boyd RL, Wilson TJ, Mitrangas K and Ward HA (1987a). Characterization of chicken thymic and bursal stromal cells. In Weber WT and Ewert DL (Eds), *Avian Immunology*. Alan R liss: New York. pp 29–40.

Boyd RL, Mitrangas K, Ramm HC, Wilson TJ, Fahey KJ and Ward HA (l987b). Chicken B lymphocyte differentiation: Ontogeny, bursal microenvironment and effect of IBD virus. In Weber WT and Ewert DL (Eds), *Avian Immunology*. Alan R Liss: New York. pp 41–52.

Brand A, Gilmour DG and Goldstein G (1976). Lymphocyte-differentiating hormone of bursa of Fabricius. *Science* **193**: 319–331.

Brand A, Galton J and Gilmour DG (1983). Committed precursors of B and T lymphocytes in chick embryonic bursa of Fabricius. *Eur J Immunol* **13**: 449–455.

Chang TS, Glick B and Winter AR (1955). The significance of bursa of Fabricius of chickens in antibody production (Abstract). *Poultry Sci* **34**: 1187.

Chen CL (1978). Ontogeny of immunoglobulin isotype diversity expressed by chicken lymphocytes (Abstract). *Fed Proc* **37**: 1395.

Chen CM and Cooper MD (1987). Identification of cell surface molecules on chicken lymphocyte with monoclonal antibodies. In Toivanen A and Toivanen P (Eds), *Avian Immunology*. CRC Press: Boca Raton, Florida. pp 137–154.

Clawson CC, Cooper MD and Good RA (1967). Lymphocyte fine structure in the bursa of Fabricius, the thymus and the germinal centers. *Lab Invest* **16**: 407–421.

Cooper MD (1986). B cell development in birds and mammals. In Cinader B and Miller RG (Eds), *Progress in Immunology VI*. Academic Press: Orlando. pp 18–32.

Cooper MD, Cain WA, van Alten PJ and Good RA (1969). Development and function of the immunoglobulin producing system. *Int Arch Allergy* **35**: 242–252.

Cooper MD, Lawton AR and Kincade PW (1972). A developmental approach to the biological basis for antibody diversity. *Cont Topics Immunobiol* **9**: 33–47.

Corbel C, Belo M, Martin C and Le Douarin NM (1987). A novel method to bursectomize avian embryos and obtain quail–chick bursal chimeras. II. Immune response of bursectomized chicks and chimeras and post-natal rejection of the grafted quail bursas. *J Immunol* **138**: 2813–2821.

Cordier A (1969). Study of the innervation of the bursa of Fabricius in the embryonic and adult chick. *Acta Anat* **73**: 38–43.

Dahan A, Reynaud C-A and Weill J-C (1983). Nucleotide sequence of the constant region of a chicken mu heavy chain immunoglobulin mRNA. *Nucl Acids Res* **11**: 5381–5389.

Dieterlen-lievre F (1975). On the origin of haemopoiesis stem cells in the avian embryo: an experimental approach. *J Embryol Exp Morphol* **33**: 607–619.

Dixon DK and Fitzsimmons RC (1980). Thymic development of the chick embryo as influenced by hormonal and early surgical bursectomy. *Dev Comp Immunol* **4**: 713–724.

Dolfi A, Lupetti M and Giannessi F (1981). Toxic effect of carrageenan on lymphoid-follicle associated epithelial cells of the bursa of Fabricius of chickens. *Cell Tissue Res* **221**: 67–75.

Dominic CJ (1962). Some remarks on the follicles of the bursa of Fabricius in birds. *Science Culture (India)* **28**: 20–21.

Donnelly N, Brand A and Gilmour DG (1975). Bursal and thymic alloantigen expression in lymphoid tissues of the chicken. *Adv Exp Med Biol* **64**: 293–302.

Dransfield JW (1945). The lymphatic system of the fowl. *Br Vet Sci* **101**: 171 ff.

Droege W (1971). Amplifying and suppressive effect of thymus cells. *Nature* **34**: 549–551.

Droege W (1976). The antigen-inexperience thymic suppressor cell: a class of lymphocytes in the young chicken thymus that inhibits antibody production and cell-mediated immune responses. *Eur J Immunol* **6**: 279–287.

Eerola E (1980). *In vitro* culture of bursal epithelium. *Cell Immunol* **53**: 162–172.

Eerola E, Lassila O, Gilmour DG and Toivanen A (1982).

Induction of B cell differentiation *in vitro* by bursal epithelium. *J Immunol* **128**: 2652–2655.

Eerola E, Jalkanen S, Granfors K and Toivanen A (1983a). Immune capacity of the chicken bursectomized at 60h of incubation. Mitogen induced cell proliferation and immunoglobulin secretion. *J Immunol* **131**: 120–124.

Eerola E, Lassila O, Gilmour DG and Toivanen A (1983b). Characteristics of chicken intraembryonic cells that express B-L (Ia-like) antigens under the influence of cultured bursal epithelium. *Scand J Immunol* **18**: 175–183.

Eerola E, Granfors K, Jalkanen S and Toivanen A (1984a). Immune capacity of the chicken bursectomized at 60h of incubation. Effect of bursal epithelial cells and bursal epithelium conditioned medium on the production of immunoglobulins and specific antibodies *in vitro. Scand J Immunol* **19**: 493–500.

Eerola E, Granfors K, Jalkanen S and Toivanen A (1984b). Immune capacity of the chicken bursectomized at 60h of incubation. Effect of adherent cells on the production of immunoglobulins and specific antibodies *in vitro. Clin Immunol Immunopathol* **31**: 202–211.

Ekino S, Matsuno K and Kotani M (1979). Distribution and role of lymph vessels of the bursa of Fabricii. *Lymphology* **12**: 247–252.

Ekino S, Nawa Y, Tanaka K, Matsuno K, Fujii H and Kotani M (1980). Suppression of immune response by isolation of the bursa of Fabricius from environmental stimuli. *Aust J Exp Biol Med Sci* **58**: 289–296.

Ekino S, Suginohara K, Urano T, Fujii H, Matsuno K and Kotani M (1985). The bursa of Fabricius: a trapping site for environmental antigens. *Immunology* **55**: 405–410.

Ewert DL and Cooper MD (1978). Ia-like alloantigens in the chicken: Serologic characterization and ontogeny of cellular expression. *Immunogenetics* **7**: 521–535.

Ewert DL and Cooper MD (1979). Effects of early embryonic bursectomy on development of $Ig^+.Ia^+$ and $Ig^-.Ia^+$ cells in chickens (Abstract). *Fed Proc* **38**: 1367.

Ewert DL, Munchus MS, Chen CLH and Cooper MD (1984). Analysis of structural properties and cellular distribution of avian Ia antigen by using monoclonal antibodies by monomorphic determinants. *J Immunol* **132**: 2524–2530.

Fitzsimmons RC, Dixon DK and Kocal EMF (1977). The bursal–thymic interrelationship and ontogeny of the immune response in the chick embryo. In Solomon JG and Horton JD (Eds), *Developmental Immunobiology.* Elsevier North-Holland Biomedical Press: Amsterdam. pp 387–394.

Fitzsimmons RC, Garrod EMF and Garnett I (1978). Immunological responses following early embryonic surgical bursectomy. *Cell Immunol* **9**: 377–383.

Fonfria J (1990). Los organos linfoides del estornino negro, *Sturnus unicolor* (Paseriforme). Doctoral Thesis. Faculty of Biology, Complutense University of Madrid.

Forbes WA (1877). On the bursa Fabricii in birds. *Proc Zool Soc London* 304–318.

Frazier J (1974). The ultrastructure of the lymphoid follicles of the chick bursa of Fabricius. *Acta Anat* **88**: 385–397.

Fredericksen TL and Gilmour DG (1988). Influence of genotypes at a non-MHC B lymphocyte alloantigen locus (Bu-l) on expression of Ia (B-L) antigen on chicken bursal lymphocytes. *J Immunol* **134**: 754–756.

Gilmore RStC and Bridges JB (1977). Studies of the bursa of Fabricius. Epithelial bud cell functions (Abstract). *J Anat* **124**: 247.

Gilmour DG, Brand A, Connelly N and Stone HA (1976). Bu-l and Th-l, two loci determining surface antigens of B or T lymphocytes in the chicken. *Immunogenetics* **3**: 549–563.

Giurgea R (1977). Developmental aspects of bursa of Fabricius and thymus during post-hatching ontogenesis in *Gallus domesticus. Ann Biol Anim Biochim Biophys* **17**: 173–178.

Glick B (1960). Extracts from the bursa of Fabricius—a lymphoepithelial gland of the chicken—stimulate the production of antibodies in bursectomized chickens. *Poultry Sci* **39**: 1097–1101.

Glick B (1977). The bursa of Fabricius and immunoglobulin synthesis. *Int Rev Cytol* **48**: 345–402.

Glick B (1979). The avian immune system. *Avian Dis* **23**: 282–289.

Glick B (1982). RES structure and function of the Aves. In Cohen N and Sigel MM (Eds), *The Reticuloendothelial System. A Comprehensive Treatise.* Vol 3. *Phylogeny and Ontogeny.* Plenum Press: New York. pp 509–540.

Glick B and Olah I (1982). The morphology of the starling (*Sturnus vulgaris*) bursa of Fabricius. A scanning and light microscope study. *Anat Rec* **204**: 341–348.

Glick B and Olah I (1984). A continuum of cells leading to an *in vivo* humoral response. *Immunol Today* **5**: 162–165.

Glick B and Olah I (1987). Contribution of a specialized dendritic cell, the secretory cell to the microenvironment of the bursa of Fabricius. In Weber WT and Ewert DL (Eds), *Avian Immunology.* Alan R Liss: New York. pp 53–66.

Glick B, Chang TS and Taap RG (1956). The bursa of Fabricius and antibody production. *Poultry Sci* **35**: 224–226.

Glick B, Holbrook KA and Perkins WD (1977). Scanning electron microscopy of the bursa of Fabricius from normal and testosterone-treated embryos. *Dev Comp Immunol* **1**: 41–46.

Granfors K, Martin C, Lassila O, Suvitaival R, Toivanen A and Toivanen P (1982). Immune capacity of the chicken bursectomized at 60h of incubation. Production of immunoglobulins and specific antibodies. *Clin Immunol Immunopathol* **23**: 459–469.

Grimpe G. (1930). Uber den Pemis von Struthio camelus L. *Zool Garten NF* **2**: 184–193.

Grossi CE, Lydyard PM and Cooper MD (1977a). Ontogeny of B cells in the chicken. II. Changing patterns of cytoplasmic IgM expression and of modulation requirements for surface IgM by anti-mu antibodies. *J Immunol* **119**: 749−756.

Grossi CE, Lydyard PM, Franzi AT and D'Anna F (1977b). Medullary localization of extracellular immunoglobulin and aminopeptidase in lymphoepithelial follicles of the chicken bursa of Fabricius and rabbit appendix. *Dev Comp Immunol* **1**: 157−164.

Hamilton HL (1952). *Lillie's Development of the Chick*. Holt, Rinehart & Winston: New York. pp 390−391.

Hodges RD (1974). *The Histology of the Fowl*. Academic Press: New York. pp 220−221.

Hoffmann-Fezer G and Lade R (1972). Postembryonale Entwicklung und involution der Bursa Fabricii beim Haushahn (*Gallus domesticus*). *Z Zellforsch* **124**: 406−418.

Holbrook KA, Perkins WD and Glick B. (1974). The fine structure of the bursa of Fabricius: 'B' cell surface configuration and lymphoepithelial organization as revealed by scanning and transmission electron microscopy. *J Ret Soc* **16**: 300−311.

Holmes KL and Haar JL (1982). Migration of chicken yolk sac cells to bursa of Fabricius supernatants. *Dev Comp Immunol* **6**: 727−736.

Hoshi S, Numoya T and Ueda S (1988). Identification of B-L antigens on reticular epithelial cells of the bursa of Fabricius. *Microbiol Immunol* **32**: 173−186.

Houssaint E. (1987). Cell lineage segregation during bursa of Fabricius ontogeny. *J Immunol* **138**: 3626−3634.

Houssaint E, Belon P and LeDouarin NM (1976). Investigations on cell lineage and tissue interactions in the developing bursa of Fabricius through interspecific chimeras. *Dev Biol* **53**: 250−254.

Houssaint E, Torano A and Ivanyi J (1983). Ontogenic restriction of colonisation of the bursa of Fabricius. *Eur J Immunol* **13**: 590−595.

Houssaint E, Diez E and Pink JRL (1987). Ontogeny and tissue distribution of the chicken Bu-Ia antigen. *Immunology* **62**: 463−470.

Huang HV and Diener WJ (1978). Bursectomy *in ovo* blocks the generation of immunoglobulin diversity. *J Immunol* **121**: 1738−1747.

Hudson L and Roitt IM (1973). Immunofluorescent detection of surface antigens specific to T and B lymphocytes in the chicken. *Eur J Immunol* **3**: 63−67.

Ivanyi J (1975a). Immunodeficiency in the chicken. I. Disparity in suppression of antibody responses to various antigens following surgical bursectomy. *Immunology* **28**: 1007−1013.

Ivanyi J (1975b). Immunodeficiency in the chicken. II. Production of monomeric IgM following testosterone treatment or infection with Bumboro disease. *Immunology* **28**: 1015−1021.

Ivanyi J (1981). Functions of the B lymphoid system in chickens. In Rose ME, Payne LN and Freeman BM (Eds), *Avian Immunology*. British Poultry Science: Edinburgh. pp 63−101.

Jalkanen S (1973). Immune capacity of the chicken bursectomized at 60h of incubation: transplantation of bone marrow cells of the bursectomized chickens into cyclophosphamide-treated newly hatched recipients. *Eur J Immunol* **13**: 779−785.

Jalkanen S, Granfors K, Jalkanen M and Toivanen P (1983a). Immune capacity of the chicken bursectomized at 60h of incubation. Surface immunoglobulin and B-L (Ia-like) antigen bearing cells. *J Immunol* **130**: 2038−2041.

Jalkanen S, Granfors K, Jalkanen M and Toivanen P (1983b). Immune capacity of the chicken bursectomized at 60h of incubation. Failure to produce immune, natural and autoantibodies in spite of immunoglobulin production. *Cell Immunol* **80**: 363−373.

Jalkanen S, Korpela R, Granfors K and Toivanen P (1984a). Immune capacity of the chicken bursectomized at 60h of incubation. Cytoplasmic immunoglobulins and histological findings. *Clin Immunol Immunopathol* **30**: 41−50.

Jalkanen S, Jalkanen M, Granfors K and Toivanen P (1984b). Defect in the generation of light-chain diversity in bursectomized chickens. *Nature* **311**: 69−71.

Jankovic BD and Isakovic K (1966). Antibody production in bursectomized chickens given repeated injections of antigen. *Nature (London)* **211**: 202−203.

Jankovic BD, Isakovic K, Markovic BM, Rajcevic M and Knezevic Z (1976). Nonbursal origin of humoral immunity: Immune capacity and cytomorphological changes in chickens bursectomized as 52−64h old embryos. *Exp Hematol* **4**: 246−255.

Jankovic BD, Isakovic K, Markovic BM and Rajcevic M (1977). Immunological capacity of the chicken embryo. II. Humoral immune responses in embryos and young chickens bursectomized and sham-bursectomized at 52−64h of incubation. *Immunology* **32**: 689−699.

Jolly J (1915). La bourse de Fabricius et les organes lympho-epitheliaux. *Arch Anat Microsc* **16**: 363−547.

Jotereau FV, Houssaint E and Le Douarin NM (1980). Lymphoid stem cell homing to the early thymic primordium of the avian embryo. *Eur J Immunol* **10**: 620−626.

Kermani-Arab V and Leslie GA (1977). Suppression of immunoglobulin synthesis by transplantation of T cells from anti-mu bursectomized chickens into normal recipients. *J Immunol* **119**: 530−536.

Kincade PW and Cooper MD (1971). Development and distribution of immunoglobulin-containing cells in the chicken. An immunofluorescence analysis using purified antibodies to mu, gamma and light chains. *J Immunol* **106**: 371−382.

Lassila O, Eskola J, Toivanen PC, Martin C and Dieterlen-Lievre F (1978). The origin of lymphoid stem cells studied in chick yolk sac embryo chimeras. *Nature* **272**: 353−354.

Lebacq AM and Ritter MA (1979). B-cell precursors in early chicken embryos. *Immunology* **37**: 123−134.

Le Douarin NM and Houssaint E (1974). L'origine des

lymphocytes de la bourse de Fabricius etudiee sur des chimeres embryonnaires de caille et de poulet. *CR Acad Sci Paris* **278**: 2975−2982.

Le Douarin NM, Houssaint E, Jotereau FV and Belo M (1975). Origin of haemopoietic stem cells in embryonic bursa of Fabricius and bone marrow studied through interspecific chimaeras. *Proc Natl Acad Sci USA* **72**: 2701−2705.

Leydig F (1857). *Lehrbuch der Histologie des Menschen und der Thiere.* Frankfurt am Main. S:321.

Lupetti M and Dolfi A (1980). Concerning bidirectional transport by the lymphoid follicle-associated epithelial cells. *Cell Molec Biol* **26**: 609−613.

Lupetti M and Dolfi A (1982). A contribution to the study of the lymphoid follicle associated epithelial cells. *Z Mikrosk Anat Forsch* **96**: 214−220.

Lupetti M, Dolfi A and Michelucci S (1983). The behavior of bursal lymphoid associated cells after treatment with testosterone. *Anat Rec* **205**: 177−183.

Lupetti M, Dolfi A, Giannessi F and Michelucci S (1986). A contribution to the study of the histogenesis of the bursal lymphoid follicles in *Gallus domesticus. Anat Anz Jena* **162**: 83−92.

Lydyard PM, Grossi CE and Cooper MD (1976). Ontogeny of B cells in the chicken. I. Sequential development of clonal diversity in the bursa. *J Exp Med* **144**: 79−97.

Mark W (1944). Die Entwicklung der Bursa Fabricii bei der Ente. *Z Mikrosk Anat Forsch* **54**: 1−95.

Mathis J (1938). Zum Feinbau der Bursa Fabricii. *Z Mikrosk Anat Forsch* **42**: 179−190.

Moore MAS and Owen JJT (1966). Experimental studies on the development of the bursa of Fabricius. *Dev Biol* **14**: 40−51.

Moore MAS and Owen JJT (1967). Chromosome marker studies in the irradiated chick embryo. *Nature* **215**: 1081−1082.

Moticka EJ (1977). The presence of immunoregulatory cells in chicken thymus: functions in B and T cell responses. *J Immunol* **19**: 987−992.

Murthy KK, Odend'hal S and Ragland WL (1984). Demonstration of T lymphocytes in the bursa of Fabricius of the chicken following cyclophosphamide treatment. *Dev Comp Immunol* **8**: 213−218.

Naukkarinen A (1982). The chicken bursa of Fabricius as a peripheral lymphoid organ. A light and electron microscopic study on the transport of colloidal carbon in the bursa. PhD Thesis, University of Kuopio (Finland).

Naukkarinen A and Sorvari TE (1982a). Cellular transport of colloidal carbon in the follicle-associated epithelium of the chicken bursa of Fabricius. *J Ret Soc* **28**: 473−482.

Naukkarinen A and Sorvari TE (1982b). Morphological and histochemical characterization of the medullary cells in the bursal follicles of the chicken. *Acta Pathol Microbiol Immunol Scand (C)* **90**: 193−199.

Naukkarinen A and Sorvari TE (1984). Involution of the chicken bursa of Fabricius. A light microscopic study with special reference to transport of colloidal carbon in the involuting bursa. *J Leukocyte Biol* **35**: 281−290.

Naukkarinen A and Syrjanen KJ (1984). Effects of anti T lymphocyte serum on immunological reactivity and on the T cell area of the cloacal bursa in the chicken. *Acta Pathol Microbiol Immunol Scand (2)* **92**: 145−151.

Naukkarinen A, Arstila AV and Sorvari TE (1978). Morphological and functional differentiation of the surface epithelium of the bursa of Fabricii in chicken. *Anat Rec* **191**: 415−432.

Niedorf HR and Wolters B (1974). Feinstrukturelle Untersuchungen an den makrophagen der Bursa Fabricii des Huhnchens. *Beitr Path Bd* **151**: 75−86.

Odend'hal S and Breazile JE (1979a). Diffusely infiltrated area of lymphoid cells in the cloacal bursa. *J Ret Soc* **25**: 315−324.

Odend'hal S and Breazile JE (1979b). Luminal lymphoid cells of the cloacal bursa. *Am J Vet Res* **40**: 1015−1018.

Odend'hal S and Breazile JE (1980). An area of T cell localization in the cloacal bursa of white Leghorn chickens. *Am J Vet Res* **41**: 255−258.

Odend'hal S and Player EC (1979). Histochemical localization of T-cells in tissue sections. *Avian Dis* **24**: 886−895.

Olah I and Glick B (1978a). The number and size of the follicular epithelium (FE) and follicles in the bursa of Fabricius. *Poultry Sci* **57**: 1445−1450.

Olah I and Glick B (1978b). Secretory cell in the medulla of the bursa of Fabricius. *Experientia* **34**: 1642−1643.

Olah I and Glick B (1981). Secretory cells in the medulla of the bursal follicles: The small lymphocyte-like cells are precursors of the secretory cells. *Dev Comp Immunol* **5**: 639−648.

Olah I, Glick B, McCorkle F and Stinson R (1979). Light and electron microscope structure of secretory cells in the medulla of bursal follicle of normal and cyclophosphamide treated chickens. *Dev Comp Immunol* **3**: 101−115.

Palladino MA, Lerman SP and Thorbecke GJ (1976). Transfer of hypogammaglobulinemia in two inbred chicken strains by spleen cells from bursectomized donors. *J Immunol* **116**: 1673−1676.

Payne LN and Rennie M (1976). The proportions of B and T lymphocytes in lymphomas, peripheral nerves and lymphoid organs in Marek's disease. *Avian Pathol* **5**: 147−154.

Pink JRL and Lassila A (1987). B-cell commitment and diversification in the bursa of Fabricius. *Curr Top Microbiol Immunol* **135**: 57−64.

Pink JRL, Lassila A and Vainio O (1987). B-lymphocytes and their self-renewal. In Toivanen A and Toivanen P (Eds), *Avian Immunology.* Vol 1. CRC Press: Boca Raton, Florida. pp 65−78.

Pink JRL, Vainio O and Rijnbeek A-M (1985). Clones of B lymphocytes in individual follicles of the bursa of Fabricius. *Eur J Immunol* **15**: 83−87.

Pintea V, Constantinescu GM and Radu C (1967). Vascular

and nervous supply of bursa of Fabricius in the hen. *Acta Vet Acad Sci Hungary* **17**: 263–268.

Potworowski EF (1972). T and B lymphocytes. Organ and age distribution in the chicken. *Immunology* **23**: 199–204.

Ratcliffe MJH, Lassila O, Reynolds J, Pink JRL and Vainio O (1987). A reevaluation of the function of the bursa of Fabricius. In Weber WT and Ewert DL (Eds), *Avian Immunology*. Alan R Liss: New York. pp 3–14.

Reynaud C-A, Dahan A and Weill J-C (1983). Complete nucleotide sequence of a chicken lambda light chain immunoglobulin derived from the nucleotide sequence of its mRNA. *Proc Natl Acad Sci USA* **80**: 4099–4103.

Reynaud C-A, Anquez V, Dahan A and Weill J-C (1985). A single rearrangement event generates most of the chicken immunoglobulin light chain diversity. *Cell* **40**: 283–291.

Romanoff AL (1960). *The Avian Embryo*. Macmillan: New York.

Romppanen T (1982). Postembryonic development of the chicken bursa of Fabricius: a light microscopic histo-quantitative study. *Poultry Sci* **61**: 2261–2270.

Ruuskanen O, Toivanen A and Raekallio J (1977). Histo-chemical characterization of chicken lymphoid tissues. *Dev Comp Immunol* **1**: 231–240.

Schaffner T, Mueller J, Hess MW, Cottier H, Sordat B and Ropke C (1974). The bursa of Fabricius: A central organ providing for contact between the lymphoid system and intestinal content. *Cell Immunol* **13**: 304–312.

Schoenwolf GC, Bell LA and Watterson RL (1981) Vasculogenesis of the bursa clocalis (Bursa of Fabricius) of the chick embryo. *J Morph* **167**: 35–42.

Sherman J and Auerbach R (1966) Quantitative characteriza-tion of chick thymus and bursa development. *Blood* **27**: 371–379.

Sorvari R and Sorvari TE (1977). Bursa Fabricii as a peri-pheral lymphoid organ transport of various materials from the anal lips to the bursal lymphoid follicles with reference to its immunological importance. *Immunology* **32**: 499–505.

Sorvari TE, Sorvari R, Ruotsalainen P, Toivanen A and Toivanen P (1975). Uptake of environmental antigens by the bursa of Fabricius. *Nature* **253**: 217–219.

Stinson R and Glick B (1978). Scanning electron microscopy of chicken lymphocytes: A comparative study of thymic, bursal and splenic lymphocytes. *Dev Comp Immunol* **2**: 311–318.

Sugimura M, Hashimoto Y and Yamada J (1975). Morpho-logy of bursa of Fabricius in bursectomized and thymec-tomized ducks. *Jap J Vet Res* **23**: 17–24.

Syrjanen KJ and Naukkarinen AHM (1982). Post-capillary venules in the T-cell area of chicken cloacal bursa with reference to the state of local immune response. In Collan Y and Romppanen T (Eds), *Morphometry in Morpho-Logical Diagnosis*. Kuopio University Press: Kuopia, Finland. pp 211–216.

Szenberg A (1976). Ontogenesis of the immune system in birds. In Marchalonis JJ (Ed), *Comparative Immunology*.

Blackwell: Oxford. pp 419–431.

Szenberg A and Warner NL (1962). Dissociation of immunological responsiveness in fowls with a hormonally arrested development of lymphoid tissues. *Nature* **194**: 146–147.

Thorbecke GJ, Warner NL, Hochwald GM and Ohanian SH (1968). Immune globulin production by the bursa of Fabricius of young chickens. *Immunology* **15**: 123–124.

Toivanen P, Toivanen A and Good RA (1972a). Ontogeny of bursal function in chicken. I. Embryonic stem cell for humoral immunity. *J Immunol* **109**: 1058–1070.

Toivanen P, Toivanen A, Linna TJ and Good RA (1972b). Ontogeny of bursal function in chicken. II. Postembryonic stem cell for humoral immunity. *J Immunol* **109**: 1071–1080.

Toivanen P, Toivanen A and Good RA (1972c). Ontogeny of bursal function in chicken. III. Immunocompetent cell for humoral immunity. *Exp J Med* **136**: 816–831.

Toivanen P, Naukkarinen A and Vainio O (1987). What is the function of bursa of Fabricius? In Toivanen A and Toivanen P (Eds), *Avian Immunology*. Vol 1. CRC Press: Boca Raton, Florida. pp 79–100.

Uyematsu T (1940). Gefassentwicklung der Bursa Fabricii der Hansente (*Anas domestica L.*). *Jap J Med Sci* **8**: 265–268.

van Alten PJ and Meuwissen HJ (1972). Production of specific antibody by lymphocytes of the bursa of Fabricius. *Science* **176**: 45–47.

Veromaa T (1988). Function of bursa of Fabricius. lympho-cyte surface antigen expression and cellular immunity in chickens bursectomized at 60h of incubation. PhD Thesis, University of Turku (Finland).

von Rautenfeld DB and Budras K-D (1980). A comparative study on the bursa (Fabricii) and tonsilla caecalis in birds. *Folia Morphol (Praha)* **28**: 168–170.

von Rautenfeld DB and Budras K-D (1982). The bursa cloacae (Fabricii) of Struthioniformes in comparison with the bursa of other birds. *J Morph* **172**: 123–138.

von Rautenfeld DB, Buddras K-D and Mitze H (1979). Morphologische Besonderheiten der Bursa cloacae (Fabricii) bei den Laufvogeln (Struthioniformes). *Verh Anato Gds* **73**: 781–783.

Waltenbaugh CR and van Alten PJ (1974). The production of antibody by bursal lymphocytes. *J Immunol* **113**: 1079–1084.

Ward JG and Middleton AL (1971). Weight and histological studies of growth and regression in the bursa of Fabricius in the mallard, *Anas platyrhynchos*. *Can J Zool* **49**: 11–14.

Weber WT and Alexander JE (1978). The potential of bursa-immigrated hematopoietic precursor cells to differentiate to functional B and T cells. *J Immunol* **121**: 653–658.

Weber WT and Mansuer R (1977). Migration patterns of avian embryonic bone marrow cells and their differentia-tion to functional T and B cells. In Benedict AA (Ed), *Avian Immunology*. Plenum Press: New York. pp 47–60.

Weill JC and Reynaud CA (1987). The chicken B cell compartment. *Science* **238**: 1094−1098.

Weill JC, Reynaud CA, Lassila O and Pink JRL (1986). Rearrangement of chicken immunoglobulin genes is not an ongoing process in the embryonic bursa of Fabricius. *Proc Natl Acad Sci USA* **83**: 3336−3340.

Wemckebach KF (1888). De ontwikkeling en de bouw der bursa Fabricii. *Tijdsch Ned Dierk Ver* **2**: 19−38.

Wolfe HR, Sheridan SA, Bilstad NM and Johnson MA (1962). The growth of lymphoidal organs and the testes of chickens. *Anat Rec* **142**: 485−493.

Woods R and Linna J (1965). The transport of cells from the bursa of Fabricius to the spleen and the thymus. *Acta Pathol Microb Immunol Scand* **64**: 470−476.

Yamada J, Sugimura M and Kudo N (1973). The weight and histological changes with age of the bursa of Fabricius in chickens. *Res Bull Obihiro Univ* **8**: 21−44.

Zucker R, Janker U and Droege W (1973). Cellular composition of the chicken thymus: effects of neonatal bursectomy and hydrocortisone treatment. *Eur J Immunol* **3**: 812−818.

5

The Thymus

INTRODUCTION

The thymus is an organ unique to vertebrates, and thus it is important to evolution of adaptive immunity. Apart from small anatomical differences and the number of pharyngeal pouches that contribute to its formation, there are no special histological variations in the organization of the thymus in all vertebrates except for the discussed presence/absence of Hassall's corpuscles in ectothermic vertebrates. Therefore, a thymus gland functioning in the production of lymphocytes occurs in all gnathostomous vertebrates. By contrast, cyclostomes (myxinoids and lampreys) apparently do not possess a thymus or any morphofunctional equivalent. In the present chapter we will review current evidence on the structure of the vertebrate thymus, with special emphasis on the presence or absence of certain cell types, mainly non-lymphoid components, and their possible role in the functioning of this gland. Moreover, the functional role of the thymus in immune reactions of ectothermic vertebrates will be emphasized in fish (mainly teleosts), amphibians and reptiles. Finally, although some histophysiological variations will be pointed out here, information on variations affecting the thymus and other lymphoid organs of ectothermic vertebrates and their relationships with exogenous and endogenous regulatory mechanisms are presented in other chapters.

THE SITUATION IN CYCLOSTOMES

Despite previous reports claiming the presence of a thymus in myxinoids and lampreys, current evidence supports its absence in Agnatha. In any case, the situation appears to be different in both groups of cyclostomes. In the Atlantic hagfish, *Myxine glutinosa*, some authors (Muller, 1845; Stannius, 1854) described a thymus gland, later shown to be the pronephros. An attempt to establish homology between the excretory system of *Amphioxus* and the vertebrate thymus was also made by Van Wijhe (1923). More recent reports accept, however, that hagfish have no thymus (Kampmeier, 1969; Papermaster *et al.*, 1964; Fange and Zapata, unpublished observations). To find a morphologically identifiable thymus, Riviere *et al.* (1975) reported lymphocyte-like cells in the muscle velar complex of the Pacific hagfish, *Eptatretus stoutii*, which indicates that this mass is a possible proto-thymus, or phylogenetic precursor of the gnathostomous thymus. The complex lies within a lymph sinus, traps particulate matter and contains antigen-binding cells not found in other muscles or in the general circulation. These workers agreed, nevertheless, that their evidence was limited and that a detailed study of their images may represent the lymphocyte-like cells which resemble satellite cells of the skeletal muscle rather than lymphoid elements. Thus, due to difficulties in capturing young hagfish where a thymus could perhaps be confirmed, there still remains doubt as to the possible early involution of the thymus in adult specimens which have been analyzed thus far. It is assumed therefore that the thymus in these cyclostomes is absent.

In lampreys, from classical light microscopical evidence, lymphoid accumulations found in the branchial region of ammocoetes were considered to be homologous to the thymus (Finstad *et al.*, 1964). However, recent ultrastructural observations and more precise knowledge of changes which occur in the lymphoid system throughout the lamprey's life cycle have conclusively rejected this possibility (Sterba, 1953; Yamaguchi *et al.*, 1979; Page and Rowley, 1982; Ardavin and Zapata, 1988a; Ardavin *et al.*, 1984). These lymphoid aggregates consist of collections of lymphocytes which are associated with blood sinuses. These aggregates are located above and below the branchial clefts, in the epipharyngeal and the hypopharyngeal folds and in the partition walls which support the branchial laminae (Figure 5.1). The histological organization of these lymphoid pharyngeal aggregates as revealed by electron microscopy is, however, similar in all locations. It consists of enlarged blood sinuses where lymphocytes and large macrophages abound (Figure 5.2). Some lymphocytes invade the pharyngeal epithelium and mitotic figures are frequent (Figure 5.2). The pharyngeal region of young adult lampreys undergoes an enormous change after metamorphosis, due principally to modifications of the branchial apparatus, resulting in the definitive, adult lamprey structure. As a consequence, those areas which formerly contained lymphoid accumulations are occupied by dense connective tissue, with accompanying signs of lymphoid aggregates. Depending on the changes which these accumulations have undergone, the cell types described in them and their histological organization, these areas might represent, at least in some life stages, lymphohemopoietic loci or blood filtering regions, but not thymic precursors. Some authors (Page and Rowley, 1982; Ardavin and Zapata, 1988a) suggest that these organs might be associated with antigen-trapping, since the pharynx itself is contiguous with the surrounding anatomical environments where microorganisms and detritus occur most abundantly.

The cavernous body is another pharyngeal formation in ammocoetes which contains lymphoid cells

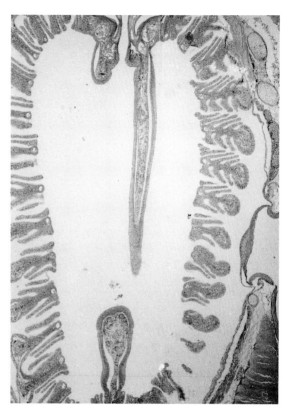

Figure 5.1 Pharyngeal region of an ammocoete, *Petromyzon marinus*, showing sinuses of the branchial cleft, the epipharyngeal fold, hypopharyngeal fold, partition wall and endostyle ($\times$ 33). (From *Acta Zool Stockh* **65**: 1, 1984, reproduced by permission.)

(Gerard, 1933; Nakao, 1978; Yamaguchi *et al.*, 1979; Ardavin and Zapata, 1988b). The gill cavernous body is a vascular structure, differentiated from the afferent artery of each gill filament. It consists of an enlarged blood sinus which is crossed by connective tissue trabeculae that are formed by reticular and collagenous fibers and lined by phagocytic endothelial cells. Numerous lymphocytes, plasmablasts and mature plasma cells occur within the lumen of the cavernous body. Yamaguchi *et al.* (1979) demonstrated the capacity of endothelial cells within the lamprey's cavernous body for trapping latex, colloidal carbon and rat erythrocytes which had been injected into the bloodstream. Moreover, Tomonaga *et al.* (1975) reported the phagocytic capacity of endothelial cells of gill efferent arterioles, thus confirming earlier findings

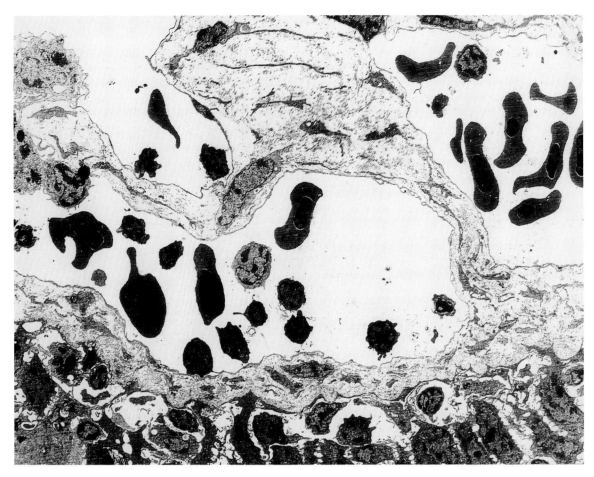

Figure 5.2 Branchial sinus in the pharynx of an ammocoete, *Petromyzon marinus*. Lymphocytes migrate into the pharyngeal epithelium and inside blood sinuses but with no characteristics similar to the thymus. Giant macrophages abound in the blood sinus (× 2920). (From *Thymus* **11**: 59, 1988, reproduced by permission.)

of phagocytic elements in the cavernous bodies of elasmobranchs (Wright, 1973). In fact, the general histology and cell types which have been observed in the lamprey's cavernous body, as in those of the pharyngeal lymphoid aggregates, resemble medullary sinuses of mammalian lymph nodes (Olah *et al.*, 1975). They probably play a role in the trapping and processing of antigens that may have gained entrance via the pharynx. In any case, it is remarkable that despite the absence of any distinguishable thymus gland in cyclostomes they are, however, able to mount immune responses typical of the T-lymphocytes of higher vertebrates (for review see Zapata, 1983).

Perhaps minimal requirements, such as the presence of circulating lymphocytes and diffuse clusters of lymphoid tissue, might be sufficient in Agnatha to elaborate immune responses.

THE THYMUS IN GNATHOSTOMES

General

Despite reports concerning the absence of a thymus gland in some gnathostomes (in the gar, *Lepisosteus platyrhincus*, Marchalonis, 1977; in adult *Sphenodon*,

Marchalonis *et al.*, 1969), it is currently assumed that the thymus is present in all vertebrates except Agnatha. Moreover, there are minimal anatomical and histological differences between the various vertebrate classes. These include principally the organ's location, number of lobes related to the pharynx, presence/ absence of well-differentiated cortex—medulla demarcation, etc. In elasmobranchs, the thymus is a multilobulated bilateral organ located near the gills (Figure 5.3). By contrast, the teleostean thymus consists of a pair of lobes located on each side of the gill cavity (Figure 5.4). A lobulated thymus has been

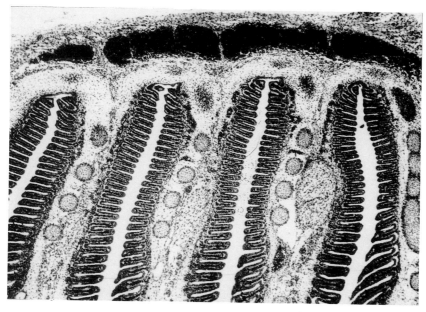

Figure 5.3 Thymus of a larva of the torpedo ray *Torpedo marmorata.* Several gill pouches contribute to the formation of the thymus (× 70).

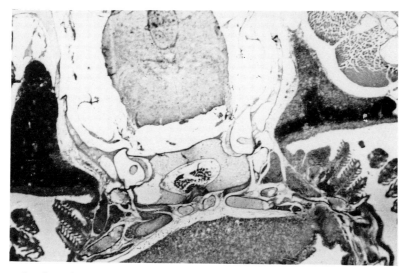

Figure 5.4 Cross-section through the anterior part of an adult fish, *Rutilus rutilus*, showing the paired thymus in continuity with the gill epithelium (× 120). (From *Dev Comp Immunol* **5**: 427, 1981, reproduced by permission.)

reported in some species of urodeles, such as *Necturus maculosus* (James, 1939) but not in others (*Notophthalmus maculosus*, Hightower and St Pierre, 1971; *Plethodon glutinosus*, Curtis *et al.*, 1979). Apodans (Garcia-Herrera and Cooper, 1968; Zapata *et al.*, 1982) and anurans (Cooper, 1976) apparently have no lobulated thymi. In the tuatara and in most lizards and snakes, there are two thymic lobes on each side of the neck, whereas the thymus of crocodilians is an elongated chain-like structure. In turtles some comparative immunologists described a single lobe (Bockman, 1970) whereas others have reported a multilobulated organ (Borysenko and Cooper, 1972; Leceta *et al.*, 1984). Glick (1982) has described a bilateral thymus in birds which consists of seven lobes. The situation is especially notable in some primitive mammals, where there are two thymus glands, one thoracic and another cervical. Although most marsupials have only a thoracic or cervical thymus, the

Macropidae, for example, the quokka *Setonix brachyurus* has both. Both thymus glands apparently have the same functions but operate at different ages (Yadav *et al.*, 1972). Yadav *et al.* (1972) have correlated the existence of a superficial thymus with an herbivorous diet, small size, long pouch life and an additional deep pouch (with closely apposed lips).

A topological relationship between the thymus and pharyngeal cavity is evident in all vertebrates, but especially in adult teleost fishes, where thymus gland and pharyngeal epithelium remain continuous (Figure 5.4). Clearly, a well-differentiated cortex and medulla are lacking in most teleosts (Figure 5.5). By contrast, three (Hafter, 1952 in *Astyanax*; Sailendri and Muthukkarruppan, 1975 in *Tilapia mossambica*; Chilmonczyk, 1983 in *Salmo gairdneri*; Gorgollon, 1983 in *Sicyases sanguineus*) or even four layers (Mulcahy, 1970 in *Esox lucius*) have been reported in the thymus of teleosts.

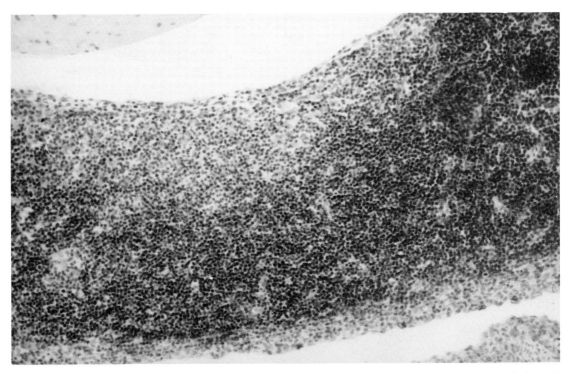

Figure 5.5 Thymus of an adult teleost fish, *Rutilus rutilus*, containing a light-staining peripheral region and a dark staining central zone. This condition in teleost fish is the reverse of that in the thymus of all other vertebrates ($\times$ 180). (From *Dev Comp Immunol* **5**: 427, 1981, reproduced by permission.)

One of us has described two regions in *Rutilus rutilus* (Zapata, 1981) although they are truly equivalent to the three found by Gorgollon (1983). An outer cortex is related to the opercular epithelium, a deep cortex is equivalent to the classical cortex of tetrapod vertebrates, and a basal region is structurally similar to the medulla. This special organization is related to the diffuse limits observed between the thymic tissue and pharyngeal epithelium and the presence of a delimiting connective tissue capsule in the teleostean thymus.

In most other vertebrates except urodelan and apodan amphibians, there is a clear separation between cortex and medulla (Figure 5.6). In primitive fishes this condition has been repeatedly confirmed (Fange and Sundell, 1969 in *Chimaera monstrosa*; Zapata, 1980 in *Raja clavata* and *Torpedo marmorata*; in the holostean bowfin, cited by Zapata, 1983), although a recent report denies it in the shark, *Scyliorhinus canicula* (cited by Fange and Pulsford, 1985). In urodeles, no distinction between thymic cortex and medulla has been clearly observed (Webster, 1934 in *Ambystoma maculosus*; James, 1939 in *Necturus maculosus*; Klug, 1967 in *Ambystoma mexicanum*; Hightower and St Pierre, 1971; Curtis *et al.*, 1979 in *Plethodon glutinosus*). A similar condition has been found in the apodan thymus (Garcia-Herrera and Cooper, 1968 in *Nectocaecilia cooperii*; Zapata *et al.*, 1982 in *Ichthyophis kohtaoensis*).

Although some investigators have attempted to relate the lack of differentiation into cortex and medulla with chronic immune reactivity in urodeles, these species do apparently contain the necessary T-like cell subpopulations to elicit quite adequate immune responses, such as rejection of skin grafts. In contrast to species differences, another important emerging concept merits brief mention here which will be elaborated extensively in a later chapter. Besides, the thymus gland of ectothermic vertebrates undergoes profound morphological variations due to age, season, stress, nutrition, etc. which can mask a clear demarcation between the two thymic areas. Thus, caution must be observed in interpreting what may be apparently precise morphology.

Anatomical Localization

The thymus, as an organ derived embryologically from the pharyngeal pouches, is related to the blood vessels and nerves of the neck, and the various pharyngeal derivatives, such as thyroid, parathyroid and ultimobranchial bodies in all vertebrates. In elasmobranchs, the thymus is located near the gills and electric organs, whereas in teleosts its relationship with the gill cavity has already been described (Figure 5.4). The thymus glands in amphibians occupy a dorsal position in relation to the mandibular joints in anurans, or lies near the posterior ends of the hyoids in urodeles (Plytycz and Bigaj, 1983). Reptilian thymus glands occur in a variable area of the neck in close relationship with large vessels and nerves. Bockman (1970) reported that, despite differences in the number and shape of thymic lobes within the major reptilian groups, a characteristic anatomical situation may be described for each. Avian thymuses are located on either side of the neck, extending from the lower jaw to the thorax. In most mammals, the thymus lies in the upper part of the thorax.

Embryonic Development

The thymus in all vertebrates develops from the pharyngeal buds, although there are differences in various classes with respect to the number and position of buds which contribute to its formation. In some elasmobranchs, the dorsal epithelium of all six embryonic pharyngeal pouches, including the spiracular pouch, can give rise to thymic lobes although they all do not contribute to the adult thymus. In the teleost *Tilapia mossambica*, the thymic rudiment is a dorsolateral derivative of the second, third and fourth pouches (Sailendri, 1973). Species of apodans retain a primitive branchiomeric arrangement of the thymic anlagen (Wiedersheim, 1879). Each pair of pharyngeal pouches develops dorsal, epithelial primordia. Of these, the first and last atrophy and the remaining four pairs produce the definitive thymic lobes. In urodeles, distinct patterns of development and differentiation in the thymus have been observed. Manning and Turner (1976) reported five initially distinct pairs of thymic buds, of which two disappear, leaving three, four and five pouches which form the adult thymus. In some newts, however, the thymus is entirely formed by the fifth pouch (Tournefier, 1973; Charlemagne, 1977). The embryological development of the thymus in several reptilian classes has been reviewed by Bockman (1970). The anterior and posterior thymic

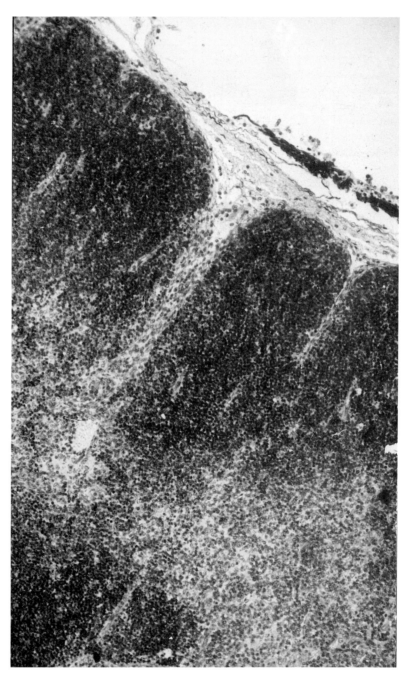

Figure 5.6 Thymus of an adult torpedo ray, *Torpedo marmorata*. Thymic lobules are separated by clearly defined connective tissue trabeculae. Note the differentiation between cortex and medulla (× 80). (From *Dev Comp Immunol* **4**: 459, 1980, reproduced by permission.)

lobes originate in lizards from the dorsal part of the second and third pharyngeal pouches. In some species, transient thymic rudiments which are associated with the first pouch have also been observed. In turtles, a third thymus originates from the corresponding pouch, while a variable fourth thymus and a transitory one develop respectively from the fourth and fifth pouches. A further caudal shift occurs in snakes, although the definitive thymus originates from the fourth and fifth pharyngeal pouches and a transitory third thymus may appear as a dorsal formation of the third pouch. Avian and mammalian thymus develop from third and fourth pharyngeal pouches (Hammond, 1954; Ruth et al., 1964), although in mammals, unlike other vertebrates, it is the ventral region of the pouch which gives rise to the developing thymus (Manning and Turner, 1976).

Apart from this diversity in the six pharyngeal pouches which contribute to the development of the vertebrate thymus, mechanisms of differentiation, origin of thymic lymphoid cells and intrathymic cell colonization appear to be similar in the various vertebrates, although information is sparse. Thus, much evidence supports the view that the thymus is the first organ to become lymphoid during ontogeny (Beard, 1900; Warner and Szenberg, 1962; Archer et al., 1964; Auerbach, 1961; Sherman and Auerbach, 1966; Cooper, 1967; Moore and Owen, 1967; Horton, 1971; Manning, 1971; Sailendri, 1973). However, in some urodeles such as the newt Triturus alpestris, the thymus appears late (7th week) and the differentiation of thymocytes still later (9th week) (Tournefier, 1973). Thymus appears ontogenically at 2 days post-hatching in Cyprinus carpio (at 22 °C) (Botham et al., 1980) and at 5 days pre-hatching in Salmo gairdneri (at 14 °C) (Grace and Manning, 1980). In carp, small lymphocytes are present at age 1 week but do not acquire surface Ig until day 14 (van Loon et al., 1981), while in Salmo salar surface Ig appears at around the time of first feeding (day 45) (Ellis, 1977). According to Clerx (1978), Ig synthesis starts at 18 days after hatching, but Ig levels are still low in month-old pike. In any case, results concerning the presence of Ig-surface-positive cells in the thymus of lower vertebrates must be viewed with some reservation. Recently Secombes et al. (1983) analyzed the ontogeny of the carp thymus using monoclonal antibodies. They found that as soon as the thymic antigen could be observed histologically, all the cells possessed the determinant which was detected by a monoclonal antibody from clone WCT4, an Ig^+ T^+ clone. At 10 – 12 days after fertilization a differential staining appeared within the thymus using this clone, but it was not until day 16 that a staining pattern similar to that of the adult thymus was observed. By contrast, the determinants detected by two Ig^- T^+ clones were not present until day 7, and the adult pattern was slower to be observed, up to 4 weeks after fertilization. Thus, those results showed that different surface determinants on thymocytes occurred on different tissues during ontogeny, reflecting, according to these authors, the appearance of distinct subpopulations during ontogeny, or the sequential acquisition of determinants which appear during differentiation.

The thymic anlage appears in anuran embryos soon after blood begins to circulate in the external gills (Nieuwkoop and Faber, 1967; Curtis et al., 1972; Nagata, 1977). The dorsal area of the pouch epithelium thickens and forms a protrusion in both the urodeles and anurans that soon loses its connection with the pharyngeal endoderm, appearing then as a small cell cluster. Nagata (1977) reported in Xenopus laevis that possible precursor lymphoid cells appear when the thymic rudiment has not detached from the pharyngeal epithelium. Moreover, the first appearance of small lymphocytes coincided with that of secretory epithelial cells (Nagata, 1977). In this regard, Henry and Charlemagne (1981) observed numerous cell contacts between the reticuloepithelial cells and developing lymphocytes during the early phase of thymic development in Pleurodeles waltlii. They concluded that the supporting cells were involved in lymphocyte multiplication and differentiation. Ultrastructural studies of thymic development in Rana pipiens revealed that once the lymphoid populations, medullary epithelial cells and myoid cells appear, later changes are basically quantitative and are accompanied by increasing numbers of cortical lymphocytes, sequential evidence of secretory activity from epithelial cells and a tendency of myoid cells to associate in clusters.

In reptiles, thymic development begins as a slight invagination of pharyngeal epithelium just medial to the branchial placode. After epithelial proliferation, a hollow, lobulated projection is formed, the connection of which to the pharyngeal pouch is broken, causing disappearance of the intermediate pouch tissue. Then, progressive cell proliferation obliterates the central cavity (Saint-Remy and Prenant, 1904; Shaner,

1921). In *Calotes versicolor*, Pitchappan and Muthukkaruppan (1977a) reported blood-borne stem cells of unknown origin which infiltrate the epithelial thymic rudiment, appearing subsequently as large and small lymphocytes. Likewise, Vasse (1983) found basophilic cells, regarded in other vertebrates as lymphoid precursors, around and among cells of the thymic epithelial anlage.

El Deeb *et al.* (1985) recently published in detail the histology of thymic development in the lizard *Chalcides ocellatus*. Thymic primordia appear by stage 30 (Zada and El Deeb, 1982) as thickenings of the posterioventral wall of pharyngeal pouch II and the posterior wall of pharyngeal pouch III. By stage 31 a slit-like fissure divides a dorsal primordium and a ventral part. Simultaneously, the anterior thymic anlage appears as a bud-like protrusion of the posterio-dorsal wall of the second visceral arch. Thereafter (stage 32) both thymic rudiments appear as epithelial cell condensations surrounded by mesenchyme, although a connective tissue capsule is not formed until stage 35. At stage 36 the thymus contains numerous undifferentiated cells and large lymphocytes among the epithelial cells. In the following stages the number of thymocytes greatly increases, the proportion of large lymphocytes diminishes as development proceeds, whereas that of medium and small lymphocytes increases. A similar sequence has been reported in the lizard *Calotes versicolor* (Kanakambika and Muthukkaruppan, 1973; Pitchappan and Muthukkaruppan, 1977a) and in turtles and alligators (Sidky and Auerbach, 1968). The cortex – medulla differentiation is accomplished at stage 41 just before hatching.

According to Le Douarin and Jotereau (1975) the avian thymus is at first populated by an influx of migrating stem cells which occurs around the 7th day of incubation. Brand *et al.* (1983), in agreement with that report, showed that initial colonization of the thymus in embryonic chickens was restricted to 6.5 – 8 days of incubation. Another migratory wave happens at the end of embryonic life which completely replaces the population of pre-existing lymphocytes that migrate to peripheral lymphoid organs (Le Douarin and Jotereau, 1975). The predominantly large lymphocytes found in the 11-day thymus are replaced progressively by smaller cells between days 11 and 13 (Sugimoto *et al.*, 1977a; Boyd and Ward, 1984) and

thus by day 18 virtually all are small lymphocytes (Boyd and Ward, 1984). Embryonic thymus-specific antigen appears at day 12 or 13, thus correlating with morphological changes in thymic lymphocytes (Sugimoto *et al.*, 1977a). At this same time reticulo-epithelial cells show electron-lucent vacuoles and dense bodies (Sugimoto *et al.*, 1977b). Abundant asymmetric division also occurs in thymocytes (Sugimoto *et al.*, 1979; Yasuda *et al.*, 1981). Their biological significance is unclear, although they are found coincidentally during a critical period when there are drastic transformations: changes in shape and motility, and the appearance of terminal deoxy-nucleotidyl transferase and thymus-specific antigens (Sugimoto *et al.*, 1977a; Schauenstein and Wick, 1977; Sugimoto and Bollum, 1979; Yasuda *et al.*, 1980); reticuloepithelial cells show electron-lucent vacuoles and dense bodies (Sugimoto *et al.*, 1977a). Using antisera raised against different B-cell markers, Boyd and Ward (1984) demonstrated minimal presence of positive cells in avian embryonic thymus. During later embryonic phases, lymphocytes expressing J chain have also been detected in the avian thymus (Moriya and Ichikawa, 1984), suggesting the presence of few B-lymphocytes in the avian embryonic thymus. In fact, several authors have reported lymphoid cell traffic between the bursa of Fabricius and thymus during the embryonic period (Hemmingsson, 1972; Albini and Wick, 1973) and adult life (Woods and Linna, 1965; Zucker *et al.*, 1973; Droege *et al.*, 1972).

Cell Types

The Thymic Capsule and Trabeculae

The vertebrate thymus is surrounded by a continuous connective tissue capsule, although some comparative immunologists have reported that the thymus of certain teleosts is relatively unprotected, without a specialized thymic membrane (Tatner and Manning, 1982). In large glands the thymic capsule projects inside the thymic parenchyma by connective tissue trabeculae carrying large blood vessels and nerves and dividing the thymic lobes into several lobules. In other cases connective tissue trabeculae in the thymus occur as short, enlarged pale areas where blood vessels and mesenchymal cells are evident (Figure 5.5). In both cases ultrastructural organization of the thymic capsule and trabeculae are similar, consisting mainly of fibroblasts and fibrocytes, together with masses of collagenous fibers (Figure 5.7). Mutual relationships between lymphocytes of the thymic parenchyma and connective tissue components of the capsule are especially remarkable. Thus reticuloepithelial processes showing a continuous basement membrane are always interposed between the lymphoid cells and connective tissue elements (Figure 5.7). It is apparently a component of the so-called blood—thymus barrier, the organization and function of which will be described later.

Reticuloepithelial Cells

The thymic parenchyma in vertebrates is formed by a network of supporting reticuloepithelial cells and free cells. Although various types of reticuloepithelial cells, sometimes with different names, have been reported in the thymus in view of their location in the cortex or medulla, electron density, more or less irregular shape, etc., all workers point out their epithelial origin and the presence of tonofilaments and desmosomes (Zapata, 1980; cited by Fange and Pulsford, 1985 in elasmobranchs; Zapata, 1981; Gorgollon, 1983 in teleosts; Kapa, 1963; Klug, 1967; Henry and Charlemagne, 1980, 1981 in urodeles;

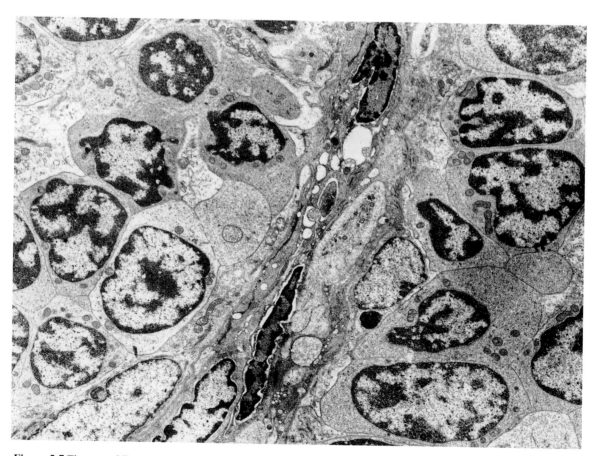

Figure 5.7 Thymus of *Torpedo marmorata*. Connective tissue trabecula formed mainly by electron-dense fibroblasts and fibrocytes separating it into thymic lobules. Reticular epithelial cells under the connective tissue capsule isolate small lymphocytes and lymphoblasts (× 2455).

Kapa *et al.*, 1968; Curtis *et al.*, 1972; Nagata, 1976, 1977; Hanzlikowa, 1979; Bigaj and Plytycz, 1981, 1984 in anurans; Bockman and Winborn, 1967, 1969 in reptiles; Frazier, 1973; Kendall and Frazier, 1979; Kendall, 1980; Fonfria *et al.*, 1983 in birds). In the thymic cortex these cells are large, irregular electron-dense elements, which contain, especially in anuran amphibians, an irregular nucleus with condensed chromatin arranged peripherally and a patent nucleolus which frequently shows striking inclusions (Figure 5.8). In the electron-dense cytoplasm, bundles of microfilaments abound as well as small mito-chondria and electron-dense granules (Figure 5.8). These cells constitute a meshwork, in whose holes lymphocytes exist, and whose numerous cell processes are joined together, thus forming a true battery of desmosomes (Figure 5.8). In the thymus of *Torpedo marmorata* and *Raja clavata* some of these cortical reticuloepithelial cells seem to have phagocytic

capacity (Zapata, 1980), although some authors (Olah *et al.*, 1975) deny this possibility, considering that only true macrophages phagocytose inside the thymus. In the medulla, supporting cells of the thymic network appear to be less electron dense and contain smaller numbers of microfilaments and desmosomes. In the thymic medulla of all vertebrates there are numerous and different epithelial cells, many of them related to secretory activity, and epithelial cysts which will be described later. In the thymus of some ectothermic vertebrates, there are cells, apparently associated with bundles of reticular fibers and surrounded by lympho-cytes, which make contacts on the surface of these cells and resemble the so-called nurse cells in the mammalian thymus.

Apart from evidence for a supporting function, the role of thymic stroma in the education of T-cells and restriction of T-cell specificities has been recently emphasized (Zinkernagel *et al.*, 1978; Longo and

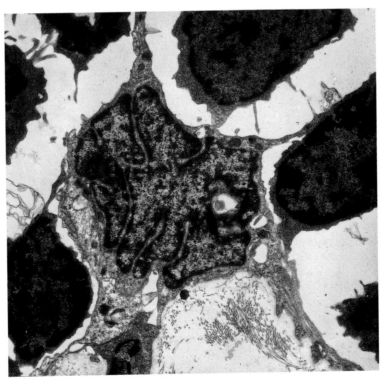

Figure 5.8 Cortical reticular epithelial cells of the thymus of *Rana perezi*. These cells containing remarkable irregular nuclei with patent inclusions are joined together by numerous desmosomes constituting the supporting apparatus of the organ (×11000).

Schwartz, 1980; Olivier and Le Douarin, 1984). Other authors, however, claimed that the thymus is not the only site for determining the range of MHC restriction (Katz *et al.*, 1979). Immunochemistry studies in the mouse thymus demonstrated that reticuloepithelial cells were the major thymic elements which expressed MHC antigens (Rouse *et al.*, 1979; van Ewijk *et al.*, 1980). Moreover, I-A and H-2K antigens have been associated with different thymic microenvironments. I-A antigens occur throughout both cortex and medulla, whereas K antigens are only found in the medulla. At present, it seems that the supporting cells of the thymic cortex express a high density of class II MHC antigens, while the medullary supporting cells express a high density of class I MHC gene products but not class II antigens (Smith, 1984). Morphological evidence of lymphostromal complexes in thymic cell suspensions (Wekerle *et al.*, 1980) has supported the relevance of thymic stroma in the differentiation of mammalian T-cells. These complexes, so-called thymic nurse cells, consist of a single epithelial cell surrounded by high numbers of intact thymocytes. They occur in the subcapsular and outer cortical areas of the thymus (Kyewski and Kaplan, 1982). Recent immunohistological characterization of these complexes indicates that they represent *in vitro* the *in vivo* association of reticuloepithelial cells with cortical thymocytes, functioning possibly in providing a cell microenvironment which guides early stages of intrathymic T-cell differentiation (van Vliet *et al.*, 1984).

Apart from certain ultrastructural images, such as those shown here, which suggest morphological resemblance with mammalian thymic nurse cells, functional evidence for this existence is lacking in ectothermic vertebrates. Nevertheless, functional studies have questioned the possible role of *Xenopus* thymus in the restriction process (Flajnik *et al.*, 1984). These authors have been unable to find a role for reticuloepithelial cells in MHC restriction, which suggests that MHC antigen presenting cells migrating inside the thymus could be cell elements implicated in this phenomenon. The possible existence of such dendritic cells in the thymus of ectothermic vertebrates will be discussed later. Flajnik *et al.* (1984) concluded that the thymus of *Xenopus laevis* does play a role in selecting MHC specificities of pre-T-cells. Moreover, this selection occurs early in life and it is not absolute.

Lymphocytes and Macrophages

Lymphocytes are obviously the most abundant cell population found in the vertebrate thymus. Thymocytes are more or less round cells, with abundant condensed chromatin and a patent nucleolus (Figure 5.7). Their size is variable and there are no morphological light and ultrastructural markers that can be used to distinguish between the different functional populations described principally in birds and mammals, although there are emerging results on the ectotherms. The assumed idea for the thymus of ectothermic vertebrates is that higher mitotic activity of large lymphocytes in the outer cortex is followed by a gradual interior deposition of small lymphocytes concomitant with their maturation (Hightower, 1975; Horton and Horton, 1975; Nagata, 1976). Sometimes pyknotic lymphocytes occur in appreciable numbers in the thymic cortex, verifying what numerous authors have concluded, i.e. most thymocytes die *in situ* (Scollay and Shortman, 1985). However, many of these pyknotic lymphocytes are related, at least in some birds, with seasonal changes affecting the thymus gland (see Kendall, 1980 for review).

Macrophages are a common component of the vertebrate thymus (Bockman, 1970; Frazier, 1973; Kendall and Frazier, 1979; Zapata, 1980; Fonfria *et al.*, 1983; Gorgollon, 1983; Bigaj and Plytycz, 1984; Leceta *et al.*, 1984), although their numbers vary according to species. They always contain cytoplasmic cell debris and their numbers are especially important in reptiles (Leceta *et al.*, 1984) and birds (Bacchus and Kendall, 1975; Kendall and Frazier, 1979), whose thymus undergoes seasonal, regressive changes. More detailed information on macrophages in the avian thymus is available in the chick and quail, where two types of accessory cells of extrinsic origin have recently been described (Olivier and Le Douarin, 1984): one expresses class II MHC determinants and is devoid of phagocytic properties; the second is a large, round phagocyte, considered as macrophages, which express no surface Ia molecules. Precursors for both cell types apparently colonize the thymic rudiment along with the first wave of lymphocytes (6.5 − 8 days fertilization in chick embryos), undergo significant expansion and differentiate early during development (a few days after the first colonization is achieved) into

accessory cells. If there are more waves of colonization, this is unknown, although current results indicate
that the first wave of accessory cells is renewed in
parallel with turnover of the first wave of thymocytes
(Olivier and Le Douarin, 1984).

Interdigitating Cells

Since their discovery in mammalian lymphoid organs
(Veldman, 1970; Veldman and Keuning, 1978;
Veldman *et al.*, 1978a, b), the presence of interdigitating cells (IDCs) has been confirmed by numerous
authors in mammals (Veldman and Kaiserling, 1980;
Villena, 1981), but information in ectothermic vertebrates is sparse (Bigaj and Plytycz, 1984; Barrutia
et al., 1985b in anurans; Leceta *et al.*, 1984 in reptiles;
Kendall and Frazier, 1979; Fonfria *et al.*, 1982 in
birds). Ultrastructural organization of thymic interdigitating cells in ectotherms appears to be similar to that
reported in mammals. Interdigitating cells occur
principally in the medulla and corticomedullary border
of the thymic parenchyma. They contain an irregularly
shaped or sometimes oval nucleus, with a peripheral
rim of condensed chromatin (Figures 5.9, 5.10). The
cytoplasm exhibits two clearly demarcated areas: a
perinuclear region which contains most of the membranous organelles, and a peripherally located electron-lucent area almost totally devoid of such
structures (Figures 5.9, 5.l0). Smooth, flattened Golgi
saccules, mitochondria and numerous tubules of
smooth endoplasmic reticulum are concentrated in a
perinuclear region (Figures 5.9, 5.10). In the thymic
interdigitating cells of the spotless starling, *Sturnus
unicolor*, rough endoplasmic reticulum is also well
developed (Fonfria *et al.*, 1982). In any case, the most
remarkable feature of interdigitating cells is their
extensive interdigitations found on the cell surface
(Figures 5.9, 5.10). Although no cell contacts generally occur between interdigitating cells and neighboring lymphocytes, they have been found in the turtle
Mauremys caspica. Small electron-dense granules are
frequently found in these cells (Figure 5.9). In addition
they sometimes contain dense bodies and cell debris,
which suggests a phagocytic capacity (Figure 5.10).
Birbeck granules reported in the IDCs of some mammals are absent in those of lower vertebrates, although
cytoplasmic granules, some with a striking morphology, often occur (Barrutia *et al.*, 1985a).

In the thymus of spotless starlings, *Sturnus
unicolor*, interdigitating cells frequently form clusters
in which the cell limits are difficult to see, thus giving
the appearance of a multinucleate formation; sometimes cytoplasmic processes of thymic myoid cells
penetrate into their cytoplasm (Fonfria *et al.*, 1983). In
addition, immature, pro-interdigitating cells exist in
the thymus of *Mauremys caspica* (Leceta *et al.*, 1984)
and *Sturnus unicolor* (Fonfria *et al.*, 1982). Presumptive pro-interdigitating cells of the thymus in the
turtle *Mauremys caspica* are especially interesting.
They are large, electron-pale dendritic cells, with
polygonal or irregular nuclei which contain a small rim
of condensed chromatin in the periphery and sometimes a small nucleolus (Figure 5.11). The cytoplasm
exhibits a characteristic pattern with scant membranous organelles arranged perinuclearly and an
empty ectoplasm which projects in numerous irregular
processes that lack cytoplasmic organelles but do
contain only some profiles of smooth, endoplasmic

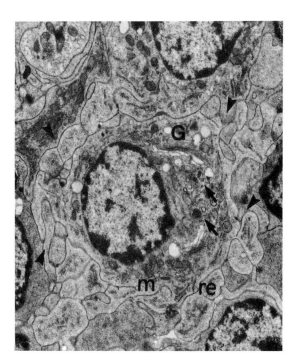

Figure 5.9 Mature interdigitating cell of the thymus of the
turtle *Mauremys caspica*. Note the perinuclear arrangement
of the cytoplasmic organelles (G = Golgi; m = mitochondria; re = reticulum) and the numerous irregular interdigitations (arrows) occurring on the cell surface (× 9500).

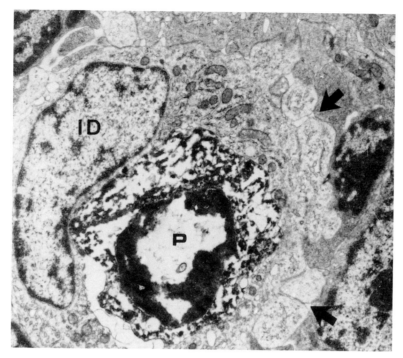

Figure 5.10 Interdigitating cell (ID) of the thymus of *Mauremys caspica* containing phagocytosed material (P) in the cytoplasm after intense cell death (× 9600).

reticulum scattered at random (Figure 5.11). In the perinuclear area, small electron-dense mitochondria, a few small granules with electron-dense areas, and abundant tubules and vesicles of smooth endoplasmic reticulum are the principal components. Sometimes a centriole, sparse profiles of rough endoplasmic reticulum and microtubules, but not microfilaments, exist also in the cytoplasm of these cells. Moreover, the numerous cell processes make contacts by cell junctions with neighboring small lymphocytes but not with reticuloepithelial cells or any other free or fixed elements of the thymic parenchyma (Figure 5.12). Birbeck granules do not occur in these pro-interdigitating cells.

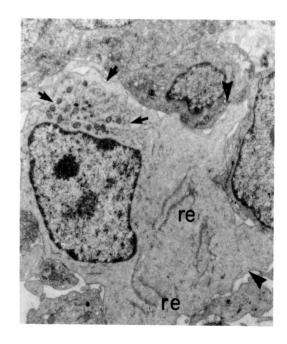

Figure 5.11 Precursor of interdigitating cell of the thymus in *Mauremys caspica*. The cell shows numerous irregular processes (arrows) making contact with neighboring lymphocytes and a small population of membranous organelles (re = endoplasmic reticulum) arranged near the nucleus (× 7600).

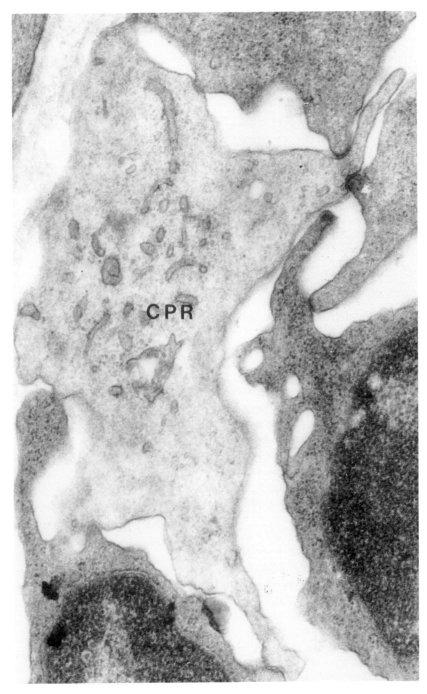

Figure 5.12 Processes (CPR) of an immature interdigitating cell making contact with lymphocytes ($\times$ 35 000). (From *Cell Tissue Res* **238**: 381, 1984, reproduced by permission.)

Studies on the functions of interdigitating cells are basically restricted to mammals. They appear to be specific microenvironmental constituents of T-dependent areas in the mammalian immune system. Close contacts between interdigitating cells and lymphocytes seem to be of fundamental importance, although nutritive or communicative functions are open to discussion. Perhaps the functional significance of IDCs in primary and secondary lymphoid organs is different. Thus, membrane contacts between both cell types have been related to adequate transfer of antigenic stimuli (Veldman and Kaiserling, 1980) and IDCs appear to be important for homing of T-cells, since in all fetal secondary lymphoid organs the development of IDCs and the appearance of T-cells occur concurrently (von Gaudecker and Muller-Hermelink, 1982). In contrast, absence of Birbeck granules in IDCs observed in ectothermic vertebrates could be considered a primitive condition; however, Thorbecke et al. (1980) suggested that interdigitating cells containing Birbeck granules in mammalian lymph nodes represent Langerhans cells or their offspring which have migrated to the lymph node paracortex after antigenic stimulation in the skin, principally during T-dependent, cellular immune reactions. Likewise, the remarkable phagocytic capacity demonstrated in the mature IDCs of the thymus in *Mauremys caspica* (Leceta et al., 1984) appears to be related to a special situation, specifically to massive (vernal) degeneration of thymic, reticuloepithelial cells. A similar phenomenon has been described in thymuses of sublethally irradiated rats, in which mature IDCs contained numerous phagocytosed necrotic lymphocytes (Duijvestijn et al., 1982a). Besides, the IDC clusters, frequently described in the thymus of *Sturnus unicolor* (Fonfria et al., 1982), show morphological similarity to those reported in the enlarged lymph nodes of humans suffering from dermatopathic lymphadenitis, a benign reactive lymphadenopathy that develops as a result of various types of chronically inflamed, dermal lesions (Kaiserling and Lennert, 1974; Rausch et al., 1977; Lennert et al., 1978).

The origin of IDCs is still a matter of conjecture. Some investigators have considered them to be macrophages involved in the presentation of antigens to T-lymphocytes (Veerman, 1974; Veerman and van Ewijk, 1975; Kamperdijk et al., 1978; Groscurth, 1981), while others (Veldman, 1970; Kaiserling and Lennert, 1974; Rausch et al., 1977) have proposed a reticular origin and function not directly associated with immunity. In vertebrates, based exclusively upon morphological evidence, both views have been suggested for ectothermic vertebrates (Fonfria et al., 1982; Leceta et al., 1984). Kamperdijk (1980) has proposed that an increase in IDCs results, at least in part, from the transformation of transitional macrophages under the influence of sensitized T-cells, which will produce macrophage inhibitory factors, since no mitotic activity has been observed in the IDCs. Duijvestijn et al. (1982b) also described the IDCs of the mammalian thymus as a specialized type of macrophage which occurs in the cortico-medullary region, the site where circulating mononuclear phagocytes enter.

Secretory Epithelial Cells—Thymic Hormones in Lower Vertebrates

Together with thymic hormones, and the supporting reticuloepithelial cells, the thymic medullary area contains a myriad of epithelial cells. Although few are known, especially from a cytochemical and functional viewpoint, these characteristics represent one of the most exciting features of the vertebrate thymus. Certain tissue cells appear as single elements, whereas others form a part of the walls of multicellular epithelial cysts. They evidently represent several different cell types: some which show morphological features of secretory, hormone-producing cells, while others are typical, glandular mucus cells. Other isolated granular cells are large, found near the medullary blood vessels. These show a few masses of condensed chromatin arranged peripherally and a cytoplasm with abundant small, round or elongated granules of different electron density, dilated profiles of rough endoplasmic reticulum, few bundles of cytoplasmic filaments and a patent basement membrane (Figure 5.13). Similar cells have been reported in the thymus of all ectotherms (Curtis et al., 1972, 1979; Frazier, 1973; Nagata, 1976, 1977; Kendall and Frazier, 1979; Bigaj and Plytycz, 1981; Henry and Charlemagne, 1981; Zapata, 1981; Gorgollon, 1983). Although many epithelial cells of the thymic medulla have numerous vacuoles and vesicles within their cytoplasm suggesting secretory activity, the functional significance of these cell types is still unclear.

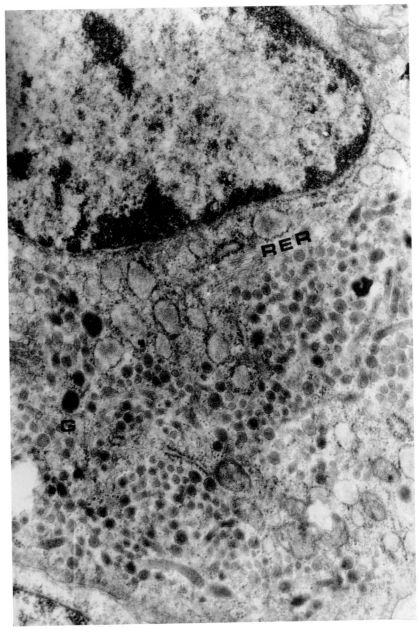

Figure 5.13 Presumptive secretory cell in thymic medulla of the lizard *Lacerta hispanica*. Numerous electron-dense granules (G) and some profiles of dilated rough endoplasmic reticulum (RER) occur in the cytoplasm (× 9400). (From *Biology of the Reptilia*, Vol. 14, 600, 1985, reproduced by permission.)

Although some workers have suggested certain roles in the production of thymic hormones, others have found their relationships only significant in the case of medullary epithelial cysts. Numerous cell types and structures have been relegated to humoral functions attributed to the thymus: 'clear vesicles' present in reticulum cells of the rat thymus (Pfoch, 1971), granular inclusions in cystic epithelial cells (Cesarini *et al.*, 1968; Chapman and Allen, 1971) or special cells (Olah *et al.*, 1975), the (self) intra- and intercellular epithelial cysts (Frazier, 1973), reticuloepithelial cells (Teodorczyk *et al.*, 1975; Sugimoto *et al.*, 1977b). Fluorescent antibody techniques have revealed the presence of thymosin-containing granules in reticuloepithelial cells (Mandi and Glant, 1973), but their relationship with the vesicles is vaguely indicated.

In two teleosts *Cyprinus carpio* and *Dicentrarchus labrax*, Froehly and Deschaux (1986) demonstrated by indirect immunofluorescence the presence of thymic serum factor in keratin-containing reticuloepithelial cells. Extracts containing hormonal properties have been recorded in the avian thymus (Brand *et al.*, 1976; Goldstein, 1984). Moreover, Coudert *et al.* (1979) found that sera from normal chickens provide mouse rosette-forming cells with a high sensitivity to azathioprine inhibition. This sensitivity was almost absent in assays using sera from thymectomized birds. In addition, the normal level of 'thymic serum factor' in sera of thymectomized chickens has been restored by injecting a synthetic thymic factor. Taken together, these results suggest that normal chicken sera contain a factor with 'thymic serum factor'-like activity which disappears after thymectomy. Similar results using the same methodology were reported previously by this same group in the urodeles *Triturus alpestris, Pleurodeles waltlii* and *Ambystoma mexicanum* (Dardenne *et al.*, 1973). Furthermore, Murthy *et al.* (1985) isolated a low-molecular-weight peptide from chicken thymus which they designated as avian thymic hormone (ATH) *in vitro*. ATH induces the expression of T-cell surface markers on bone marrow precursor cells and functional maturation of thymocyte subpopulations, while *in vivo* administration of ATH (1 mg/day) to day-old chicks for 1 week and week-old chicks for 3 weeks resulted in significant ($p < 0.05$) increase in PHA-induced proliferation of peripheral blood mononuclear cells.

Erickson-Viitanen *et al.* (1983) found thymosin beta 4, one of several peptides isolated from thymosin fraction 5, in tissues of all vertebrate classes, including bursa of Fabricius and liver, except bony fish, which contained yet another related peptide designated thymosin beta 11. Finally the presence of thymosin alpha, another group of peptides, related to maturation and differentiation of T-cells, has been recently investigated in chicken and trout spleen (Yialouris *et al.*, 1988). In rats and humans, prothymosin alpha and parathymosin alpha show similar size, amino acid composition and limited homology at their N-terminus but differential tissue distribution (Haritos *et al.*, 1984) and opposing biological activities (Haritos *et al.*, 1985a, b). Thymosins alpha 1 and alpha 2 represent N-terminal fragments of prothymosin alpha with sequences corresponding to segments $1-28$ and $1-35$, respectively. In both species, Sephacryl S-200 gel filtration separation combined with radioimmunoassay showed a major immunoreactive peak, the elution volume of which corresponds to that of rat prothymosin alpha for chicken tissues, whereas trout corresponds to a significant higher molecular weight (Yialouris *et al.*, 1988). No detectable levels of shorter fragments, including thymosin alpha 1, were observed in either of the two species (Yialouris *et al.*, 1988). Further structural analysis of vertebrate thymic hormones will illuminate their molecular evolution, biological significance and cellular origin.

Epithelial Cysts and Hassall's Corpuscles

Epithelial cysts are always present in the thymic medulla of vertebrates. They occur as unicellular structures which develop from large intracytoplasmic vacuoles (Figure 5.14), large vacuoles surrounded by a single layer of electron-dense vacuolated reticuloepithelial cells (Figure 5.15) or multicellular structures formed by several layers of cells whose significance is variable (Figure 5.16). A similar classification of three different types has been reported in the avian thymus by Isler (1976). The origin of thymic epithelial cysts appears to be from large, pale epithelial cells which develop intracytoplasmic vacuoles that exhibit mucous material and cell debris (Figure 5.14). These cells also contain numerous small mitochondria, several dictyosomes and electron-dense granules (Figure 5.14). Nagata (1976) has provided evidence using cytochemical techniques that the medullary

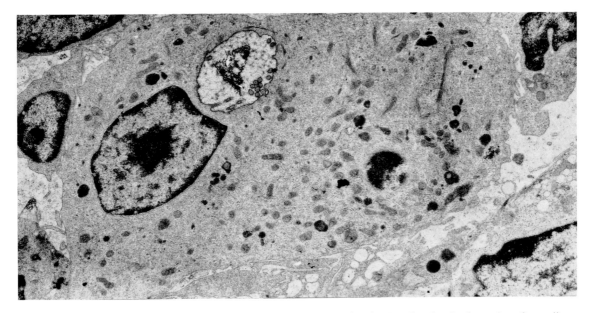

Figure 5.14 Medullary epithelial cell of the thymus of the natterjack, *Bufo calamita*, showing the formation of a small cyst in the cytoplasm ($\times$ 7560).

epithelial cells which comprise the thymic cysts in *Xenopus laevis* produce and secrete carbohydrates into the cystic lumens. In multicellular cysts, cells which immediately surround the lumen are frequently extremely electron dense and contain microvilli and cilia (Figure 5.17) projecting into the lumen, where degenerated material is found (Figure 5.15) (Bigaj and Plytycz, 1984). Epithelial cells which form the layer of multicellular cysts are joined together by desmosomes and show abundant evidence of active secretion such as the presence in the cytoplasm of electron-dense granules, Golgi apparatus, profiles of rough endoplasmic reticulum and numerous mitochondria (Figure 5.15) (Bigaj and Plytycz, 1984).

Moreover, granular and mucus cells are numerous in the walls of medullary epithelial cysts (Figure 5.16). Some of these mucus cells are apparently in different stages of their secretory cycle, which suggests a contribution to the content of the cyst lumen (Figure 5.16). Numerous mucus cells have been reported in thymic cysts of *Plethodon glutinosus* (Curtis *et al.*, 1979). Especially remarkable are isolated mucus cells found in the thymic medulla of certain anurans (Figure 5.18) or others forming a part of the cyst walls (Figure 5.16). In this instance, they resemble morphologically cell

components of skin glands. These mucus cells are characterized by numerous granules which fill the cytoplasm and consist of large round or polygonal granules with a pale or moderate, electron-dense material which contains a smaller electron-dense inclusion (Figures 5.16, 5.18).

Clothier and Balls (1985) have reported TRH (thyrotropin-releasing hormone) and 5'-hydroxytryptamine (5-HT) in the thymus of *Xenopus laevis*. From the resemblance between the thymic gland cells and skin glands, which contain such pharmacologically biological molecules, it may be inferred that gland cells in the thymus contain TRH and 5-HT. However, it must be considered that other cell populations present in the thymus, such as mast cells, also contain large amounts of 5-HT. This interesting finding of biologically active compounds has focused attention on the derivation of these granular cells and their mechanisms of action. In this regard, it is important to emphasize the apparent common embryological derivation of some cell populations in the skin, thymus and gastrointestinal tract (Pearse, 1977).

In an earlier study, Clothier *et al.* (1983) reported that the various types of granules or stages in granule development which are characteristic of the skin

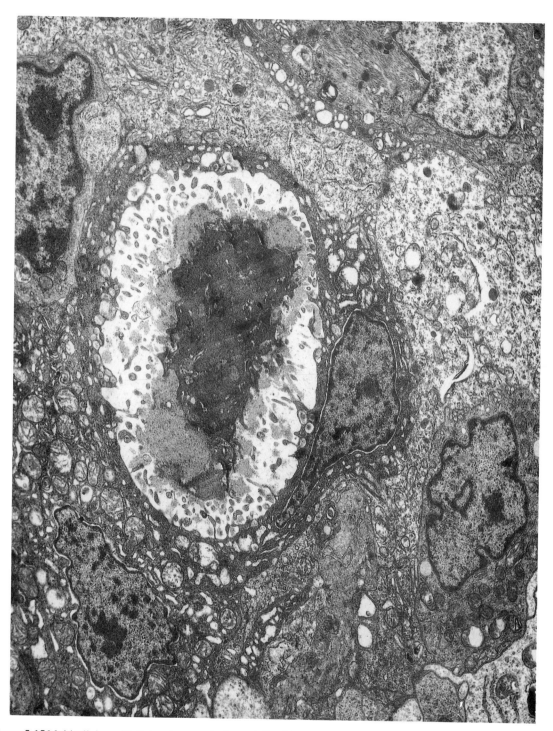

Figure 5.15 Multicellular epithelial cyst present in the medulla of the spotless starling, *Sturnus unicolor*. Abundant cell debris occurs in the cyst (× 10 450).

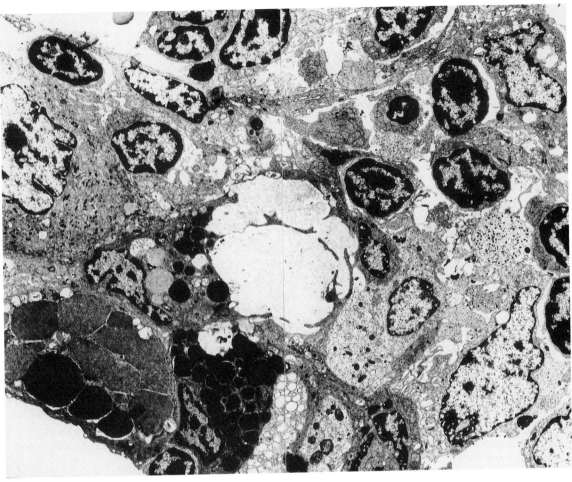

Figure 5.16 Mucus cell forming a part of the wall of a multicellular epithelial cyst in the thymus of the natterjack, *Bufo calamita*. Note the various sizes and densities of the cytoplasmic granules of these cells. Note lymphocytes ($\times$ 5250) (From *Tissue and Cell* **21**: 69–81, reproduced by permission.)

glands were also present in granular cells of the thymus in *Xenopus laevis*. Granular cells are not found in the larval thymus, but they appear as isolated cells during metamorphosis from larva to adult, when the 5-HT content of the skin also increases markedly (Vanable, 1964), as does its caerulein content (Inselvini, 1975). Granular cells in the thymic medulla of a metamorphosing toad (stage 62) contain relatively fewer granules than those from older animals. This suggests that there is a slow accumulation of contents within thymic granular cells, as in dermal granular glands. No TRH has been found in stage 59 thymus glands, but significant amounts of TRH and 5-HT have been observed in thymus glands from toadlets six months

after metamorphosis. Apart from the internal, functional significance that some elements of the epithelial cystic walls can have, the significance of thymic epithelial cysts is unknown. Preliminary reports relating them to the production and secretion of thymic hormonal factors (Trainin, 1974; Curtis *et al.*, 1979) seem no longer acceptable. Shier (1963) has suggested that they are manifestations of the original endodermal epithelial tubules from which the thymus develops, whereas other workers consider them to be associated with degenerative processes.

Another puzzling feature of the thymus is the presence and functional significance of the so-called Hassall's corpuscles or bodies found in the medulla.

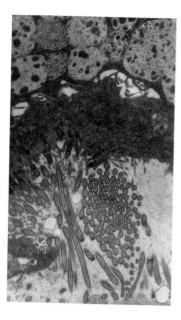

Figure 5.17 Presence of cilia in the lumen of a multicellular, epithelial cyst in the medulla of *Rana perezi* (× 5400).

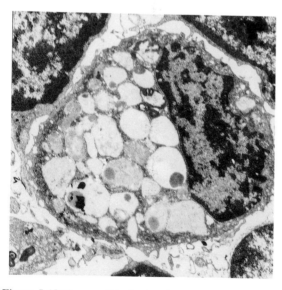

Figure 5.18 Mucus cell in the thymic medulla of the natterjack, *Bufo calamita*. Note the cytoplasmic granules (× 10 200). (From *Tissue and Cell* **21**: 69–81, reproduced by permission.)

From a phylogenetic perspective, the first point to consider is the presence or absence of structures morphologically identifiable as Hassall's bodies in ectothermic vertebrates. They have been reported in several species (Good *et al.*, 1966 in *Polyodon spathula*; Gorgollon, 1983 in *Sicyases sanguineos*; Curtis *et al.*, 1979 in urodeles; Fabrizio and Charipper, 1941; Sterba, 1950; Kapa, 1963; Curtis and Volpe, 1971; Bigaj and Plytycz, 1984 in anurans) but many workers consider that Hassall's bodies are lacking, although groups of medullary reticuloepithelial cells (Fange and Sundell, 1969) or degenerative epithelial cysts, frequent in the thymic medulla of all ectotherms (Frazier, 1973), can be considered morphologically similar to Hassall's bodies. Even in the chick thymus, it seems likely that the large cysts which contain degenerating cells may be an early stage in the formation of Hassall's corpuscles, especially since some of them which form these large cysts contain many intracytoplasmic fibrils (Frazier, 1973).

The most detailed descriptions of presumptive Hassall's bodies in lower vertebrates have revealed 'cell complexes formed by apposition of two or more large or hypertrophied medullary epithelial cells' (Gorgollon, 1983), or 'degenerative epithelial cells grouped with tonofibrillae' (Bigaj and Plytycz, 1984). As a summary, in our opinion, Hassall's corpuscles occur exclusively in the thymus of endothermic vertebrates, especially mammals. Reports of their existence in ectothermic vertebrates correspond to identifiable clusters of medullary reticuloepithelial cells or giant, epithelial cysts which are more or less modified.

One of us found unicellular Hassall's bodies in the thymic medulla of the spotless starling, *Sturnus unicolor*. They appear as pale reticuloepithelial cells which contain numerous bundles of keratin filaments that are surrounded in successive layers by a central irregular nucleus (Figure 5.19). Frazier (1973) reported similar cells in the chick thymus and proposed that they might be related to the formation of Hassall's corpuscles. Our own observations also agree with those of Frazier on the possible origin of Hassall's bodies from degenerated large epithelial cysts. Kendall and Frazier (1979) have described small Hassall's corpuscles of chick thymus as structures which develop from the coalescence of pale cells to form a loose 'ball', and as the corpuscles enlarge the cells then become flattened as more are gradually

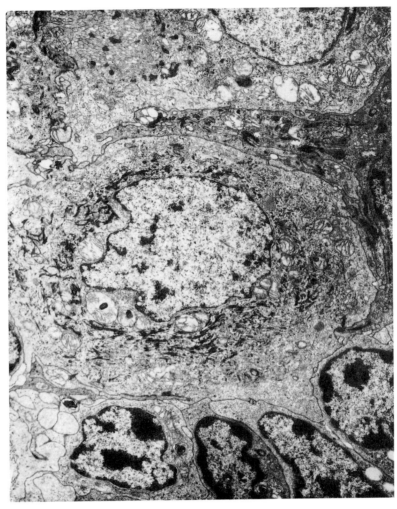

Figure 5.19 Unicellular Hassall's corpuscle in the thymic medulla of the spotless starling, *Sturnus unicolor*. Numerous keratin filaments occur in the cytoplasm surrounding the nucleus (× 8000).

incorporated. Large Hassall's bodies consist of several concentric layers of flattened cells, some of which become densely filled with tracts of tonofilaments around the nucleus or along the apical cell surfaces. Some of the constituent cells have electron-dense inclusions within the apical region (Frazier, 1973; Kendall and Frazier, 1979). The central mass is usually keratinized, may give a positive reaction with PAS, and appears to contain dead cells believed to have been desquamated from the walls of the corpuscle and other cells.

The functions of Hassall's bodies, if they have any, are unknown, although relevant information is available. In some mammals there is apparently a correspondence between the onset of humoral immune competence and the appearance of Hassall's corpuscles in the developing thymus (Ashman and Papadimitriou, 1975 in the quokka; Block, 1964; Rowlands *et al.*, 1964 in the opossum; Bryant and Shifrine, 1972; Jacoby *et al.*, 1969 in dogs; Chapman and Allen, 1971 in monkey; Norris, 1938, Solomon, 1971 in humans). On the other hand, in the Australian echidna, *Tachyglossus aculeatus*, Diener and Ealey (1965) demonstrated numerous Hassall's corpuscles, which selectively take up ^{125}I-labeled flagella antigen 24 hours after its injection. Finally, Hassall's bodies have been involved in mechanisms related to the development of self-tolerance to antigens of epithelial or ectodermal origin (Beletskaya and Gnesditskava, 1980).

In some cases, multinucleated giant cells appear in the thymic medulla of some vertebrates. These cells, which one of us found in the thymus of the natterjack, *Bufo calamita*, seem to be equivalent to others reported previously in the spleen of this toad (Barrutia *et al.*, 1983, 1985b). They are giant cells with four or five nuclei, abundant small mitochondria, electron-dense granules and many profiles of rough endoplasmic reticulum arranged in a parallel fashion in the periphery of the cell (Figure 5.20) and surrounded by numerous small lymphocytes. Multinucleated giant cells have been described in cell cultures of human thymic tissue and in age-involuted adult human thymus (von Gaudecker, 1978). Workers have suggested that multinucleated giant cells are formed by a confluence of macrophages. From an ultrastructural aspect, these cells appear to be giant cells with a phagocytic capacity of obscure function. If these cells reported in the thymus of *Bufo calamita* are confirmed as equivalent to those described as antigen-presenting cells in the spleen (Barrutia *et al.*, 1985b) they might play a role in MHC restriction which occurs in the thymus, according to the hypothesis proposed for *Xenopus laevis* (Flajnik *et al.*, 1984).

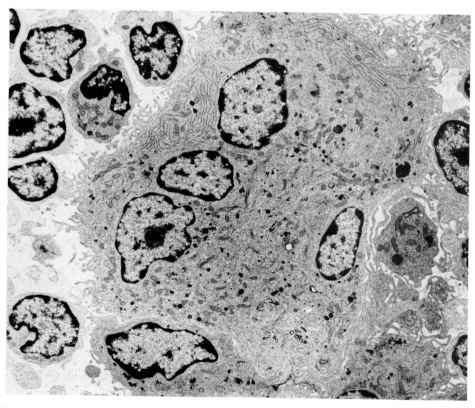

Figure 5.20 Giant epithelial cell in the thymic medulla of *Bufo calamita*. Note the fine nuclei contained within the same cell and abundant endoplasmic reticulum ($\times$ 4210). (From *Tissue and Cell* **21**: 69–81, reproduced by permission.)

Granular, Endocrine-like Cells

Epithelial cells with the appearance of endocrine cells occur in the thymic medulla of many vertebrates. They have a nucleus with small amounts of condensed chromatin and small nucleoli. In the cytoplasm, the most remarkable feature is a homogeneous population of small, round electron-dense granules (Figure 5.21). Apart from the TRH- and 5-HT-containing cells of the thymus of *Xenopus laevis*, in the thymic medulla of *Plethodon glutinosus*, Curtis *et al.* (1979) described a type III cell which closely resembles endocrine cells associated with the gastrointestinal epithelium. A cell type which has a similar appearance to the beta cells of pancreatic islands has also been found in the thymus of various reptiles (Bockman and Winborn, 1967; Bockman, 1970; Leceta, 1984). In the avian thymus, Payne (1971), using the light microscope, observed the presence of granular, argentaffin cells, and Hakanson *et al.* (1974) reported various endocrine cells in the chick thymus; one stores 5-HT which increases in amounts with age. Other cell types contain dopamine and various peptides and amines. Intense activities of glucose 6-phosphate and lactate dehydrogenase observed in the juxtacortical medulla of the chick thymus (Ruuskanen *et al.*, 1977) also suggest the occurrence of endocrine-like cells. In the mammalian thymus, van Ewijk *et al.* (1980) using monoclonal antibodies, have demonstrated reticuloepithelial cells which form the major MHC-positive elements. According to Smith (1984) a new monoclonal antibody that appears specific for neuroendocrine cells stains many supporting cells at the corticomedullary junction. All these examples suggest a role for endocrine cells in the regulation of immunological functions in the thymus, although further research is necessary to confirm this possibility.

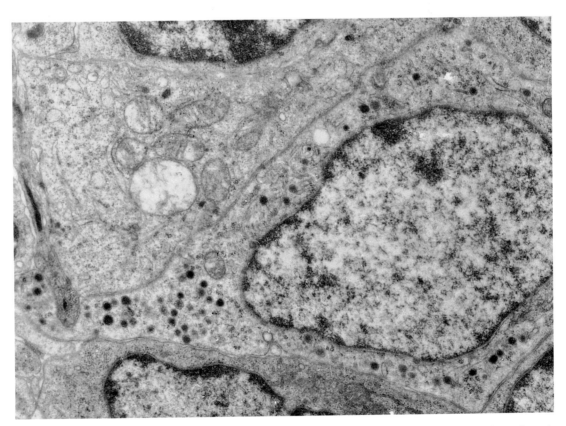

Figure 5.21 Granular cell in the thymic medulla of *Sturnus unicolor*. Granules are electron dense and different from those described in Figure 5.13 ($\times$ 14040).

Myoid Cells

Immature, mature and degenerative myoid cells are frequent in the thymus of all ectothermic vertebrates, although some authors have been unable to find them (Fange and Pulsford, 1985 in *Scyliorhinus canicula*; Klug, 1967 in *Ambystoma mexicanum*; Hightower and St Pierre, 1971 in *Notophthalmus viridescens*). From the very first descriptions by Mayer (1888) and Hammar (1905), myoid cells have been investigated in most vertebrates, although their functional significance still remains obscure. Truly significant differences appear to be in the numbers of myoid cells in various vertebrates. Some workers have indicated that myoid cells occur in greatest numbers and most representatively in ectotherms (van de Velde and Friedman, 1966b; Bockman and Winborn, 1967; Toro *et al.*, 1969), while others, by contrast, found few in certain fish (Hill, 1935; Dulzetto, 1968; Gorgollon, 1983). In our own work, myoid cells are especially abundant in certain amphibians and reptiles (Figure 5.22), where they form large clusters (Bockman and Winborn, 1967; Curtis *et al.*, 1972). Earlier suggestions that

myoid cells increase in number throughout life (Raviola and Raviola, 1967) or undergo seasonal variations, offering a possible explanation for these disputed results (Muthukkaruppan *et al.*, 1982), still need further confirmation.

Both mature and immature myoid cells are covered by a continuous basement membrane. Degenerated myoid cells, also found in the vertebrate thymus, exhibit subsarcolemmal vacuolization with loss of cross-striations, condensation and hyalinization of contractile material and dilatation of sarcoplasmic cisterns. From a histochemical point of view, Hanzlikova (1979) reported that the enzymatic characteristics of mature myoid cells of *Rana esculenta* were apparently similar to those of fast muscle fibers of the frog, although the histochemical reactions of individual myoid cells differed in intensity due to variations in the amount and developmental maturity of contractile and sarcoplasmic material during different stages of the myoid cell's life cycle. Mature myoid cells, found predominantly in the medulla, are round or oval, large cells showing an irregular, light electron-dense nucleus, with scant condensed chromatin arranged peripherally and a patent nucleolus (Figure 5.23). The

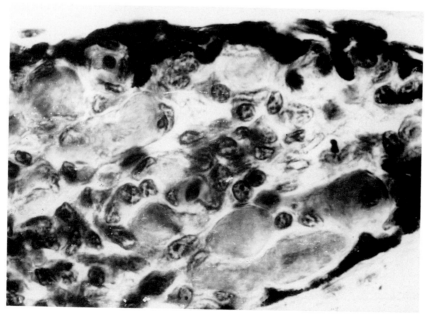

Figure 5.22 Mature myoid cells completely fill the thymus of the lizard *Lacerta hispanica* ($\times$ 750).

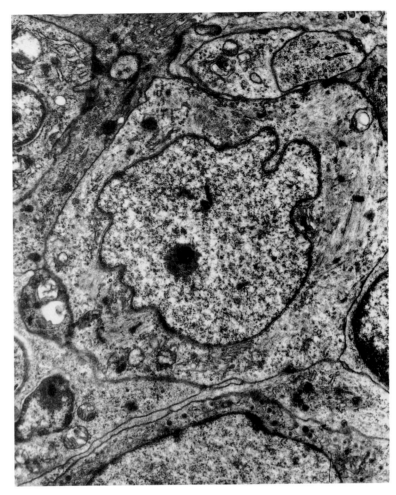

Figure 5.23 Mature myoid cell in the thymus of the natterjack, *Bufo calamita*. Note the cytoplasmic sarcomeres and small electron-dense granules ($\times$ 12 200).

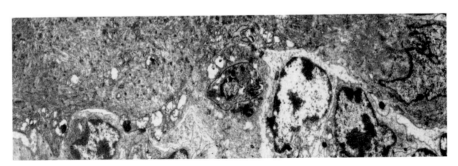

Figure 5.24 Immature myoid cell in the thymus of the spotless starling, *Sturnus unicolor*. Myofilaments are not fully developed ($\times$ 7500).

cytoplasm appears to be filled by large myofibrils, comparable to those in skeletal muscle. Straight and narrow Z-lines and prominent M-lines occur in the sarcomeres, although the course of myofibrils remains disorganized, frequently showing a tendency to circular orientations (Figure 5.23). Developing, immature myoid cells show appreciable numbers of cytoplasmic ribosomes and scant myofibrils composed of few sarcomeres radially oriented around one large Z-line (Figure 5.24). Small mitochondria and some electron-dense granules are also evident in the cytoplasm (Figure 5.24).

The origins and functions of myoid cells are also a matter of discussion. On the question of the embryonic origin, some workers suppose that they are accidental inclusions left from embryogenesis (van de Velde and Friedman, 1966a; Mandel, 1968), muscle elements of mesodermal origin which migrate into the thymus and persist as myoid cells (Pensa, 1905; Weissenberg, 1907; Wassjutatschkin, 1913), or they are the progeny of adventitial cells which invade the thymus via blood vessels (Dustin, 1909). Others believe that they originated from the reticuloepithelial cells of the thymic parenchyma (Hammar, 1905). Evidence supporting an intrinsic origin comes from ultrastructural observations of desmosomes between immature myoid cells and neighboring thymic reticular cells in amphibians, reptiles and humans (Raviola and Raviola, 1967; Toro et al., 1969; Henry, 1966) and from tissue culture experiments demonstrating that myogenic stem cells may be generated in vitro from cultures of murine thymus reticulum (Ketelsen and Wekerle, 1976). By contrast, studies using immunofluorescence staining with antibodies against striated or smooth muscle myosin have demonstrated conclusively that myoid and reticuloepithelial cells of the thymus are two entirely separate entities (Drenckhahn et al., 1979).

Recently, myoid cells have been reported to originate from neural crest, results obtained using the quail−chick chimera model (Nakamura et al., 1986). Fibrocytes in the interlobular region and in the medulla of the thymus also originate from the neural crest (Nakamura et al., 1986). The neural crest cells are reported to reach the thymus anlage before the 10th day of incubation (Nakamura et al., 1986) but we do not know whether they are already committed as myoid cells or as fibrocytes by that time. With independence of the embryonic origin of thymic myoid cells, the presence of both immature and degenerative stages of these cells suggests a turnover of myoid cells in the adult thymus, whose cell precursors and significance are indeed obscure.

Finally, another unclear point on the biology of myoid cells is their significance in the thymus. First, there is apparently no muscular function due to the lack of innervation (Bockman and Winborn, 1967; Raviola and Raviola, 1967; Kapa et al., 1968); nevertheless, Terni (1929) described many nerve arborizations on myoid cells. Other authors have therefore suggested contraction without innervation, by means of diffusive substances (Taxi, 1965), or by a similar mechanism of autocontraction as in Purkinje fibers (Hammar, 1905; Raviola and Raviola, 1966). Under in vitro conditions, rat thymic myoid cells form myotubes (Ketelsen and Wekerle, 1976) which contract, both spontaneously and in response to electrical stimulation (Kao and Drachman, 1977).

Other evidence presents thymic myoid cells as a source of muscle-specific self-antigens (Toro et al., 1969; Rimmer, 1980). Thus, serum gamma globulins in patients with myasthenia gravis react in vitro like an antibody against antigens of mammalian skeletal and cardiac muscle and thymic myoid cells (Strauss et al., 1967). These human globulins also reacted with reptilian myoid cells (Strauss et al., 1966). In this sense, Henry (1966) and Bockman and Winborn (1967) proposed that myoid cells play a central role in the sensitization and subsequent formation of anti-muscle antibodies. Other experiments have demonstrated that, during the differentiation of myogenic stem cells from murine thymic reticulum in culture, developing muscle clones exhibit transient, high-density expression of acetylcholine receptors with localized 'hotspots' where acetylcholine receptors are even more concentrated (Wekerle et al., 1978). These authors suggest that if such cells were in some way arrested or 'frozen' at this stage of differentiation (perhaps by viral infection) then they might be necessary and appropriate in the presentation of antigen for autoimmune sensitization. This evolutionary persistence might be, however, difficult to explain, if they are indeed a primary cause of such an autoimmune disease. The role of myoid cells in myasthenia gravis is obscure as well as the role of the thymus and T-lymphocytes in the etiology of the disease (Levinson et al., 1985).

Plasma Cells

Plasma cells occur in the thymic parenchyma of many vertebrates, mainly in the perivascular spaces or connective tissue septa. The function of this intrathymic antibody-producing cell population might be important despite its low frequency of appearance. Intrathymic, mature plasma cells show the typical round, electron-dense nucleus with abundant condensed chromatin arranged peripherally and a patent nucleolus (Figure 5.25). The cytoplasm is filled with enlarged profiles of rough endoplasmic reticulum which are electron dense. Small granules and an incipient Golgi apparatus are obvious in the more immature plasmacytes (Figure 5.25). Plasma cells in the avian thymus increase in number and maturity while the bursa of Fabricius matures. The bursa shows a further increase in number until it begins to involute at about 8 months of age (Thorbecke et al., 1957; Hoffmann-Fezer, 1973).

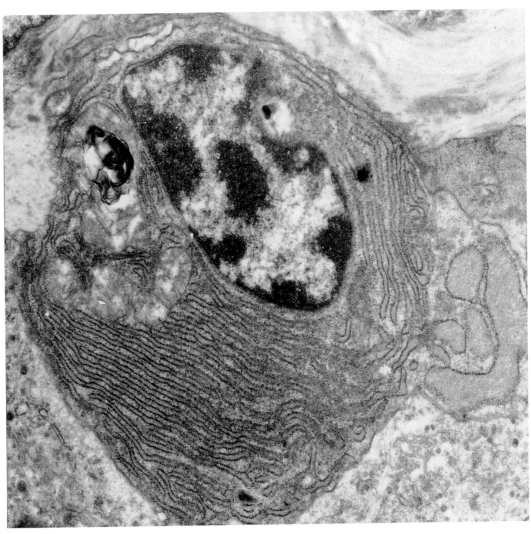

Figure 5.25 Mature plasma cell in the thymus of the turtle *Mauremys caspica* ($\times$ 11 250).

Du Pasquier and Horton (1982) recently reviewed the condition of plasma cells in *Xenopus laevis*, and according to their observations the low numbers of plasma cells cannot be considered insignificant. Thus, in a parallel analysis comparing *Xenopus* and mouse thymus populations, only $0.2-0.9\%$ of mouse thymocytes are Ig^+. These populations, however, contained Ig-secreting cells comparable to those found in the spleen when corrected for B-cell (Ig^+) content. Moreover, thymic B-cells appear to be, in some respects, the same subsets as those of splenic B-cells. Primed to a T-dependent antigen (DNP-KLH), both subsets require the presence of T-helper cells which are carrier-specific and both produce IgM and LMW Ig. In addition, SDS gel patterns of Ig molecules, precipitated by a rabbit anti-*Xenopus* Ig, revealed no differences between surface or biosynthetically labeled Ig produced by nylon wool-adherent splenic and thymic B-cells. Thymic B-cells differ, however, from splenic B-cells in their capacity to synthesize large amounts of LMW Ig antibodies after they have been purified from the original thymic cell suspensions and helped (the T-cell helper function) by splenic T-cells. Thymic B-cells may represent, according to Du Pasquier and Horton (1982), a subset of lymphocytes resting in or passing through the thymus as a necessary step in their later function in the regulation of immune responses. It is possible that many of the cells are suppressed in the thymus, and that what is detected are those which escape suppression. Alternatively, the existence of B-cells in the thymus which produce antibodies independently of T-cell help must be considered.

Erythrocytes

One interesting observation concerns erythrocytes which, of course, are always present in bone marrow, which is mainly a generator of myeloid cells as a primary organ of the immune system. Erythrocytes usually occur in the thymic parenchyma; however, erythropoietic capacity in the thymus gland is less frequent, where it is mainly reported in birds and is apparently a cyclic phenomenon (Kendall, 1980; Fonfria *et al.*, 1983). Some free erythrocytes found among stromal elements of the thymic parenchyma have been reported in some fish (Hafter, 1952; Gorgollon, 1983), but these authors were unable to find precursor erythroblastic islets (Gorgollon, 1983).

In anuran amphibians, mainly in senescent individuals, erythroid cells have also been found (Cooper and Hildemann, 1965; Bigaj and Plytycz, 1984). The capacity of the embryonic thymus to support low levels of erythropoiesis has been observed in birds by Romanoff (1960), and it occurs also in adults (Kendall and Ward, 1974; Bacchus and Kendall, 1975; Kendall, 1975a, b; 1979, 1980; Fonfria *et al.*, 1983). Intrathymic erythropoiesis has also been observed in mammals: the mouse (Albert *et al.*, 1965a, b), the bank vole, *Clethrionomys glareolus* (Kendall, 1980), human fetuses and children (Albert *et al.*, 1966; Taylor and Skinner, 1976) and adults (Kendall and Singh, 1980). The morphology of this process is clear in Figure 5.26. Erythroid cells, including the earliest developmental stages, occur in enlarged thymic lobules where they occupy the cortical areas which also house numerous pyknotic cells and degenerated reticuloepithelial cells. Within these enlarged lobules, there are, in addition, abundant, large epithelial cysts which are localized in the medulla and corticomedullary border. As erythroid clusters, they consist of erythroblasts, immature and mature erythrocytes. At the periphery, many free polysomes and rhopheocytic vesicles have been observed.

The significance of intrathymic, cyclic (seasonal) erythropoiesis may result from an increased demand for blood (as during molt) or following a period of physiological stress (Ward and Kendall, 1975). Recent experimental reports by Fonfria *et al.* (1983) of intrathymic erythropoiesis in the spotless starling, *Sturnus unicolor*, suggest roles played by sex hormones and the cellular microenvironment in the regulation of erythropoiesis. Fonfria and his colleagues concluded that: (1) intrathymic erythropoiesis is a cyclic process related to the sexual reproductive cycle; (2) avian intrathymic erythropoiesis may be preceded by changes in the thymic cellular microenvironment. Alterations are accompanied by an increased number of pyknotic lymphoid cells and macrophages and degeneration of the cortical reticuloepithelial cells. Thus, they were able to observe a relationship between appearance and disappearance of intrathymic erythropoiesis, and degeneration/regeneration of lymphoid components and of the reticuloepithelial microenvironment. Relating these results to the reproductive cycle, the maximum size of the testes in this bird occurs in April, when thymic degeneration commences, lead-

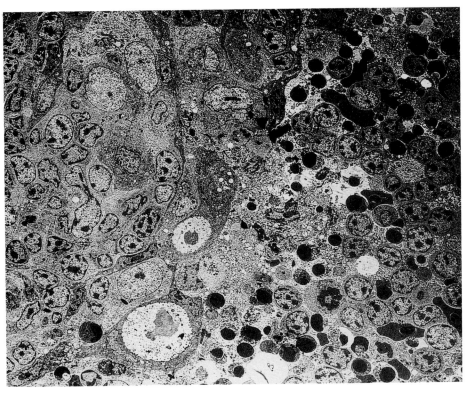

Figure 5.26 Cortico-medullary junction of an enlarged thymic lobule of the spotless starling, *Sturnus unicolor*, showing extensive lymphoid degeneration, erythropoietic activity and increased numbers of epithelial cysts ($\times$ 2020). (From *Cell Tissue Res* **232**: 445, 1983, reproduced by permission.)

ing to the appearance of intrathymic erythropoiesis in May–June (mating period) or July (post-juvenile molt). Moreover, in adult *Sturnus unicolor* (1–2 years old) the ovary is not appreciably large in January, but it reaches its full development in April and May. Although in other birds degeneration of reticulo-epithelial cells has not been reported, the hormonal effects are perhaps similar and intrathymic erythropoiesis in it may be regulated, at least in part, by these physiological modulators.

Other Cell Types

Granulocytes, although few in number, are generally frequent in the vertebrate thymus, especially in association with connective tissue of the capsule and septa. They have been found in fish (Gorgollon, 1983), amphibians (Klug, 1967; Kapa *et al.*, 1968; Csaba *et al.*, 1970; Kapa and Csaba, 1972; Curtis *et al.*, 1979), reptiles (Bockman, 1970) and birds (Hohn,

1947; Lucas and Jamroz, 1961; Bacchus and Kendall, 1975; Kendall, 1975a; Kendall and Frazier, 1979). Mature and immature mast cells have been found in the thymus of *Lacerta hispanica* and *Elaphe scalaris* (Zapata, 1973). The origin of intrathymic mast cells is unclear. While some investigators have pointed out that they originate within the thymus, others have considered that they penetrate into it from the bloodstream after having been formed in other sites. In addition to granulocytes, the thymus of some vertebrates contains a lipid-laden cell type which is usually localized in the cortex. These cells show numerous electron-lucent large vacuoles, whose morphology suggests a lipid nature (Figure 5.27). These cells also contain numerous phagosomes which contain cell debris. Similar cells have been observed in the mammalian thymus (Dung, 1973). Actually, their significance is obscure, although they may represent a different form of macrophage or a modified reticuloepithelial cell.

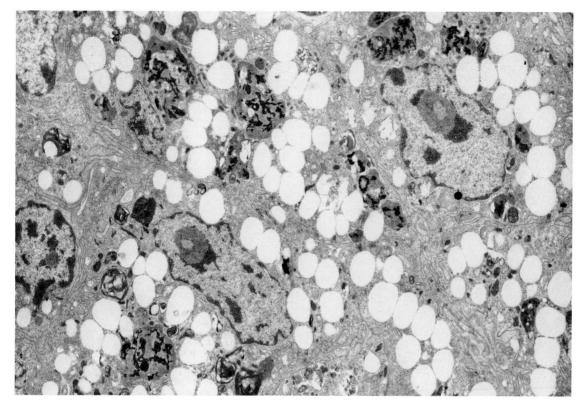

Figure 5.27 Lipid-laden cell in the thymus of the spotless starling, *Sturnus unicolor*. The presence of these cells appears to be dependent upon the season (× 7475).

Vascularization and Innervation—On the Existence of a Blood–Thymus Barrier

Few recent reports are available on the blood supply and innervation of the vertebrate thymus apart from classical anatomical descriptions. Large blood vessels enter the thymic parenchyma with connective tissue septa. Ramifications from these vessels invade the thymic stroma, being always, at least in the cortical area, surrounded by a continuous layer of processes of reticuloepithelial cells which constitutes the morphological basis of the so-called 'hemato-thymic' barrier. Such a histological organization has been reported in the blood vessels of various lower vertebrates (Zapata, 1981; Bigaj and Plytycz, 1984), although Tatner and Manning (1982) reported that the thymus of *Salmo gairdneri* is relatively unprotected, and the antigens could gain entrance directly into the embryonic thymus from the gill cavity. Thus, the thymic blood vessels

appear to provide a certain selective permeability for circulating tracers. Unmyelinated nerves usually coursing along with the large blood vessels occur in connective tissue septa of the thymus (Figure 5.28). They contain small electron-dense vesicles suggesting a sympathetic nature (Figure 5.28). No information is currently available on the nature of the innervation in the thymus of lower vertebrates.

Functional Aspects of the Thymus in Ectothermic Vertebrates

Although previous descriptions of the histology and cell types which occur in the thymus of non-mammalian vertebrates have usually included information on the avian thymus, the following description of thymic functions will emphasize ectothermic vertebrates, fish, amphibians and reptiles, since the

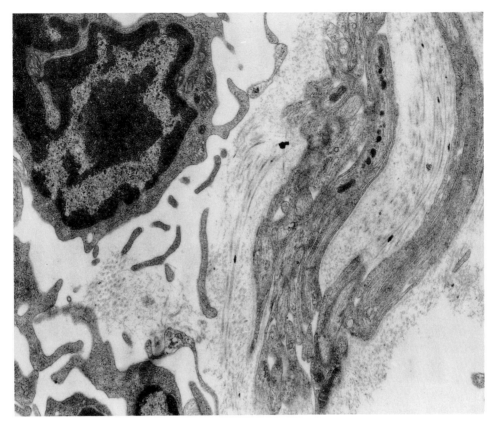

Figure 5.28 Nerve ending in a connective tissue trabeculae of the thymus of *Mauremys caspica* (× 4860).

functions of the avian immune system have been reported more extensively in books, monographs and reviews. In general, functions of the thymus are related to T-dependent immune responses, effected by T-lymphocytes which are produced and undergo differentiation in the thymus gland.

Fish

The role of the thymus in fish immune reactions is derived almost exclusively from teleosts (see review by McCumber *et al.*, 1982; Zapata, 1983). Sigel *et al.* (1968) suggested that sharks lack T-helper cells and that B-like cells are able to respond to mammalian thymus-dependent antigens in a T-independent manner. Moreover, the cellular immune capacity is controversial in cartilaginous fish and positive mixed lymphocyte reactions have not been demonstrable in

sharks (McKinney *et al.*, 1976, 1981). By contrast, sharks possess lymphocytes capable of responding to mitogens which are stimulators of mammalian T-cells (Lopez *et al.*, 1974), thus suggesting the presence of suppressor cells in nurse sharks (Sigel *et al.*, 1968). Information concerning functions of the teleost thymus in immunoreactivity is derived mainly from studies on relationships between thymic ontogeny, appearance of certain immune responses and the effects of earlier thymectomy on immune reactivity.

In *Salmo gairdneri*, responses to foreign histo-incompatible tissue appear to be correlated with histological maturation of the thymus, lymphocytic differentiation in the kidney and presence of small lymphocytes in the peripheral blood (Secombes and Manning, 1982). According to Secombes and Manning, scale grafts transplanted in 5-day-old rainbow trout did not show lymphocytic infiltrations until

14–20 days, when the lymphoid organs, principally the thymus, were more mature. Under these conditions, the grafts were not rejected until 30 days after transplantation. At 5 days, thymus and kidney contained only large undifferentiated cells and splenic development still had not begun. Grafts transplanted on day 14 showed lymphocytic infiltration 4 days later, reaching a maximum at 12 days, followed by rejection on day 30. At 14 days, the thymus and kidney already contained many small lymphocytes. The spleen, although present, was mainly erythropoietic. In other experiments, trout grafted on day 21 showed lymphocytes in the graft region 4 days post-transplantation, and the graft was completely rejected after 20 days. At 21 days, the thymus and kidney were histologically mature and the spleen, although predominantly erythroid, already contained small lymphocytes.

The effects of adult thymectomy have been analyzed in *Tilapia mossambica* (Sailendri, 1973) and *Salmo gairdneri* (Botham et al., 1980). In *Tilapia*, adult thymectomy had no effects on primary graft rejection or antibody production against T-independent antigens, such as polyvinylpyrrolidone. However, the responses to sheep erythrocytes (SRBC), a typical T-dependent antigen, were reduced. In *Salmo gairdneri* there were no effects on primary and secondary graft rejection. By contrast, thymectomy in 2-month-old *Tilapia* induced total suppression of the response against SRBC, and the rejection of primary allografts in 4-month-old fish. In *Cymatogaster aggregata*, intraovarian embryos do not respond to allografts but grafts transplanted after birth are rejected. Times of rejection are inversely related to the age of fish (Triplett and Barrymore, 1960). *Xiphophorus maculatus* rejects allografts 23 days after fertilization, a time which is slower than that which occurs in the adults (Kallman, 1970). In *Tilapia mossambica* the mean survival time of scale allografts was longer in 0.5-month-old fish than in those of 4.5 months or adults (Sailendri, 1973). *Cyprinus carpio* responds to allografts 16 days after hatching. In addition, an allograft transplanted on day 16 can induce specific anamnestic responses 1 month later (Botham et al., 1980).

The effects of embryonic thymectomy on cell proliferation in peripheral lymphoid organs, allograft rejection and antibody production have also been analyzed in *Salmo gairdneri* (Secombes and Manning, 1982). Trout thymectomized at day 14 post-hatching,

injected with human gamma globulin (HGG) in Freund's complete adjuvant 1 month later and killed at 4 or 6 weeks after immunization, showed a proliferative response in the spleen and kidney. Skin grafts placed on trout thymectomized at 2 months and grafted 1 month later all showed graft rejection but the process was delayed when compared to that of non-thymectomized, control specimens. These and other results suggest that in *Salmo gairdneri* the anti-T-independent antigen response (for example, against *Aeromonas salmonicida*) appears earlier than that against T-dependent antigens (for example, HGG). Thus, Etlinger et al. (1978) found that the anti-T-independent antigen response was the same in young as in adult trout, whereas responses against T-dependent antigens were weaker in young fish. Some evidence suggests that T-dependent antigens can induce tolerance in young fish, although the specificity of suppressed responses is unknown. Moreover, the presence of suppressor cells in the carp thymus has been suggested. Thus, carp immunized with formalin-killed *Aeromonas salmonicida*, after adult thymectomy, show higher antibody titers on day 7 than control unimmunized fish.

Reactivity to mitogens has also been tested in the teleost thymus, although results are contradictory. Etlinger et al. (1976) concluded that in *Salmo gairdneri* lymphocytes from the thymus respond only to Con A, from the pronephros to LPS and to both mitogens in the spleen and peripheral blood. By contrast, Cuchens and Clem (1977) experimenting with *Lepomis macrochirus* reported that the pronephros contains Con A and LPS-responding cells, whereas thymocytes responded only to LPS. Finally, a clear response to Con A and LPS has been recently reported in lymphoid organs (thymus, spleen, pronephros) and peripheral blood of *Salmo gairdneri* (Warr and Simon, 1983).

Amphibians

Amphibians, due to their key position in phylogeny, the relative simplicity of manipulating their larval stages, and the striking phenomenon of metamorphosis, represent excellent models for analyzing the evolution of immune responses. Thus, salamanders, frogs and toads are among the best known lower vertebrates, in our opinion, from the viewpoint of comparative immunology. These species have been useful models by providing information on at least three interesting immunological subjects: the origin of antibody diversity, the immunological role of the thymus, and generation of tolerance to self. Numerous reports on immunoreactivity in adult amphibians are available but there is additional information on immunological ontogeny and the role of the thymus gland. The immune capacity of urodeles and anurans exhibits remarkable differences which become evident when thymic function in immune responses is analyzed. In the third group— the apodans or caecilians— although they reject skin allografts chronically, how the thymus influences the process has not been determined (Cooper, 1976).

Thymectomy, during anuran larval life, profoundly abrogates allograft rejection (Cooper and Hildemann, 1965; Du Pasquier, 1965, 1968; Horton and Manning, 1972; Tochinai and Katagiri, 1975; Curtis and Volpe, 1971). Some discrepancies, however, have arisen probably due to different genetic relationships between donors and hosts used in each laboratory. According to Tochinai and Katagiri (1975), thymectomy in *Xenopus* must be performed as early as stage 45 to completely prevent allograft rejection. By contrast, Horton and his coworkers concluded that there is a T-independent component associated with allograft rejection. However, both these research teams agree that after stage 48 thymectomy has no effect whatsoever on the fate of a subsequent allograft. Kaye and Tompkins (1983) reported recently no evidence for a thymus-independent source of alloreactive T-cells. According to these authors, the period of time in which thymectomy is effective occurs when there is stem cell immigration into the thymus, and the ability of thymectomized animals to reject allogeneic grafts is dependent upon the population of cells already processed by the thymus and released prior to thymectomy.

Finally, a striking point concerning ontogeny of allograft rejection in amphibians, mainly anurans, is that during metamorphosis reactivity of host animals or antigenicity of donor grafts may change, resulting in prolonged survival of some transplants In summary, during metamorphosis larvae pass through a transient stage when they cannot reject certain grafts. The duration of this period depends on the immunogenetic disparity between donor and host, the size of the graft and the MHC haplotype dose (Di Marzo and Cohen,

1979). The tolerance is due to an active suppression exerted by some lymphocytes during this period. The process is obviously unresolved and further studies might consider influences of extra-immune mechanisms, especially endocrine parameters.

Mixed lymphocyte reactions can be detected between lymphocytes from stage 55−56 of *Xenopus* by using standard thymidine uptake protocols. In *Rana catesbeiana* positive MLR has been demonstrated in mixed suspensions of tadpole cells (Du Pasquier, 1982). Larval amphibians respond to T-mitogens (Pross and Rowland, 1975) but thymectomy does not abrogate the ability of *Xenopus* lymphocytes to respond to *E. coli* lipopolysaccharide (Manning *et al.*, 1976). Effects of early thymectomy on both phenomena show minor contradictory results. Some investigators have reported total abrogation of both functions (Du Pasquier and Horton, 1976), others only impairment (Manning *et al.*, 1976; Green and Cohen, 1979). This residual activity, sometimes detected, might be due to T-cells that have already migrated out of the thymus, to T-cells with an alternative pathway of differentiation, or even to B-cells (Du Pasquier, 1982).

Thymic regulation of antibody responses has been investigated repeatedly in anurans using sequential thymectomy. No LMW Ig can be detected in the serum of thymectomized *Xenopus*, whereas the level of IgM is normal or higher than in sham thymectomized (Weiss *et al.*, 1973; Manning, 1975). Thymectomy in *Xenopus* causes different responses relative to the antigens. In the case of T-dependent antigens it abrogates the IgG response but fails to modify IgM responses, and in T-independent antigens, such as PVP or LPS, the response which consists essentially of IgM antibody production is not abrogated (Turner and Manning, 1974; Collie *et al.*, 1975; Tochinai, 1976). These observations in *Xenopus* agree with previous reports using *Rana*, where late larval thymectomy also impaired antibody responses to soluble proteins (Cooper *et al.*, 1964).

In contrast, the existence of T-cell subpopulations has been demonstrated in some anurans. The thymus appears to generate a population of helper T-cells that exert a collaborative role in antibody production. Thus, in the classic hapten (TNP)-carrier (foreign erythrocyte) experiment, a good anti-hapten response requires low-dose, carrier-specific priming (Ruben and Edwards, 1979). The morphology and kinetics of

RFC in spleen and thymus suggest that helper cells arose from the thymus (Ruben, 1975). TNP−SRBC reactivity is abolished after thymic removal in larval and adult life (Horton *et al.*, 1979; Gruenewald and Ruben, 1979). In contrast, anti-TNP RFC reactivity following injection of the same hapten conjugated to a thymus-independent carrier (LPS) is unaffected by thymus removal. Ig production *in vitro* against the hapten DNP also requires (as in *in vivo* conditions) collaboration of primed B- and T-like lymphocytes (Blomberg *et al.*, 1980). Blomberg and her colleagues have also demonstrated that carrier-primed *Xenopus* T-helper cells will collaborate efficiently with hapten-primed B-cells *in vitro* to produce a secondary Ig 'G' antibody response, only if the two lymphocyte types share at least one allele associated with the MHC, the so-called XLA (Blomberg *et al.*, 1980). Studies on the effects of late thymectomy on antibody production suggest that the thymus is necessary to provide helper cells during the entire larval period. There is no evidence as to whether this help is similar to that necessary in adults. Although thymic function is evident in larvae, it may not be fully differentiated. Thus, since to some extent larval lymphocytes appear to lack MHC antigens, Du Pasquier (1982) suggested that T−B collaboration cannot be optimal during larval stages. The end of the period when thymectomy can efficiently prevent antibody responses to T-dependent antigens is practically coincident with the onset of histocompatibility antigen expression on the surface of lymphocytes.

In vitro experiments in *Xenopus* using nylon-wool-passed thymus cells suggest some suppressive activity since the addition of thymic T-cells to splenic B-cells, largely depleted of helper T- cells, resulted in a three- to tenfold reduction of antibody output, as measured by the phage inactivation assay (Du Pasquier and Bernard, 1980). When 'suppressor' T-cells were added to unfractionated spleen cells little or no suppression was observed. Du Pasquier and Bernard concluded that T-cells seem to be compartmentalized in *Xenopus*, with most helper cells in the spleen and the majority of suppressor cells in the thymus. On the other hand, Manning (1975) reported that splenic antigen-trapping in *Xenopus* is a thymus-dependent process. Likewise, Klempau and Cooper (1984) suggest a thymic origin for *Rana pipiens* E-rosetting receptor until the cells leave the thymus, and larval,

weak E-rosettes as well as adult thymic weak E-rosettes seem to be immature T-cells (Klempau and Cooper, 1983).

Finally, we will comment on different periods of functional maturation which occur in the anuran thymus. Sequential thymectomy has revealed that allograft rejection, MLR, PHA responsiveness and T-helper functions do not mature at the same time, suggesting sequential generation of different T-cell subsets. The thymus is only necessary for a short period to establish a full complement of peripheral cells capable of effecting normal alloimmune responses and mixed lymphocyte culture reactivity, but it is necessary for a considerably longer period to establish normal antibody production and T-mitogen reactivity (Horton *et al.*, 1977; Horton and Sherif, 1977; Manning and Collie, 1977).

The capacity to respond to TNP−Ficoll (a T-independent 2 antigen in mammals) arises with the development of a thymic medulla (Ruben *et al.*, 1984). Also, the suppressor function has been related to the thymic medulla since injection of a N-methyl-N-nitrosourea (NMU), a powerful alkylating lymphocytotoxic agent (Clothier *et al.*, 1980; James *et al.*, 1982), selectively destroys the cortex and retains the suppressor capacity (Ruben *et al.*, 1984). On the contrary, the cells engaged in helper function in *Xenopus* could reside in and be derived from the cortical region of the thymus (Clothier *et al.*, 1984)

Reptiles

Information concerning immune functions of the thymus in reptiles is less complete than in amphibians. Lizards (*Chalcides ocellatus*), 3−5 months after adult thymectomy, show depleted lymphocytes in the periarteriolar regions of the spleen, slightly prolonged skin allograft survival and enhanced anti-RRBC antibody responses (El Masri, 1979). Antibody responses to HSA and PVP produced no effects (El Masri, 1979). Results in *Calotes versicolor* also demonstrate the importance of the thymus in anti-T-dependent antigen responses. Thymectomized *Calotes versicolor* treated with an anti-T serum (ATS) shows abrogation of PFC responses to SRBC. Moreover, a definitive recovery of anti-SRBC responses after ATS treatment occurs in the presence of the thymus (Pitchappan and Muthukkaruppan, 1976, 1977b; Muthukkaruppan *et al.*, 1976). Bilateral thymectomy performed one month before immunization significantly reduces the PFC response to optimal doses of SRBC, but the response to supra-optimal doses is not altered (Jayaraman, 1976). Furthermore, as in *Chalcides ocellatus*, the periarteriolar region of the splenic white pulp in *Calotes versicolor* becomes depleted of lymphocytes one month after adult thymectomy (Pitchappan and Muthukkarappan, 1977c). By contrast the antibody response to PVP, a known T-independent antigen, was not affected by adult thymectomy performed 1 month before immunization (Muthukkaruppan *et al.*, 1982). Finally, Ramila (1978) found that helper-carrier functions are impaired in adult lizards 1 month after ablation of the thymus.

FINAL COMMENT

The thymus is an essential organ that enables vertebrates to mount immune responses. Its universal presence, except in cyclostomes, an enigma which is still unresolved, during vertebrate phylogeny with only minor variations in structure, supports its importance. Further experiments must be performed to analyze satisfactorily the peculiar situation of cyclostomes—primitive vertebrates which are able to mount immune responses in the apparent absence of a functional thymus or an identifiable morphofunctional equivalent. Without suitable phenotypic markers, a fine analysis of different lymphoid and non-lymphoid cell populations in ectothermic vertebrates has been slow to emerge. These reagents would help to reveal the T- and B-cell dichotomy and their respective lymphocyte subtypes. Production of specific monoclonal antibodies and biochemical analysis of the molecular components of lymphocytic membranes will be tools of extreme importance for these objectives. Likewise, obtaining histocompatible clones in those animals with known haplotypes is essential. With the acquisition of this new technology we can analyze the numerous inductive processes which occur inside the embryonic and neonatal thymus and plays a role in the differentiation of various functional lymphocyte subsets.

REFERENCES

Albert S, Wolf PL and Pryjma I (1965a). Evidence of erythropoiesis in the thymus of mice. *J Ret Soc* **2**: 30–39.

Albert S, Wolf PL, Pryjma I and Vazquez J (1965b). Variations in morphology of erythroblasts of normal mouse thymus. *J Ret Soc* **2**: 158–171.

Albert S, Wolf PL, Pryjma I and Vazquez J (1966). Erythropoiesis in the human thymus. *Am J Clin Pathol* **45**: 460–464.

Albini B and Wick G (1973). Immunoglobulin determinants on the surface of chicken lymphoid cells. *Int Arch Allergy* **44**: 804–822.

Archer OK, Sutherland DE and Good RA (1964). The developmental biology of lymphoid tissue in the rabbit. Consideration of the role of thymus and appendix. *Lab Invest* **13**: 259–271.

Ardavin CF and Zapata A (1988a). The pharyngeal lymphoid aggregates of lampreys: a morpho-functional equivalent of the vertebrate thymus? *Thymus* **11**: 59–65.

Ardavin CF and Zapata A (1988b). Lymphoid components in the branchial cavernous body of the ammocoete of *Petromyzon marinus*. *Acta Zool Stockh* **69**: 23–28.

Ardavin CF, Gomariz RP, Barrutia MG, Fonfria J and Zapata A (1984). The lymphohemopoietic organs of the anadromous sea lamprey *Petromyzon marinus*. A comparative study throughout its life span. *Acta Zool Stockh* **65**: 1–15.

Ashman RB and Papadimitriou JM (1975). Evidence of erythropoiesis in the thymus of mice. *J Ret Soc* **2**: 30–39.

Auerbach R (1961). Experimental analysis of the origin of cell types in the development of the mouse thymus. *Dev Biol* **3**: 336–354.

Bacchus S and Kendall MD (1975). Histological changes associated with enlargement and regression of the thymus glands of the red-billed *Quelea quelea* L. (Plocidae: weaver birds). *Phil Trans Roy Soc B* **273**: 65–78.

Barrutia MG, Leceta J, Fonfria J, Garrido E and Zapata A (1983). Non-lymphoid cells of the anuran spleen: an ultrastructural study in the natterjack *Bufo calamita*. *Am J Anat* **167**: 83–94.

Barrutia MG, Villena A, Razquin B, Gomariz RP and Zapata A (1985a). Presence of presumptive interdigitating cells in the spleen of the natterjack *Bufo calamita*. *Experientia* **41**: 1393–1394.

Barrutia MG, Villena A, Gomariz RP, Razquin B and Zapata A (1985b). Ultrastructural changes in the spleen of the natterjack *Bufo calamita*, after antigenic stimulation. *Cell Tissue Res* **239**: 435–441.

Beard J (1900). The source of leucocytes and the true function of the thymus. *Anat Anz* **18**: 550–560.

Beletskaya LV and Gnesditskava EV (1980). Detection of squamous epithelial intercellular substance antigen(s) in Hassall's corpuscles of human and animal thymus. *Scand J Immunol* **12**: 93–98.

Bigaj J and Plytycz B (1981). Ultrastruktura komorek grasiczych zaby. *Przeglad Zoologiczny* **25**: 489–494.

Bigaj J and Plytycz B (1984). Cytoarchitecture of the thymus gland of the adult frog *Rana temporaria*. *Folia Histochem Cytobiol* **22**: 63−70.

Bigaj J and Plytycz B (1987). Interdigitating cells in the thymus of the frog *Rana temporaria*. *Folia Histochem Cytobiol* **24**: 65−68.

Block M (1964). The blood forming tissues and the blood of the newborn opossum *Didelphys virginiama*. *Ergeb Anat Entw* **37**: 237−366.

Blomberg B, Bernard CCA and Du Pasquier L (1980) *In vitro* evidence for T−B lymphocyte collaboration in the clawed toad *Xenopus laevis*. *Eur J Immunol* **10**: 869−876.

Bockman DE (1970). The thymus. In Gans C and Parsons TS (Eds), *Biology of the Reptilia*. Vol 3. Academic Press: London. pp 111−133.

Bockman LM and Winborn WB (1967). Electron microscopy of the thymus in two species of snakes *Crotalus atrox* and *Lampropeltis getulus*. *J Morph* **121**: 277−294.

Bockman LM and Winborn WB (1969). Ultrastructure of thymic myoid cells. *J Morph* **129**: 201−210.

Borysenko M and Cooper EL (1972). Lymphoid tissue in the snapping turtle *Chelydra serpentina*. *J Morph* **138**: 487−498.

Botham JW, Grace MF and Manning MJ (1980). Ontogeny of first set and second set alloimmune reactivity in fishes. In Manning MJ (Ed.), *Phylogeny of Immunological Memory*. Elsevier/North-Holland Biomedical Press: Amsterdam. pp 83−92.

Boyd RL and Ward HA (1984). Lymphoid antigenic determinants of the chicken: Ontogeny of bursa-dependent lymphoid tissue. *Dev Comp Immunol* **8**: 149−168.

Brand A, Galton J and Gilmore DG (1976). Lymphocyte-differentiating hormone of bursa of Fabricius. *Science* **193**: 319−321.

Brand A, Galton J and Gilmore DG (1983). Committed precursors of B and T lymphocytes in chick embryonic bursa of Fabricius. *Eur J Immunol* **13**: 449−455.

Bryant BJ and Shifrine M (1972). Histogenesis of lymph nodes during development of the dog. *J Ret Soc* **12**: 96−107.

Cesarini JP, Benkoel L and Bonneau H (1968). Ultrastructure comparée du thymus chez le hamster jeune et adulte. *CR Soc Biol (Paris)* **162**: 1975−1979.

Chapman Jr WL and Allen JR (1971). The fine structure of the thymus of the fetal and neonatal monkey *Macaca mulatta*. *Z Zellforsch* **114**: 220−233.

Charlemagne J (1977). Thymus development in amphibians: colonization of thymic endodermal rudiments by lymphoid stem-cells of mesenchymal origin in the urodele *Pleurodeles waltlii* Michah. *Ann Immunol* **128C**: 897−904.

Chilmonczyk S (1983). The thymus of the rainbow trout *Salmo gairdneri*. Light and electron microscopic study. *Dev Comp Immunol* **7**: 59−68.

Clerx JPM (1978). Studies on pike fry rhabdovirus and the immunoglobulin of pike *Esox lucius*. Doctoral thesis, University of Utrecht.

Clothier RH and Balls M (1985). Structural changes in the thymus glands of *Xenopus laevis* during development. In Balls M and Bownes M (Eds), *Metamorphosis*. Clarendon Press: Oxford. pp 332−359.

Clothier RH, Balls M, Hodgson RM and Horn NJ (1980). Effects of *N*-methyl-*N*-nitrosourea on the lymphoid tissues and skin allograft response of *Xenopus laevis*. *Dev Comp Immunol* **4**: 265−272.

Clothier RH, Balls M, Water AD, Marsden CA and Bennett GW (1983). Location and synthesis of thyrotropin releasing hormone and 5-hydroxytryptamine in the skin and thymus of *Xenopus laevis*. In Griffiths EC and Bennett GW (Eds), *Thyrotropin Releasing Hormone*. Raven Press: New York. pp 203−216.

Clothier RH, Ruben HS, James HS and Balls M (1984). TNP−Ficoll response in *Xenopus laevis*: substitution and reconstitution in thymectomized animals. *Immunology* **52**: 483−489.

Collie H, Turner RJ and Manning MJ (1975). Antibody production to lipo-polysaccharide in thymectomized *Xenopus*. *Eur J Immunol* **5**: 426−427.

Cooper EL (1967). Lymphomyeloid organs of amphibia. I. Appearance during larval and adult stages of *Rana catesbeiana*. *J Morphol* **122**: 381−398.

Cooper EL (1976). Immunity mechanisms. In Lofts B (Ed), *Physiology of the Amphibia*. Vol 3. Academic Press: New York. pp 163−272.

Cooper EL and Hildemann WH (1965). Allograft reactions in bullfrog larvae in relation to thymectomy. *Transplantation* **3**: 446−448.

Cooper EL, Pinkerton W and Hildemann WH (1964). Serum antibody synthesis in larvae of the bullfrog *Rana catesbeiana*. *Biol Bull* **127**: 232−238.

Coudert RH, Cavechy L and Dambrine G (1979). Evidence for a thymic factor in sera of chickens. *Folia Biol (Praha)* **25**: 317−318.

Csaba G, Olah I and Kapa E (1970). Phylogenesis of the mast cells. II. Ultrastructure of the mast cells in the frog. *Acta Biol Acad Sci Hung* **21**: 255−264.

Cuchens MA and Clem LW (1977). Phylogeny of lymphocyte heterogeneity. II. Differential effects of temperature on fish T-like and B-like cells. *Cell Immunol* **34**: 219−227.

Curtis SK and Volpe EP (1971). Modification of responsiveness to allografts in larvae of the leopard frog by thymectomy. *Dev Biol* **24**: 177−197.

Curtis SK, Volpe EP and Cowden RR (1972). Ultrastructure of the developing thymus of the leopard frog *Rana pipiens*. *Z Zellforsch* **127**: 323−346.

Curtis SK, Cowden RR and Nagel JW (1979). Ultrastructural and histochemical features of the thymus glands of the adult lungless salamander *Plethodon glutinosus* (Caudata: Plethodontidae). *J Morph* **160**: 241−274.

Dardenne M, Tournefier A, Charlemagne J and Bach J-F (1973). Studies on thymic products. VII. Presence of thymic hormone in urodele serum. *Ann Immunol* **124C**: 465−469.

Diener E and Ealey EH (1965). Immune system in a monotreme: studies on the Australian echidna *Tachyglossus aculeatus*. *Nature* **208**: 950−953.

DiMarzo S and Cohen N (1979). Ontogeny of alloimmunity to major histo-compatibility (MHC) antigens in the frog *Xenopus* (Abstract). *Am Zool* **19**: 856.

Drenckhahn D, von Gudecker B, Muller-Hermelink HK, Unsicker K and Groschel-Stewart U (1979). Myosin and actin containing cells in the human postnatal thymus. Ultrastructural and immunohistochemical findings in normal thymus and in myasthenia gravis. *Virchows Arch Cell Pathol* **32**: 33−45.

Droege W, Malchow D and Strominger JL (1972). Cellular heterogeneity in the thymus. I. Electrophoretic analysis of lymphoid cell populations from chickens. *Eur J Immunol* **2**: 156−161.

Duda PL and Gupta A (1980). Hassall's corpuscles in chelonian thymus. *Corr Sci* **49**: 202−203.

Du Pasquier L (1965). Aspects cellulares et humoraux de l'intolerance aux homogreffes de tissu musculaire chez le tetard d'*Alytes obstetricans*: role du thymus. *CR Acad Sci Paris* **261**: 1144−1147.

Du Pasquier L (1968). Les proteines seriques et le complex lymphomyeloide chez le tetard d'*Alytes obstetricans* normal et thymectomise. *Ann Inst Pasteur* **114**: 490−502.

Du Pasquier L (1982). Ontogeny of immunological functions in amphibians. In Cohen N and Sigel MM (Eds), *The Reticuloendothelial System. A Comprehensive Treatise.* Vol 3. *Phylogeny and Ontogeny*. Plenum Press: New York. pp 633−658.

Du Pasquier L and Bernard CC (1980). Active suppression of the allogeneic histocompatibility reactions during the metamorphosis of the clawed toad *Xenopus*. *Differentiation* **16**: 1−7.

Du Pasquier L and Horton JD (1976). The effect of thymectomy on the mixed leukocyte reaction and phytohemagglutinin responsiveness in the clawed toad *Xenopus laevis*. *Immunogenetics* **3**: 105−112.

Du Pasquier L and Horton JD (1982). Restoration of antibody responsiveness in early thymectomized *Xenopus* by implantation of major histocompatibility complex−mismatched larval thymus. *Eur J Immunol* **12**: 546-551.

Duijvestijn AM, Kohler YG and Hoefsmit ECM (1982a). Interdigitating cells and macrophages in the acute involuting rat thymus. An electron microscopy study on phagocytic activity and population development. *Cell Tissue Res* **224**: 291−301.

Duijvestijn AM, Sminia T, Kohler YG, Jause EM and Hoefsmit ECM (1982b). Rat thymus micro-environment. An ultrastructural and functional characterization. In Nieuwenhuis P, van der Broek AA and Hanna Jr MG (Eds), *In vivo Immunology. Histophysiology of the Lymphoid System*. Plenum Press: New York. pp 441−446.

Dulzetto F (1968). Timo. In: *Anatomia Comparata dei Vertebrati*. Edizioni Calderini: Bologna. pp 2148−2153.

Dung HC (1973). Electron microscopic study in involuting thymus of 'lethargic' mutant mice. *Anat Rec* **177**: 585−602.

Dustin AP (1909). Contributions a l'etude du thymus des reptiles cellules epithelioides, cellules myoides et corps de Hassall. *Archs Zool Exp Gen* **2**: 43−227.

El Deeb S, Zada S and El Ridi R (1985). Ontogeny of hemopoietic and lymphopoietic tissues in the lizard *Chalcides ocellatus* (Reptilia, Saura, Scincidae). *J Morph* **185**: 241−253.

El Masri N (1979). Role of thymus and spleen in immune response of the lizard *Chalcides ocellatus*. MSc thesis, Faculty of Sciences, Cairo University.

Ellis AE (1977). Ontogeny of the immune response in *Salmo salar*. Histogenesis of lymphoid organs and appearance of membrane immunoglobulin and mixed leucocyte reactivity. In Solomon JB and Horton JD (Eds), *Developmental Immunobiology*. Elsevier/North-Holland Biomedical Press: Amsterdam. pp 225−231.

Erickson-Viitanen S, Ruggieri S, Natalini P and Horecker BL (1983). Distribution of thymosin B_4 in vertebrate classes. *Arch Biochem Biophys* **221**: 570−574.

Etlinger HM, Hodgins HO and Chiller JM (1976). Evolution of the lymphoid system. I. Evidence for lymphocyte heterogeneity in rainbow trout revealed by the organ distribution of mitogenic responses. *J Immunol* **116**: 1547−1553.

Etlinger HM, Hodgins HO and Chiller JM (1978). Evolution of the lymphoid system. III. Morphological and functional consequences of mitogenic stimulation of rainbow trout lymphocytes. *Dev Comp Immunol* **2**: 263−276.

Fabrizio M and Charippa HA (1941). The morphogenesis of the thymus gland of *Rana sylvatica* as correlated with certain stages of metamorphosis. *J Morphol* **68**: 179−195.

Fange R and Pulsford A (1985). The thymus of the angler fish *Lophius piscatorius* (Pisces: Teleostei): a light and electron microscopic study. In Manning MJ and Tatner MF (Eds), *Fish Immunology*. Academic Press: London. pp 293−311.

Fange R and Sundell G (1969). Lymphomyeloid tissues, blood cells and plasma proteins in *Chimaera monstrosa* (Pisces, Holocephali). *Acta Zool Stockh* **50**: 155−168.

Finstad J, Papermaster BW and Good RA (1964). Evolution of the immune response. II. Morphologic studies on the origin of the thymus and organized lymphoid tissue. *Lab Invest* **13**: 490−512.

Flajnik MF, Kaufman JF, Hsu E and Du Pasquier L (1984). The major histocompatibility complex of amphibians. In Cooper EL and Wright RK (Eds), *Aspects of Developmental and Comparative Immunology II. Dev Comp Immunol* Suppl **3**: 9−12.

Fonfria J, Barrutia MG, Villena A and Zapata A (1982). Ultrastructural study of interdigitating cells in the thymus of the spotless starling *Sturnus unicolor*. *Cell Tissue Res* **225**: 687−691.

Fonfria J, Barrutia MG, Garrido E, Ardavin CF and Zapata A (1983). Erythropoiesis in the thymus of the spotless starling *Sturnus unicolor*. *Cell Tissue Res* **232**: 445−455.

Frazier JA (1973). Ultrastructure of the chick thymus. *Z Zellforsch* **136**: 191−205.

Frohely MF and Deschaux PA (1986). Presence of tonofilaments and thymic serum factor (FTS) in thymic epithelial cells of a fresh water fish (Carp *Cyprinus carpio*) and a sea water fish (Bass *Dicentrarchus labrax*). *Thymus* **8**: 235–244.

Garcia-Herrera F and Cooper EL (1968). Organos linfoides del amfibio apodo *Typhlonectes compressicauda*. *Acta Med* **4**: 157–160.

Gerard P (1933). Sûr le systeme athrophagocytaire chez l'ammocoete de la *Lampetra planeri* (Bloch). *Arch Biol Paris* **44**: 327–346.

Glick B (1982). RES structure and function of the aves. In Cohen N and Sigel MM (Eds), *The Reticuloendothelial System. A Comprehensive Treatise*. Vol 3. *Phylogeny and Ontogeny*. Plenum Press: New York. pp 509–568.

Goldstein AL (Ed) (1984). *Thymic Hormones and Lymphokines*. Plenum Press: New York.

Good RA, Finstad J, Pollara B and Gabrielsen AE (1966). Morphological studies on the evolution of the lymphoid tissues among the lower vertebrates. In Smith RT, Miescher PA and Good RA (Eds), *Phylogeny of Immunity*. University of Florida Press: Gainesville. pp 149–168.

Gorgollon P (1983). Fine structure of the thymus in the adult cling fish *Sicyases sanguineus* (Pisces Gobiesocidae). *J Morph* **177**: 25–40.

Grace MF and Manning MJ (1980). Histogenesis of the lymphoid organs in rainbow trout *Salmo gairdneri*. Richardson 1836. *Dev Comp Immunol* **4**: 255–264.

Green (Donnelly) N and Cohen N (1979). Phylogeny of immunocompetent cells. III. Mitogen response characteristics of lymphocyte subpopulations from normal and thymectomized frogs *Xenopus laevis*. *Cell Immunol* **48**: 59–70.

Groscurth P (1980). Non-lymphatic cells in the lymphoid node cortex of the mouse. I. Morphology and distribution of the interdigitating cells and the dendritic reticular in the enteric node of the adult IRC mouse. *Pathol Res Pract* **169**: 212–234.

Gruenewald DA and Ruben LN (1979). The effect of adult thymectomy upon helper function in *Xenopus laevis*, the South African clawed toad. *Immunology* **38**: 191–194.

Hafter E (1952). Histological age changes in the thymus of the telost *Astyanax*. *J Morph* **90**: 555–581.

Hakanson R, Larsson L-I and Sundler F (1974). Peptide and amine-like cells in the chicken thymus. A chemical, histochemical and electron microscopic study. *Histochemistry* **39**: 25–34.

Hammar JA (1905). Zur histogenese und involution der thymusdruse. *Anat Anz* **27**: 23–30, 41–89.

Hammond WS (1954). Origin of thymus in the chick embryo. *J Morph* **95**: 501–521.

Hanzlikova V (1979). Histochemical and ultrastructural properties of myoid cells in the thymus of the frog. *Cell Tissue Res* **197**: 105–112.

Haritos AA, Goodall GJ and Horecker BL (1984). Prothymosin alpha: isolation and properties of the major immunoreactive form of thymosin alpha 1 in rat thymus. *Proc Natl Acad Sci USA* **81**: 1008–1011.

Haritos AA, Caldarella J and Horecker BL (1985a). Simultaneous isolation and determination of prothymosin alpha, parathymosin alpha, thymosin beta 4, and thymosin beta 10. *Anal Biochem* **144**: 436–440.

Haritos AA, Salvin SB, Blacher R, Stein S and Horecker BL (1985b). Parathymosin alpha: a peptide from rat tissues with structural homology to prothymosin alpha. *Proc Natl Acad Sci USA* **82**: 1050–1053.

Hemmingsson EJ (1972). Ontogenic studies on lymphoid cell traffic in the chicken. II. Cell traffic from the bursa of Fabricius to the thymus and the spleen in the embryo. *Int Arch Allergy* **42**: 764–774.

Henry K (1966). Mucin secretion and striated muscle in the human thymus. *Lancet* **i**: 183–185.

Henry M and Charlemagne J (1980). Development of amphibian thymus. I. Morphological differentiation, multiplication, migration and lysis of thymocytes in the urodele *Pleurodeles waltlii*. *J Embryol Exp Morphol* **57**: 219–232.

Henry M and Charlemagne J (1981). Development of amphibian thymus. II. Sequential occurrence of two epithelial cell types in the urodele *Pleurodeles waltlii*. *Dev Comp Immunol* **5**: 449–460.

Hightower JA (1975). DNA synthesis in the thymus of the adult newt *Notophthalmus viridescens*. *Acta Anat* **92**: 454–466.

Hightower JA and St Pierre RL (1971). Hemopoietic tissue in the adult newt *Notophthalmus viridescens*. *J Morph* **135**: 299–308.

Hill BH (1935). The early development of the thymus glands of *Amia calva*. *J Morph* **57**: 61–89.

Hoffmann-Fezer G (1973). Histologische untersuchungen an lymphatischen organen des huhnes (*Gallus domesticus*) wahrend des ersten lebensjahres. *Z Zellforsch* **136**: 45–58.

Hohn EO (1947). Seasonal cyclical changes in the thymus of the mallard. *J Exp Biol* **24**: 184–191.

Horton JD (1971). Histogenesis of the lymphomyeloid complex in the larval leopard frog *Rana pipiens*. *J Morphol* **134**: 1–20.

Horton JD and Horton TL (1975). Development of transplantation immunity and restoration experiments in thymectomized amphibians. *Am Zool* **15**: 73–84.

Horton JD and Manning MJ (1972). Response to skin allografts in *Xenopus laevis* following thymectomy at early stages of lymphoid organ maturation. *Transplantation* **14**: 141–154.

Horton JD and Sherif NEHS (1977). Sequential thymectomy in the clawed toad: Effect on mixed leucocyte reactivity and phytohemagglutinin responsiveness. In Solomon JB and Horton JD (Eds), *Developmental Immunobiology*. Elsevier/North-Holland: Amsterdam. pp 283–290.

Horton JD, Rimmer JJ and Horton TL (1977). Critical role of the thymus in establishing humoral immunity in amphibians: Studies on *Xenopus* thymectomized in larval and adult life. *Dev Comp Immunol* **1**: 119–130.

Horton JD, Edwards BF, Ruben LN and Mette S (1979). Use of different carriers to demonstrate thymic-dependent and thymic-independent anti-trinitrophenyl reactivity in the amphibian *Xenopus laevis*. *Dev Comp Immunol* **3**: 621−633.

Inselvini M (1975). First appearance of caerulein during the development of *Xenopus laevis*. *Gen Pharmacol* **6**: 215−217.

Isler H (1976). Fine structure of chicken thymic epithelial vesicles. *J Cell Sci* **20**: 135−147.

Jacoby RD, Dennis RA and Griesemer RA (1969). Development of immunity in fetal dogs: humoral responses. *Am J Vet Res* **30**: 1503−1510.

James ES (1939). The morphology of the thymus and its changes with age in the amphibian *Necturus maculosus*. *J Morphol* **64**: 445−481.

James HS, Clothier RH, Ferrer IR and Balls M (1982). Effects of *N*-methyl-*N*-nitrosourea on carrier-primed anti-hapten responses in *Xenopus laevis*. *Dev Comp Immunol* **6**: 499−507.

Jayaramen S (1976). Modulation of humoral and cell-mediated immune response to sheep erythrocytes in the lizard *Calotes versicolor*. PhD thesis, Madurai University, Tamilnadu (India).

Kaiserling E and Lennert K (1974). Die interdigitierende reticulumzellem in menschlichen lymphknoten. *Virchows Arch Abt B* **16**: 51−61.

Kaiserling E, Stein H and Muller-Hermelink HK (1974). Interdigitating reticulum cells in the human thymus. *Cell Tissue Res* **155**: 47−55.

Kallman K (1970). Genetics of tissue transplantation in teleostei. *Transplant Proc* **2**: 262−271.

Kamperdijk EWA (1980). Lymph node macrophages and reticulum cells in the immune response. PhD thesis, University of Amsterdam.

Kamperdijk EWA, Raamayers EM, de Leeuw JHS and Hoefsmit EMC (1978). Lymph node macrophages and reticulum cells in the immune response. I. The primary response of paratyphoid vaccine. *Cell Tissue Res* **192**: 1−23.

Kampmeier OF (1969). *Evolution and Comparative Morphology of the Lymphatic System*. Charles C Thomas: Springfield.

Kanakambika P and Muthukkaruppan VR (1973). Lymphoid differentiation and organization of the spleen in the lizard *Calotes versicolor*. *Proc Indian Acad Sci* **78**: 37−44.

Kao I and Drachman DB (1977). Thymic muscle cells bear acetylcholine receptors: possible relation to myasthenia gravis. *Science* **195**: 64−75.

Kapa E (1963). Histological and histochemical analysis of the thymus in tailless amphibians. *Acta Morphol* **12**: 1−8.

Kapa E and Csaba G (1972). Phylogenesis of mast cells. III. Effect of hormonal induction on the maturation of mast cells in the frog. *Acta Biol Acad Sci Hung* **23**: 47−54.

Kapa E, Olah I and Toro I (1968). Electron-microscopic investigation of the thymus of adult frog *Rana esculenta*. *Acta Biol Acad Sci Hung* **19**: 203−123.

Katz DH, Katz LR, Bogowitz CA and Skidmore BJ (1979). Adaptive differentiation of murine lymphocytes. II. The thymic micro-environment does not restrict the cooperative partner cell preference of helper T cells differentiating on $F_1 F_1$ thymic chimeras. *J Exp Med* **149**: 1360−1370.

Kaye C and Tompkins R (1983). Allograft rejection in *Xenopus laevis* following larval thymectomy. *Dev Comp Immunol* **7**: 287−294.

Kendall MD (1975a). Sizes and numbers of nuclei in the cortex of thymus glands of the red-billed weaver *Quelea quelea*. *Cell Tissue Res* **164**: 233−249.

Kendall, MD (1975b). EMMA-4 analysis of iron in the cells of the thymic cortex of weaver-bird *Quelea quelea*. *Phil Trans Roy Soc B*. **273**:79−82.

Kendall MD (1979). Ultrastructural studies on erythropoiesis in avian thymus glands. II. A stereological analysis on the lymphoid and erythroid cells. *Cell Tissue Res* **199**: 63−74.

Kendall MD (1980). Avian thymus glands: a review. *Dev Comp Immunol* **4**: 191−210.

Kendall MD and Frazier JA (1979). Ultrastructural studies on erythropoiesis in the avian thymus. I. Description of cell types. *Cell Tissue Res* **199**: 37−61.

Kendall MD and Singh J (1980). The presence of erythroid cells in the thymus gland of man. *J Anat* **130**: 183−199.

Kendall MD and Ward P (1974). Erythropoiesis in an avian thymus. *Nature (London)* **249**: 366−367.

Ketelsen, U-P and Wekerle H (1976). Thymus-derived striated muscle clones. An ultrastructural analysis of cell differentiation. *Differentiation* **5**:185−187.

Klempau AE and Cooper EL (1983). T-lymphocyte and B-lymphocyte dichotomy in anuran amphibians. I. T-lymphocyte proportions, distribution and ontogeny, as measured by E-rosetting, nylon wool adherence, post-metamorphic thymectomy and non-specific esterase staining. *Dev Comp Immunol* **7**: 99−110.

Klempau AE and Cooper EL (1984). T-lymphocyte and B-lymphocyte dichotomy in anuran amphibians. III. Further investigations on the E-rosetting lymphocyte by using monoclonal antibody, azathioprine inhibition and mitogen-induced polyclonal expansion. *Dev Comp Immunol* **8**: 323−338.

Klug H (1967). Submikroskopische zytologie des thymus von *Ambystoma mexicanum*. *Z Zellforsch Mikrosk Anat* **78**: 388−401.

Kyewski BA and Kaplan HS (1982). Lymphoepithelial interactions in the mouse thymus: phenotypic and kinetic studies on thymic nurse cells. *J Immunol* **128**: 2287−2294.

Leceta J (1984). Cambios estacionales en el sistema immune de *Mauremys caspica*. Papel regulador del sistema neuroendocrino. PhD thesis, Complutense University, Madrid.

Leceta J, Villena A, Razquin B, Fonfria J and Zapata A (1984). Interdigitating cells in the thymus of the turtle *Mauremys caspica*. Possible relationships to macrophages. *Cell Tissue Res* **238**: 381−385.

LeDouarin N and Jotereau F (1975). Tracing of cells of the avian thymus through embryonic life in interspecific chimeras. *J Exp Med* **142**: 17−40.

Lennert K, Stein H, Morhi N, Kaiserling E and Muller-Hermelink HK (1978). *Malignant Lymphomas other than Hodgkin's Disease*. Springer-Verlag: New York.

Levinson AI, Lisak RP, Zweiman B and Korstein M (1985). Phenotypic and functional analysis of lymphocytes in myasthenia gravis. *Springer Semin Immunopathol* **8**: 209–233.

Longo DL and Schwartz RH (1980). T-cell specificity for H-2 and Ir gene phenotype correlates with the phenotype of thymic antigen presenting cells. *Nature* **287**: 144–146.

Lopez DM, Sigel MM, and Lee JC (1974). Phylogenetic studies on T cells. I. Lymphocytes of the shark with differentiated response to PHA and Con A. *Cell Immunol* **10**: 287–293.

Lucas AM and Jamroz C (1961). Atlas of avian haematology. *Agric Monogr 25*. USDA: Washington.

Mandel T (1968). Ultrastructure of epithelial cells in the cortex of guinea pig thymus. *Z Zellforsch* **92**: 159–168.

Mandi B and Glant T (1973). Thymosin-producing cells of the thymus. *Nature New Biol* **246**: 25.

Manning MJ (1971). The effect of early thymectomy on histogenesis of the lymphoid organs in *Xenopus laevis*. *J Embryol Exp Morphol* **26**: 219–229.

Manning MJ (1975). The phylogeny of thymic dependence. *Am Zool* **15**: 63–71.

Manning MJ and Collie MH (1977). The ontogeny of thymic dependence in the amphibian *Xenopus laevis*. In Solomon JB and Horton JD (Eds), *Developmental Immunobiology*. Elsevier/North-Holland: Amsterdam. pp 241–298.

Manning MJ and Turner RJ (1976). *Comparative Immunobiology*. Blackie: Glasgow.

Manning MJ, Donnelly N and Cohen N (1976). Thymus-dependent and thymus-independent components of the amphibian immune system. In Wright RK and Cooper EL (Eds), *Phylogeny of Thymus and Bone Marrow—Bursa Cells*. Elsevier/North-Holland: Amsterdam. pp 123–132.

Marchalonis JJ (1977). *Immunity in Evolution*. Arnold: London.

Marchalonis JJ, Ealey EHM and Diener E (1969). Immune response of the tuatara *Sphenodon punctatum*. *Aust J Exp Biol Med Sci* **47**: 367–380.

Mayer S (1888). Concerning the study of the thyroid gland and thymus in amphibians. *Anat Anz* **3**: 97.

McCumber LJ, Sigel MM, Tranger RJ and Cuchens MA (1982). RES structure and function of the fishes. In Cohen N and Sigel MM (Eds), *The Reticuloendothelial System. A Comprehensive Treatise*. Vol 3. *Phylogeny and Ontogeny*. Plenum Press: New York. pp 393–422.

McKinney EC, Ortiz G, Lee JC, Sigel MM, Lopez DM, Epstein RS and McLeod TF (1976). Lymphocytes of fish: multipotential or specialized? In Wright RK and Cooper EL (Eds), *Phylogeny of Thymus and Bone Marrow—Bursa Cells*. Elsevier/North-Holland: Amsterdam. pp 73–82.

McKinney EC, McLeod TF and Sigel MM (1981). Allograft rejection in a holostean fish *Lepisosteus platyrhynchus*. *Dev Comp Immunol* **5**: 65–75.

Moore MAS and Owen JJT (1967). Chromosome marker studies in the irradiated chick embryo. *Nature* **215**: 1081–1082.

Moriya O and Ichikawa Y (1984). J chain-positive cells in bursectomized chicks. *Immunol Letters* **7**: 289–291.

Mulcahy MF (1970). The thymus glands and lymphosarcoma in the pike *Esox lucius* L. (Pisces; Esocidae) in Ireland. In Dutcher RM (Ed), *Comparative Leukemia Research 1969*. Karger: Basel.

Muller J (1845). General description of the viscera of *Myxine* and *Bdellostoma*. *Abh Ak Berlin* 109.

Muthukkaruppan VR, Pitchappan RM and Ramila G (1976). Thymic dependence and regulation of the immune response to sheep erythrocytes in the lizard. In Wright RK and Cooper EL (Eds), *Phylogeny of Thymus and Bone Marrow—Bursa Cells*. Elsevier/North-Holland: Amsterdam. pp 185–194.

Muthukkaruppan VR, Borysenko M and El Ridi R (1982). RES structure and function of the reptilia. In Cohen N and Sigel MM (Eds), *The Reticuloendothelial System. A Comprehensive Treatise*. Vol 3. *Phylogeny and Ontogeny*. Plenum Press: New York. pp 461–507.

Nagata S (1976). An electron microscopic study on the thymus of larval and metamorphosed toads *Xenopus laevis* Daudin. *J Fac Sci Hokkaido Univ Ser VI Zool* **20**: 263–271.

Nagata S (1977). Electron microscopic study on the early histogenesis of thymus in the toad *Xenopus laevis*. *Cell Tissue Res* **179**: 87–96.

Nakamura H, Nakayo KE and Yasuda M (1986). The ontogeny of thymic myoid cells in the chicken. *Dev Growth Differ* **8**: 185–190.

Nakoa T (1978). An electron microscopic study of the cavernous bodies in the lamprey gill filament. *Am J Anat* **151**: 316–366.

Nieuwkoop PD and Faber J (1967). *Normal Table of Xenopus laevis (Daudin)*. North-Holland: Amsterdam.

Norris E (1938). The morphogenesis and histogenesis of the thymus gland in man in which the origin of the Hassall's corpuscles of the human thymus is discovered. *Contrib Embryol Carnegie Inst* **27**: 191–208.

Olah I, Rohlich P and Toro I (1975). *Ultrastructure of Lymphoid Organs*. Masson: Paris.

Oliver PD and Le Douarin NM (1984). Avian thymic accessory cells. *J Immunol* **132**: 1748–1755.

Page M and Rowley AF (1982). A morphological study of pharyngeal lymphoid accumulations in larval lampreys. *Dev Comp Immunol* Suppl **2**: 35–40.

Papermaster BW, Condie RM, Finstad J and Good RA (1964). Phylogenetic development of adaptive immunologic responsiveness in vertebrates. *J Exp Med* **119**: 105–130.

Payne LN (1971). The lymphoid system. In Bell DJ and Freeman BM (Eds), *Physiology and Biochemistry of the Domestic Fowl*. Vol 2. Academic Press: London. pp 985–1037

Pearse AG (1977). The diffuse neuroendocrine system and the APUD concept: related 'endocrine' peptides in brain, intestine, pituitary, placenta, and anuran cutaneous glands. *Med Biol* **55**: 115−125.

Pensa A (1905). Osservazioni sulla struttura del timo. *Anat Anz* **27**: 529−541.

Pfoch M (1971). Vergleichende elektronenmikroskipische Untersuchung an entodermalen Thymus-Retikulumzellen neugeborener und alter Wistar-Ratten. *Z Zellforsch Mikrosk Anat* **114**: 271−280.

Pitchappan R and Muthukkaruppan VR (1976). Procedure for thymectomy in the lizard *Calotes versicolor*. *Proc Indian Acad Sci Sect B* **84**: 42−49.

Pitchappan R and Muthukkaruppan VR (1977a). Analysis of the development of the lizard *Calotes versicolor*. II. Histogenesis of the thymus. *Dev Comp Immunol* **1**: 217−230.

Pitchappan R and Muthukkaruppan VR (1977b). Role of the thymus in the immune response to sheep erythrocytes in the lizard *Calotes versicolor*. *Proc Indian Acad Sci Sect B* **85**: 25−33.

Pitchappan R and Muthukkaruppan VR (1977c). Thymus-dependent lymphoid regions in the spleen of the lizard *Calotes versicolor*. *J Exp Zool* **199**: 177−188.

Plytycz B and Bigaj J (1983). Seasonal cyclic changes in the thymus gland of the adult frog *Rana temporaria*. *Thymus* **5**: 327−344.

Pross SH and Rowlands Jr DT (1975). Immunity in the developing amphibian. *Adv Exp Med Biol* **64**: 373−382.

Ramila G (1978). Studies on cellular interactions in the immune response and antigenic competition in the lizard *Calotes versicolor*. PhD thesis, Madurai University, Tamilnadu (India).

Rausch E, Kaiserling E and Goos M (1977). Langerhans cells and interdigitating reticulum cells in the thymus-dependent regions in human dermatophic lymphoadenitis. *Virchows Arch B* **25**: 327−343.

Raviola E and Raviola G (1966). Fine structure of the myoid cells of the reptilian and avian thymus (Abstract). *Anat Rec* **154**: 483.

Raviola E and Raviola G (1967). Striated muscle cells in the thymus of reptiles and birds: An electron microscopic study. *Am J Anat* **121**: 623−645.

Rimmer JJ (1980). Myoid cells and myasthenia gravis: a phylogenetic overview. *Dev Comp Immunol* **4**: 385−394.

Riviere HB, Cooper EL, Reddy AL and Hildemann WH (1975). In search of the hagfish thymus. *Am Zool* **15**: 39−49.

Romanoff AL (1960). *The Avian Embryo. Structural and Functional Development*. Macmillan: New York.

Rouse RV, van Ewijk W, Jones PP and Weissman IL (1979). Expression of MHC antigens by mouse thymic dendritic cells. *J Immunol* **122**: 2508−2515.

Rowlands Jr DT, La Via MF and Block MH (1964). The blood forming tissues and the blood of the newborn opossum *Didelphys virginiana*. II. Ontogenesis of antibody formation to flagella of *Salmonella typhi*. *J Immunol* **3**: 157−164.

Ruben LN (1975). Ontogeny, phylogeny and cellular co-operation. *Am Zool* **15**: 93−106.

Ruben LN and Edwards BF (1979). The phylogeny of the emergence of 'T−B' collaboration in humoral immunity. In Cohen N and Marchalonis JJ (Eds), *Contemporary Topics in Immunobiology*. Vol 9. Plenum Press: New York. pp 55−89.

Ruben LN, Clothier RH, James HS and Balls M (1984). Immunologic reactivity to TNP−Ficoll during development and aging in *Xenopus laevis*, the South African clawed toad. *Cell Differ* **14**: 1−5.

Ruth RF, Allen CP and Wolfe HR (1964). The effect of thymus on lymphoid tissue. In Good RA and Gabrielsen AE (Eds), *The Thymus in Immunobiology*. Harper & Row: New York. pp 183−206.

Ruuskanen O, Toivanen A and Raekallio J (1977). Histochemical characterization of chicken lymphoid tissue. *Dev Comp Immunol* **1**: 231−239.

Sailendri K (1973). Studies on the development of lymphoid organs and immune responses in the teleost *Tilapia mossambica* (Peters). Doctoral thesis, Madurai University. p 106.

Sailendri K and Muthukkaruppan VR (1975). Morphology of lymphoid organs in a cichlid teleost *Tilapia mossambica* (Peters). *J Morphol* **147**: 109−122.

Saint-Remy G and Prenant A (1904). Recherches sur le developpement des derives branchiaux chez les sauriens et les ophidiens. *Arch Biol Paris* **20**: 145−216.

Schauenstein K and Wick G (1977). Surface antigens of chicken white blood cells detected by heterologous antisera. In Solomon JB and Horton JD (Eds), *Developmental Immunobiology*. Elsevier/North-Holland: Amsterdam. pp 363−369.

Scollay R and Shortman K (1985). Cell traffic in the adult thymus. Cell entry and exits. Cell birth and death. In Watson JD and Marbrook J (Eds), *Recognition and Regulation in Cell-Mediated Immunity*. Marcel Dekker: New York. pp 3−30.

Secombes CJ and Manning MJ (1982). Histological changes in lymphoid organs of carp following injection of soluble or particulate antigens. *Dev Comp Immunol* Suppl **2**: 53−58.

Secombes CJ, Van Groningen JJM, Van Muiswinkel WB and Egberts E (1983). Ontogeny of the immune system in carp *Cyprinus carpio* L. The appearance of antigenic determinants on lymphoid cells detected by mouse anti-carp thymocyte monoclonal antibodies. *Dev Comp Immunol* **7**: 455−464.

Shaner RF (1921). The development of the pharynx and aortic arches of the turtle, with a note on the fifth and pulmonary arches of mammals. *Am J Anat* **29**: 407−409.

Sherman J and Auerbach R (1966). Quantitative characteristics of chicken thymus and bursa development. *Blood* **27**: 371−379.

Shier KJ (1963). The morphology of the epithelial thymus. Observations on lymphocyte depleted and fetal thymus. *Lab Invest* **12**: 316−326.

Sidky Y and Auerbach R (1968). Tissue culture analysis of immunological capacities of snapping turtles. *J Exp Zool* **167**: 187−196.

Sigel MM, Acton RT, Evans EE, Russell WJ, Wells TG, Painter B and Lucas AH (1968). T2 bacteriophage clearance in the lemon shark. *Proc Soc Exp Biol Med* **128**: 977–979.

Smith K (1984). Inside the thymus. *Immunol Today* **5**: 83–84.

Solomon JB (1971). *Foetal and Neonatal Immunology*. North-Holland: Amsterdam.

Stanley NF, Yadau M, Waring H and Eadie M (1972). The effect of thymectomy on response to various antigens of a marsupial *Setonix brachyurus* (quokka). *Aust J Exp Biol Med Sci* **50**: 689–702.

Stannius F (1854). General anatomy of myxinoids. *Zootomie d Fische*.

Sterba G (1950). Uber die morphologischen und histogenetischen thymus probleme bei *Xenopus laevis* Daudin nebst einigen beinerkungen uber die morphologie der kaulquapper. *Abh Sachs Akad Wiss* **44**: 1–54.

Sterba G (1953). Die physiologie und histogenese der schilddruse und des thymus beim bactineunauge (*Lampetra planeri* Bloch = *Petromyzon marinus* Bloch) als grundlagen phylogenetischer studien uber die evolution der innersekretorischen kiemendarmderivate. *Wiss Z Friedrich Schiller Univ Jena Math Naturwiss* **2**: 239–298.

Strauss AJL, Kemp Jr PG and Douglas SD (1966). Myasthenia gravis. *Lancet* **i**: 771–773.

Strauss AJL, Kemp Jr PG and Douglas SD (1967). An immunohistological delineation of striated muscle cells in the thymus. In Smith RT, Good RA and Miescher PA (Eds), *Ontogeny of Immunity*. University of Florida Press: Gainesville. pp 180–185.

Sugimoto M and Bolloni FJ (1979). Terminal deoxynucleotidyl transferase (TdT) in chick embryo lymphoid tissue. *J Immunol* **122**: 392–397.

Sugimoto M, Yasuda T and Egashira Y (1977a). Development of the embryonic chicken thymus. I. Characteristic synchronous morphogenesis of lymphocytes accompanied by the appearance of an embryonic thymus-specific antigen. *Dev Biol* **56**: 281–292.

Sugimoto M, Yasuda T and Egashira Y (1977b). Development of the embryonic chicken thymus. II. Differentiation of the epithelial cells studied by electron microscopy. *Dev Biol* **56**: 293–305.

Sugimoto C, Kodama H and Mikami T (1979). Complement-dependent antibody cytoxicity test of chicken antibody with duck complement used against cells of a Marek's disease lymphoma-derived cell line (MSB-1). *Avian Dis* **23**: 229–234.

Tatner MF and Manning MJ (1982). The morphology of the trout *Salmo gairdneri* Richardson thymus: some practical and theoretical considerations. *J Fish Biol* **21**: 27–32.

Taxi J (1965). Contribution a l'etude des connexions des neurones moteurs de systeme nerveux autonome. *Ann Sci Nat Zool Paris* **7**: 413–674.

Taylor CR and Skinner JM (1976). Evidence for significant hematopoiesis in the human thymus. *Blood* **47**: 305–313.

Teodorczyk JA, Potworowski EF and Suiculis A (1975).

Cellular localization and antigenic species specificity of thymic factors. *Nature (London)* **258**: 617–619.

Terni T (1929). Richerche istologische sull' innervazione del timo dei sauropsidi. *Z Zellforsch Mikrosk Anat* **9**: 377–424.

Thorbecke CJ, Silberberg-Synakin I and Flotte TJ (1980). Langerhans cells as macrophages in skin and lymphoid organs. *Invest Dermatol* **75**: 32–43.

Thorbecke GJ, Gordon HA, Wostman B, Wagner M and Reyniers JA (1957). Lymphoid tissue and serum gamma globulin in young germfree chickens. *J Infect Dis* **101**: 237–251.

Tochinai S (1976). Demonstration of thymus independent immune system in *Xenopus laevis*. Response to polyvinylpyrrolidone. *Immunology* **31**: 125–128.

Tochinai S and Katagiri CH (1975). Complete abrogation of immune response to skin allografts and rabbit erythrocytes in the early thymectomized *Xenopus*. *Dev Growth Differ* **17**: 383–394.

Tomonaga S, Sakai K, Tashiro J and Awaya K (1975). High-walled endothelium in the gills of the hagfish. *Zool Mag* **84**: 151–155.

Toro I, Olah I, Rohlich P and Viragh SZ (1969). Electron microscopic observations on myoid cells of the frog's thymus. *Anat Rec* **165**: 329–342.

Tournefier A (1973). Developpement des organes lymphoides chez l'amphibien urodele *Triturus alpestris* Laur: tolerance des allogreffes apres la thymectomie larvaire. *J Embryol Exp Morphol* **29**: 383–396.

Trainin N (1974). Thymic hormones and the immune response. *Physiol Rev* **54**: 272–315.

Tripplett EL and Barrymore S (1960). Tissue specificity in embryonic and adult *Cymatogaster aggregata* studied by scale transplantation. *Bio Bull* **118**: 463–471.

Turner RJ and Manning MJ (1974). Thymic dependence of amphibian antibody response. *Eur J Immunol* **4**: 343–346.

van de Velde RL and Friedman NB (1966a). The thymic 'myoidzellen' (thymoma) and myasthenia gravis. *J Am Med Assoc* **198**: 287–288.

van de Velde RL and Friedman NB (1966b). Muscular elements of the thymus. *Fed Proc* **25**: 661.

van Ewijk W, Rouse RV and Weissman IL (1980). Distribution of H-2 microenvironments in the mouse thymus. Immuno-electron microscopic identification of I-A and H-2K bearing cells. *J Histochem Cytochem* **28**: 1089–1099.

van Loon JJA, van Oosterum R and van Muiswinkel WB (1981). Development of the immune system in the carp *Cyprinus carpio*. In Solomon JB (Ed), *Aspects of Developmental and Comparative Immunology I*. Pergamon Press: New York. pp 469–471.

van Vliet E, Melis M and van Ewijk W (1984). Monoclonal antibodies to stromal cell types of the mouse thymus. *Eur J Immunol* **14**: 524–529.

Van Wijhe JW (1923). Thymus spiracular sense organ and fenestra vestibuli (ovalis) in a 63mm long embryo of *Heptanchus cinereus*. *Proc Sci Akad Wetensch*

Amsterdam **26**: 727.

Vanable JW (1964). Granular gland development during *Xenopus laevis* metamorphosis. *Dev Biol* **10**: 331–357.

Vasse J (1983). Transplantation of turtle embryonic thymus into quail embryo: colonization by quail cells. *J Embryol Exp Morphol* **77**: 309–322.

Veerman AJP (1974). On the interdigitating cells in the thymus-dependent area of the rat spleen: a relationship between the mononuclear phagocyte system and T lymphocytes. *Cell Tissue Res* **156**: 416–441.

Veerman AJP and van Ewijk W (1975). White pulp compartments in the spleen of rats and mice. *Cell Tissue Res* **156**: 416–441.

Veldman JE (1970). Histophysiology and electron microscopy of the immune response. Part 1 and 2. PhD thesis, Groningen.

Veldman JE and Kaiserling E (1980). Interdigitating cells. In Carr I and Daems WT (Eds), *The Reticuloendothelial System. A Comprehensive Treatise*. Vol 1. *Morphology*. Plenum: New York. pp 381–416.

Veldman JE and Keuning FJ (1978). Histophysiology of cellular immunity reactions on B-cell deprived rabbits. An x-irradiation model for delineation of an isolated T-cell system. *Virchows Arch Abt B* **28**: 203–216.

Veldman JE, Keuning FJ and Molenaar I (1978a). Site of initiation of the plasma cell reaction in the rabbit lymph node. Ultrastructural evidence for two distinct antibody forming cell predecessors. *Virchows Arch Abt B* **28**: 187–202.

Veldman JE, Molenaar I and Keuning FJ (1978b). Electron microscopy of cellular immunity reactions in B-cell deprived rabbits. Thymus derived antigen reactive cells, their microenvironment and progeny in the lymph node. *Virchows Arch Abt B* **28**: 217–228.

Villena A (1981). Influencia de los microambientes en el desarrollo postnatal del ganglio linfatico de tata. Doctoral thesis, Facultad de Ciencias, Universidad del Pais Vasco, Bilbao.

von Gaudecker B (1978). Ultrastructure of the age-involuted adult human thymus. *Cell Tissue Res* **186**: 507–525.

von Gaudecker B and Muller-Hermelink HK (1982). The development of the human tonsilla pallatina. *Cell Tissue Res* **224**: 579–600.

Ward P and Kendall MD (1975). Morphological changes in the thymus of young and adult red-billed queleas *Quelea quelea* (Aves). *Phil Trans R Soc B* **273**: 55–64.

Warner NL and Szenberg A (1962). Dissociation of immunological responsiveness in fowls with a hormonally arrested development of lymphoid tissues. *Nature* **194**: 146–147.

Warr GW and Simon RC (1983). The mitogen response potential of lymphocytes of the rainbow trout *Salmo gairdneri* re-examined. *Dev Comp Immunol* **7**: 379–384.

Wassjutatschkin A (1913). Untersuchungen uber die histogenese des thymus. I. Uber den Ursprung der myoiden elemente des thymus der huhnerembryos. *Anat Anz* **43**: 349–366.

Webster WD (1934). The development of the thymus bodies in *Necturus maculosus*. *J Morph* **56**: 295–323.

Weiss N, Horton JD and Du Pasquier L (1973). The effect of thymectomy on cell surface associated and serum immunoglobulin in the toad *Xenopus laevis* (Daudin): A possible inhibitory role of the thymus on the expression of immunoglobulins. In Panijel J and Liacopoulos P (Eds), *L'etude Phylogenique et Ontogenique de la Response Immunitaire et Son Apport a la Theorie Immunologigue*. INSERM: Paris. pp 165–174.

Weissenberg E (1907). Uber die quergestreiften zellen des thymus. *Arch F Mikr Anat* **70**: 193–226.

Wekerle H, Ketelsen U-P, Zurn AD and Fulpius BW (1978). Intrathymic pathogenesis of myasthenia gravis: transient expression of acetylcholine receptors on thymus-derived myogenic cells. *Eur J Immunol* **8**: 579–582.

Wekerle H, Ketelsen U-P and Ernst M (1980). Thymic nurse cells. Lymphoepithelial complexes in murine thymuses: morphological and serological characterization. *J Exp Med* **151**: 925–944.

Wiedersheim R (1879) cited by Pischinger A (1933). In Bolk L, Goppert E, Kallius E and Lubosch W (Eds), *Handbuch der Vergleichenden Anatomie der Wirbeltiere*. Vol III. Urban & Schwarzenberg: Munich. pp 279–348.

Woods R and Linna J (1965). The transport of cells from the bursa of Fabricius to the spleen and the thymus. *Acta Pathol Microbiol Scand* **64**: 470–476.

Wright DE (1973). The structure of the gills of the elasmobranch *Scyliorhinus canicula* L. *Z Zellforsch* **144**: 489–509.

Yadav M, Stanley NF and Waring H (1972). The thymus glands of marsupial *Setonix brachyurus* (quokka) and their role in immune processes. Structure and growth of the thymus glands. *Aust J Exp Biol Med Sci* **50**: 347–356.

Yamaguchi K, Tomonaga S, Ihara K and Awaya K (1979). Electron microscopic study of phagocytic lining cells in the cavernous body of the lamprey gill. *J Electron Microsc* **28**: 106–116.

Yasuda T, Sugimoto M and Egashira Y (1980). Development of the embryonic chicken thymus. IV. Motile activity of immature lymphoid cells studied by time-lapse films and electron microscopy. *Thymus* **2**: 5–18.

Yasuda T, Sugimoto M and Egashira Y (1981). Asymmetric division of lymphoid cells of the embryonic chicken thymus. An ultrastructural study with the use of serial sectioning method. *Immunol Letters* **2**: 311–316.

Yialouris PP, Evangelatos GP, Soteriadis-Vlahos C, Heimer EP, Felix AM, Tsitsiloni OE and Haritos AA (1988). The identification of prothymosin alpha-like material in vertebrate lymphoid organs by a radioimmunoassay for the N-terminal decapeptide. *J Immunol Methods* **106**: 267–275.

Zada S and El Deeb S (1982). Normal table of development of the lizard *Chalcides ocellatus*. *Bull Fac Sci Cairo Univ* (in press). Cited in El Deeb *et al.* (1985) *J Morph* **185**: 241–253.

Zapata A (1973). Contribucion al estudio de la estructura y ultraestructura del timo de algunos reptiles. Master dissertation, Complutense University, Madrid.

Zapata A (1980). Ultrastructure of elasmobranch lymphoid tissue. I. Thymus and spleen. *Dev Comp Immunol* **4**: 459–472.

Zapata A (1981). Lymphoid organs of teleost fish. I. Ultrastructure of the thymus of *Rutilus rutilus*. *Dev Comp Immunol* **5**: 427–436.

Zapata A (1983). Phylogeny of the fish immune system. *Bull Inst Pasteur* **81**: 165–186.

Zapata A, Gomariz RP, Garrido E and Cooper EL (1982). Lymphoid organs and blood cells of the caecilian *Ichthyophis kohtaoensis. Acta Zool Stockh* **63**: 11–16.

Zinkernagel RM, Callahan GN, Althage A, Cooper S, Klein PA and Klein J (1978). On the thymus in the differentiation of H-2 self-recognition by T cells: evidence for dual recognition? *J Exp Med* **147**: 882–911.

Zucker R, Jauker V and Droege W (1973). Cellular composition of the chicken thymus: effects of neonatal bursectomy and hydrocortisone treatment. *Eur J Immunol* **3**: 812–818.

6

The Spleen

INTRODUCTION

The spleen is a large blood-filtering organ which evolved an increasingly important role throughout phylogeny in generating both T and B immune responses. In addition, erythropoiesis, granulopoiesis and/or thrombopoiesis occur in the spleen of some vertebrates. During vertebrate phylogeny, the spleen undergoes anatomical, histological and functional variations which reflect strategies necessary in order to diversify and specialize splenic functions. In this regard, the roles played by distinct splenic cell compartments in immune reactions seem to be of differential importance in various vertebrate groups. Thus, the presence or absence of a sharply delimited white pulp, the possibility to differentiate T and B areas and the presence or absence of germinal centers and marginal zones are important stages in defining the histophysiological evolution of the vertebrate spleen.

In this chapter we will present the structure and function of the spleen in ectothermic vertebrates and birds. We will focus special attention on its role in the trapping and processing of antigen, the structural changes after antigenic stimulation and modifications which have occurred in its vascularization patterns which helped splenic efficiency in immune reactions. Because the spleen is so intimately associated with the circulatory system, its gross morphology will be presented in some depth in contrast to other lymphomyeloid organs. For it is via the blood, perhaps in all species that most antigens can be trapped and processed for antibody formation.

PRIMITIVE FISH: CHONDRICHTHYES— GANOIDS, DIPNOI

General Appearance— Gross and Light Microscopic Observations

Although other comparative immunologists have considered that lymphoid masses in the hagfish intestine and typhlosole in lampreys represent primitive phylogenetic precursors of the spleen, our opinion as presented in Chapter 3 on bone marrow differs. Both of these lymphohemopoietic tissues are blood-forming organs, functionally related to bone marrow, and for this reason they deserve no more attention in this chapter.

Little information is available on the spleen of holosteans (gar, bowfin) and chondrosteans (sturgeons, paddlefish) (Good *et al.*, 1966), polypterids (bichirs) (Yoffey, 1929) and the coelocanth (*Latimeria*) (Millot *et al.*, 1978). Ganoids (chondrosteans and holosteans) possess a spleen with red and white pulp. The white pulp in holosteans consists of dense collections of lymphocytes and mature plasma cells which appear as small lymphoid nodules scattered at random throughout the splenic parenchyma (Figure 6.1). Extensive immunization of paddlefish causes a marked increase in numbers of splenic plasma cells (Good *et al.*, 1966).

The spleen of representative Dipnoi is located in a remarkable position, within the stomach wall and in the anterior intestinal region (Yoffey, 1929; Jordan and Speidel, 1923a; Rafn and Wingstrand, 1981). Because of its anatomical location, it is classified as the

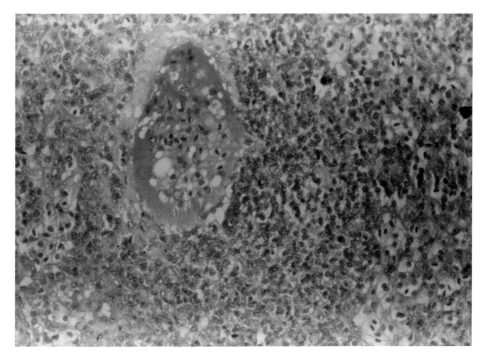

Figure 6.1 Collections of lymphoid cells constitute the splenic white pulp of the gar, *Lepisosteus platyrhynchus* (× 600).

so-called intra-enteric type (Yamada, 1951). Yoffey (1929) pointed out that the structure of the spleen in *Calamoichthys* is strikingly primitive. Splenic arteries and veins run parallel to each other within lymphoid tissue which is surrounded by red pulp. Jordan and Speidel (1931) noted three regions in spleens of the African lungfish, *Protopterus ethiopicus*: a central area of lymphoid cells surrounded by a region of pulp cords and sinuses, and a thin peripheral capsular region. The central mass appears to be active in lymphopoiesis while the splenic pulp is erythropoietic.

Saito (1984) has recently studied the anatomical relationships between spleen and enteric blood vessels during development in the Australian lungfish *Neoceratodus forsteri*. Apparently the blood vascular dynamics of the foregut and the yolk gut are intimately involved in formation of the spleen. Although four anatomical stages in splenic development have been described, there are no indications of cellular or histological modifications, including: (1) appearance of the

splenic primordium as a mesenchymal condensation in a limited portion of the region supplied by the third and fourth vitelline arteries in both sites; (2) development of splenic sinuses within the primordium; (3) formation of the 'gastric' and enteric splenic portal systems; and (4) growth of the spleen along the anterior extremity of the spinal valve.

In holocephalans (*Chimaera*, *Hydrolagus*), mesenteries are strongly reduced and the spleen is situated in the peritoneal cavity free from the stomach and intestine but firmly associated with the pancreas (Fange, 1984). The spleen in *Chimaera monstrosa* consists of lymphoid foci which comprise the white pulp and a red pulp where erythropoiesis and thrombopoiesis occur (Figure 6.2) (Mattison, personal communication). Moreover, large ellipsoids appear as pale structures throughout the splenic parenchyma (Figure 6.3). The white pulp and ellipsoids in Holocephali reveal a general structural similarity with that of elasmobranchs, at least by light and electron microscopy.

Figure 6.2 Spleen of *Chimera monstrosa* formed by areas of lymphoid tissue surrounding an ellipsoid and red pulp (× 150).

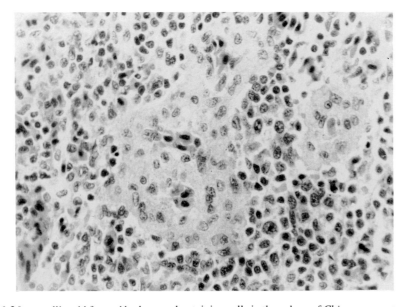

Figure 6.3 Large ellipsoid formed by large pale-staining cells in the spleen of *Chimera monstrosa* (× 750).

In selachians the spleen is an elongated, lobate mass situated in the duodenum. In the trasher shark, *Alopias vulpes*, it is more than 1 m long and is supplied by numerous arteries and veins (Hemmeter, 1926). In rays and skates, by contrast, the spleen is a round, compact, only slightly lobed organ. In elasmobranchs the arterial supply arrives from the lienogastric artery. (Fange and Nilsson, 1985) and the splenic veins join the hepatic portal system. The spleen is innervated by sympathetic nerves that reach it via the middle splanchnic nerves (Nilsson, 1983). There are no descriptions of ganglion cells within the spleen.

Apart from classical light microscopic observations (Phisalix, 1885; Maximow, 1923; Tait, 1927; Yoffey, 1929; Kanesada, 1956; Fey, 1965), the ultrastructure of spleens in elasmobranchs has been reported for the shark *Ginglymostoma cirratum* (Fange and Mattison, 1981), dogfish *Scyliorhinus canicula* (Pulsford *et al.*, 1982;) and rays *Torpedo marmorata* and *Raja clavata* (Zapata, 1980). There is a recent classification of vertebrate spleens (Hartwig and Hartwig, 1985; Tischendorf, 1985) as either a place for storage or immunodefense, based upon the supporting apparatus which they contain (trabeculae and muscle elements); the elasmobranch spleen belongs to the second type.

In all elasmobranchs thus far studied, the spleen appears to be similar histologically although the development of splenic follicles is variable (Figures 6.4, 6.5). In all of them a white pulp, lymphoid in nature, is distinguishable from a red pulp where erythropoiesis and thrombopoiesis occur in sinusoids (Figure 6.4). No marginal zone which separates the white from the red pulp has been found. Thus in some species the limits between these two areas are difficult to define (Zapata, 1980; Pulsford *et al.*, 1982). Morrow (1978), however, found lymphoid areas sharply demarcated in the dogfish spleen which had been previously challenged by antigen. Moreover, clear ellipsoidal blood vessels are prominent (Figures 6.5, 6.6).

White Pulp

Immunoglobulin-producing Cells

The white pulp is composed of lymphocytic elements: small, medium and large lymphocytes and mature and immature plasma cells scattered among parenchymal reticular processes (Figure 6.7). The presence of plasma cells in the spleen of cartilaginous fishes was first described by Engle *et al.* (1958) in the smooth dogfish, spiny dogfish, dusky shark, torpedo and the skate. Later, Good *et al.* (1966) also found plasma cells in antigen-stimulated fish, including the sting ray, leopard shark, nurse shark, lemon shark and brown shark. The numbers of plasma cells seem to be highly variable: they are reported to be numerous in *Torpedo marmorata* (Zapata, 1980), *Ginglymostoma cirratum* (Fange and Mattisson, 1981) and *Raja kenojei* (Tomonaga *et al.*, 1984), whereas plasma cells are few in *Raja clavata* (Zapata, 1980), *Etmopterus spinax* (Mattison and Fange, 1982) and *Scyliorhinus canicula* (Pulsford *et al.*, 1982).

Both high-molecular-weight (HMW) and low-molecular-weight (LMW) Ig have been detected in cells of the spleen in *Raja kenojei* (Tomonaga *et al.*, 1984). Immunofluorescence double staining revealed two cell types: HMW Ig-forming cells and LMW Ig-forming cells. There was no overlap between the two cell populations and the ratio between them was approximately even, with only slight fluctuations

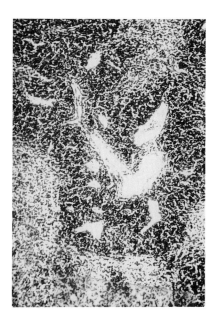

Figure 6.4 White pulp surrounding a large blood vessel in the spleen of the torpedo ray *Torpedo marmorata*. A sharp demarcation occurs between the red and the white pulp (× 300). (From *Dev Comp Immunol* **4**: 459, 1980, reproduced by permission.)

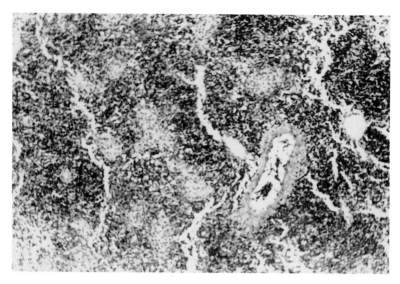

Figure 6.5 White pulp of the spleen of the dogfish *Scyliorhinus canicula* showing abundant lymphoid tissue related to arterial and ellipsoidal blood vessels (× 150).

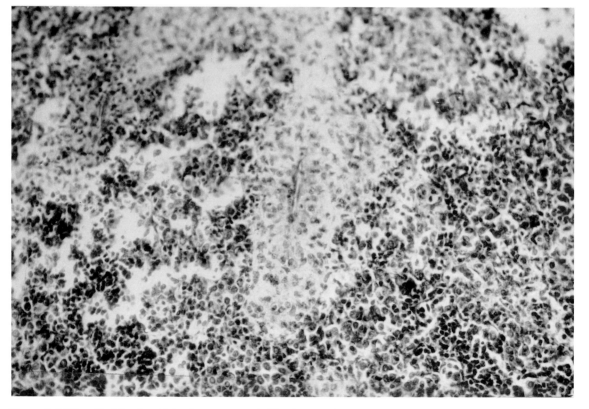

Figure 6.6 Ellipsoid of the skate *Raja clavata* surrounded by abundant lymphoid tissue (× 760). (From *Dev Comp Immunol* **4**: 459, 1980, reproduced by permission.)

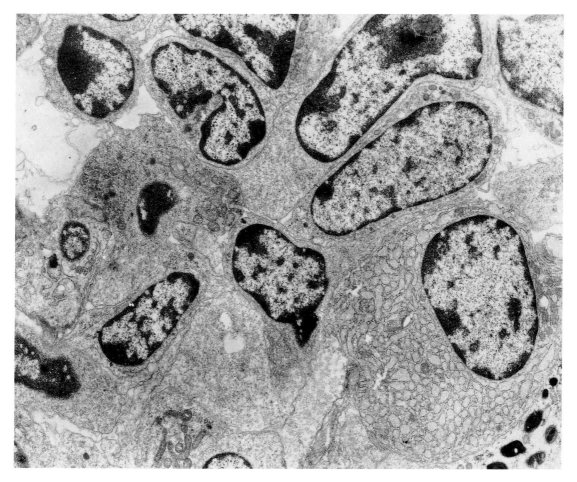

Figure 6.7 Lymphoid component of the splenic white pulp which consists of lymphocytes of differing sizes and plasma cells in *Torpedo marmorata* (× 3230).

between individual fish and spleens. Additional preliminary information revealed that antibody-containing cells first appear in the spleen during ontogeny. Although Ferren (1967) reported that splenectomy failed to diminish immune responses of the lemon shark, *Negaprion brevirostris*, and the nurse shark, *Ginglymostoma cirratum*, Morrow (1978) and Zapata (1980) considered the spleen to be the main site of antibody synthesis in elasmobranchs based on morphological evidence. Recent results by Tomonaga and his associates support this hypothesis (1984).

Relationship Between Macrophages and Lymphocytes

Another important structural feature is the remarkable association between macrophages and lymphocytes found in white pulp and red pulp dogfish spleens (Pulsford *et al.*, 1982). These associations in the red pulp are probably involved in phagocytosis in most vertebrates (Weiss, 1972), but in the white pulp they are probably related to immunological exchange, a rather common feature in other ectotherms (Zapata,

1982 in teleosts; Barrutia *et al.*, 1983 in anurans; Zapata *et al.*, 1981a in reptiles). Farr and de Bruyn (1975) found specially arranged cluster formations between macrophages and lymphocytes. These rosette formations provide a morphological substrate for interactions which are necessary for primary and secondary immune responses to occur (Pierce and Benacerraf, 1969; Nielsen *et al.*, 1974).

The main function of the lymphoid system is to offer an *in situ* opportunity for immune reactions to develop *in vivo*. The interaction between antigen, T-lymphocytes, B-lymphocytes and mononuclear phagocytes takes place within a framework of reticular cells in peripheral lymphoid organs. The consequences of these interactions are likely to be determined by the precise microenvironment in which they occur

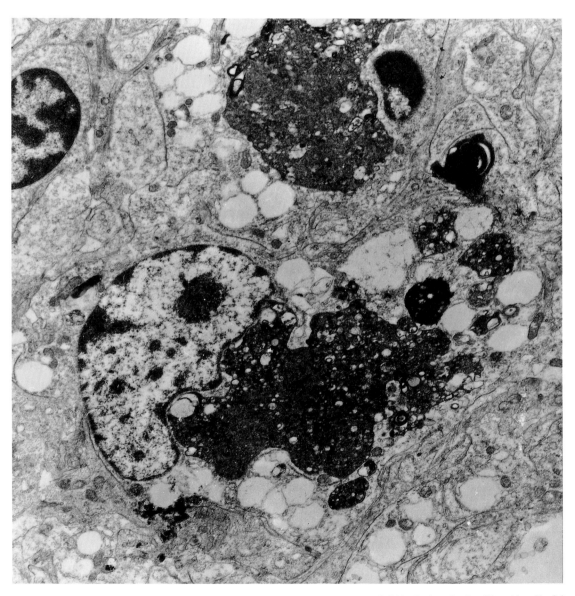

Figure 6.8 Large macrophages containing enormous amounts of cell debris and lipid inclusions in the ellipsoid wall of the spleen of *Torpedo marmorata* (× 10000). (From *Dev Comp Immunol* **4**: 459, 1980, reproduced by permission.)

(Parrott *et al.*, 1966; Veerman and van Ewijk, 1975; Hoefsmith *et al.*, 1980). This idea of microenvironment, although perhaps not entirely unique, has been recently expressed by Eikelemboom *et al.* (1985), who emphasize the importance of cell−cell associations to effect immune responses mainly in ectothermic vertebrates, including elasmobranchs, where there are no germinal centers.

Ellipsoids

At this point, it is appropriate to consider additional aspects of splenic morphology. By definition, ellipsoids are terminal branches of splenic arteries with a sheath consisting of cell aggregates and fibers (Figure 6.6). Ellipsoids of the dogfish spleen (Pulsford and Zapata, unpublished observations) are remarkably similar to the so-called 'periarterial macrophage sheaths' observed by Blue and Weiss in the mammalian spleen (Weiss *et al.*, 1985). Both the elasmobranch and mammalian structures possess: (1) a continuous basement membrane beneath the endothelial lining; (2) adventitial reticular cells, which by branching into the surrounding cords hold the arterial terminal in the splenic reticulum; (3) associated macrophages. In the elasmobranch spleen, some of these macrophages contain lipid inclusions and ingested cellular debris (Figure 6.8). Dustin (1939, 1975) observed accumulations of lipids in the cells of ellipsoids from birds and mammals and has suggested that ellipsoids may function as lipid storage depots. The intracytoplasmic deposition of lipid within sheaths of humans has also been demonstrated in cases of hyperlipemia. We wish to emphasize that ellipsoidal macrophages from dogfish are free cells in the mammalian spleen, which suggests that their function is to trap various materials (see description later). They can also migrate throughout the splenic parenchyma (Weiss *et al.*, 1985). Obviously modern views on the status of macrophages differ from older reports (Wislocki, 1917; Tait, 1927; Yoffey, 1929). According to these views, cells which form the ellipsoidal walls are sessile and fixed.

Melanomacrophages

Isolated melanomacrophages are additional cell types found in the elasmobranch spleen. In the dogfish, mainly in red pulp, certain melanomacrophages contain inclusions of lipofucsin and melanin, which are the most abundant pigments. Although melanin appears in varying amounts in the melanomacrophages of all fish, melanin seems to be especially frequent in trout and dogfish (Agius and Agbede, 1984). Melanin in melanomacrophages from dogfish spleen appears to be derived from phagocytosis of melanin granules or their precursors which normally occur in melanocytes (Pulsford and Zapata, unpublished observations). Agius and Agbede (1984) speculate that this kind of phagocytosis might occur in order to eliminate potentially toxic pigment from ruptured or degenerated melanocytes or to neutralize the activity of free radicals formed invariably during lipid peroxidation reactions (Edelstein, 1971). More information on melanomacrophages of fish will be described later.

ADVANCED FISH: TELEOSTS

General Characteristics

The spleen has been studied in several teleosts by light microscopy (Yoffey, 1929; Jordan and Speidel, 1930; Rasquin, 1951; Tamura and Honma, 1970; Pontius and Ambrosius, 1972; Anderson, 1974; Ellis and de Sousa, 1974; Sailendri and Muthukkaruppan, 1975; Grace and Manning, 1980; Secombes and Manning, 1980). Ultrastructural studies, however, are somewhat scant (Ellis *et al.*, 1976; Graf and Schulns, 1979; Zapata, 1982; Fulop and McMillan, 1984). Splenic lymphoid tissue is not highly developed in teleosts (Figure 6.9). It surrounds small arteries (Jordan and Speidel, 1930; Pontius and Ambrosius, 1972; Sailendri and Muthukkaruppan, 1975), appears diffuse in the splenic parenchyma (Yoffey, 1929; Rasquin, 1951; Ellis and de Sousa, 1974; Ellis *et al.*, 1976) and is related to melanomacrophage centers (Sailendri and Muthukkaruppan, 1975; Ellis *et al.*, 1976; Ferguson, 1976; Zapata, 1982). Indeed, the entire spleen may even be mainly red pulp (Anderson, 1974; Grace and Manning, 1980; Secombes and Manning, 1980) or the dominant cells are lymphoid cells and macrophages, as in the icefish, *Chaenocephalus aceratus*, a teleost which possesses practically no erythrocytes (Walvig, 1958).

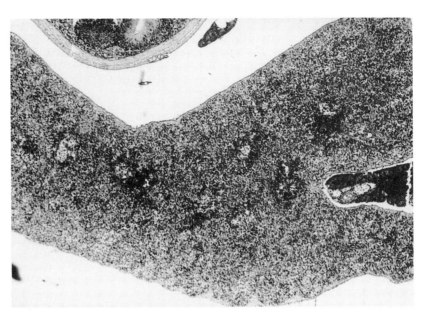

Figure 6.9 Spleen of the teleost fish *Rutilus rutilus*. Small aggregates of lymphoid cells surrounding blood vessels and melanomacrophage centers constitute the white pulp ($\times$ 60).

The teleost spleen is encapsulated by connective tissue from which small septa project into the parenchyma. By electron microscopy the white pulp is composed of lymphoid cells, mainly small, medium and large lymphocytes arranged between supporting elements composed of irregular reticular cells (Figure 6.10). Macrophages occur in both red and white pulp. In the red pulp, they appear to be associated with blood sinusoids containing large, engulfed bodies (Figure 6.11). In the white pulp, large ramified macrophages form clusters with small lymphocytes, lymphoblasts and plasma cells (Figure 6.12). The importance of these clusters in immune responses has already been presented for the elasmobranchs.

Ellipsoids

The other component of the teleost spleen which is important in immune function is the ellipsoid. In all vertebrates, splenic ellipsoids consist of stellate reticular cells and macrophages within a framework of reticular fibers which surround arterial capillaries (Figure 6.13). They vary in size and shape in different vertebrates; they are absent in rodents and largest in fish and birds (Klemperer, 1938; Dustin, 1975).

Ellipsoids have been reported often in teleosts (Yoffey, 1929; Dustin, 1939; Ellis *et al.*, 1976; Ferguson, 1976; Graf and Schulns, 1979; Fulop and McMillan, 1984; Herraez and Zapata, 1986). However, ellipsoids are considered to be absent by Zwillenberg (1964), who investigated their presence in *Salmo gairdneri* by electron microscopy, and Haider (1966), who observed them by light microscopy in various fish, including carp. Macrophages which occur in ellipsoidal walls are undoubtedly the most conspicuous elements which form the ellipsoids and they probably serve to determine how these splenic regions function. They are irregular elements which contain electron-dense granules (Figure 6.14). The phagocytic nature of macrophages in ellipsoidal walls has been confirmed by histochemical studies of carp spleen, which has revealed high lysosomal enzyme activity (Graf and Schulns, 1979).

Many contradictory theories concerning the function of ellipsoids suggest that they are poorly understood. Apparently they can trap various substances which are antigenic, or even non-antigenic ones, including pathogens and degenerated erythrocytes, as Yoffey (1929) observed in fish. In mammals some

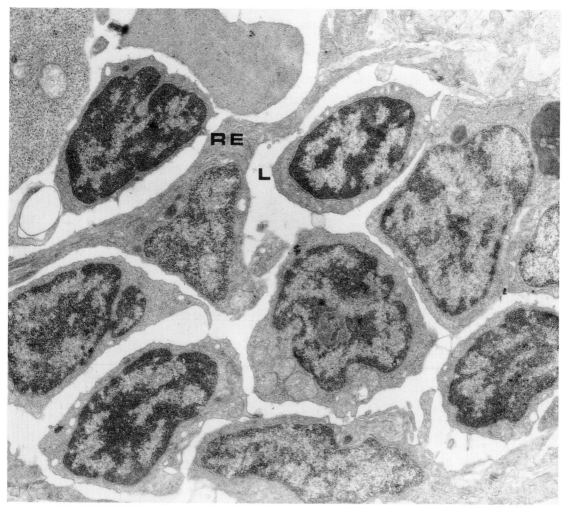

Figure 6.10 Splenic white pulp of *Rutilus rutilus*. Reticular cell (RE) containing filaments and desmosomes which constitute a network that supports free lymphocytes (L), macrophages and plasma cells (× 6300).

investigators have considered ellipsoids to be sites of breakdown of effete erythrocytes (Solnitzky, 1937; Dustin, 1975). Graf and Schulns (1979) provided evidence for the passage of erythrocytes and granulocytes through the endothelial lining of sheathed vessels in carp. They have also reported that the macrophages in ellipsoidal walls show high activity for beta-*N*-acetylglucosamine, an enzyme involved in the disintegration of glycoproteins which occur on erythrocyte surfaces. Perhaps this enzyme is involved in digesting senescent or phagocytosed erythrocytes. However, no passage of such cells has been observed in ellipsoids of sunfish

(Fulop and McMillan, 1984) or goldfish (Herraez and Zapata, 1986).

Regarding clearance of foreign particles, observations have revealed that injected India ink and trypan blue are taken up initially by ellipsoids (Tait, 1927 in *Raja batis*; Dustin, 1934 in *Protopterus*; Dragotoiu-Untu, 1970 in *Tinca tinca*; Ellis *et al.*, 1976 in *Pleuronectes platessa*; Ferguson, 1976 in *Scopthalmus maximus*; Fulop and McMillan, 1984 in *Lepomis* sp.; Herraez and Zapata, 1986 in *Carassius auratus*). This same activity has been reported in mammals (Solnitzky, 1937; Dustin, 1975). Moreover,

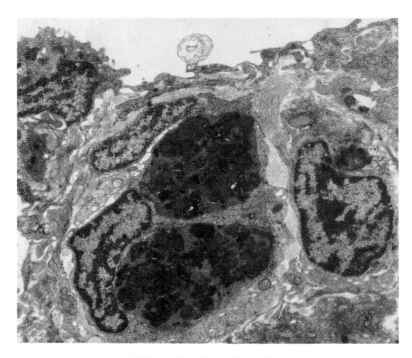

Figure 6.11 Macrophages in the red pulp of *Gobio gobio*. The cell located near blood sinusoids contains remarkably large dense bodies in the cytoplasm which represent engulfed degenerated cells (× 11 800).

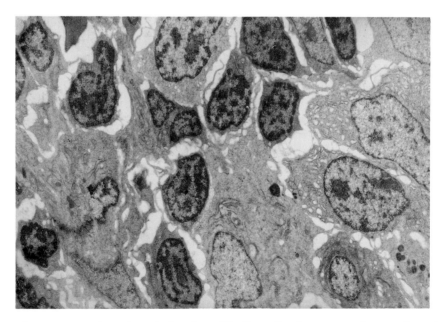

Figure 6.12 Lymphocyte − macrophage cluster in the spleen of *Rutilus rutilus*. Large macrophages make contacts on surface membranes of neighboring lymphocytes, developing and mature plasma cells (× 4200). (From *Dev Comp Immunol* **6**: 87, 1982, reproduced by permission.)

ellipsoids in teleosts appear to be involved in antigen trapping (see description later) (Ellis, 1980; Secombes and Manning, 1980; Maas and Bootsma, 1982; Secombes et al., 1982a; Lamers, 1985; Herraez and Zapata, 1986). Infection with *Aeromonas hydrophila* produces important changes in ellipsoids (Bach et al., 1978). Finally, the presence of cytoplasmic filaments in the endothelial cells of ellipsoids of fish and mammals (Hatae, 1978; Blue and Weiss, 1981a) suggests a sphincteric function regulating blood flow into the splenic sinuses, or they may even function as a cytoskeletal support for the endothelial cells of capillaries.

T- and B-cells

Attempts to demonstrate the spatial distribution of T- and/or B-cells in the teleostean spleen have failed (Ellis and de Sousa, 1974) but this is based upon limited information. Tatner (1985) has demonstrated a preferential migration of thymocytes in trout to the spleen, confirming previous results of Ellis and de Sousa (1974), who used plaice. Thus, apparently, lymphocytes in teleosts, as in mammals, home specifically to certain sites in peripheral lymphoid organs (a phenomenon called ecotaxis by de Sousa). After immunization, the spleen of *Tilapia mossambica* shows considerably increased amounts of lymphoid cells which form aggregations of small lymphocytes and overcrowd the red pulp with lymphocytes (Sailendri and Muthukkaruppan, 1975). There is also an increase in vascularization, in the numbers of dividing cells and in the frequency of plasma cells.

With respect to primary and secondary responses, Secombes et al. (1982b), using the carp spleen, demonstrated its apparently greater involvement in secondary responses. Primary intraperitoneal injections of human gamma globulin (HGG) in saline or Freund's complete adjuvant (FCA) produced little change in the spleen. After injecting *Aeromonas salmonicida*, the main changes affect melanomacrophage centers (MMCs) which after 6 weeks begin to form, particularly in the axilla of branching ellipsoids. A second challenge with HGG in FCA causes a peak at day 7. Numerous pyroninophilic cells occur within the ellipsoids but they accumulate mainly in such large numbers that they cause a bulging of the sheath to form a nodule. In contrast, a secondary immunization with HGG in saline has little effect on the spleen. Obviously adjuvant is necessary in the overall immunological protocol as is usually the case.

Function of the Spleen

Ontogeny

Functions of the spleen are also controversial because information is sparse and different species may have different immunological capacities which seem to reflect the amounts of splenic lymphoid tissue. Thus, results from ontogenetic studies in salmon (Ellis, 1977), carp (Grace and Manning, 1980) and trout (Tatner and Manning, 1983) suggest that the spleen is not essential for immunological maturation since lymphocytes of thymus and kidney carry surface Ig and display mixed leukocyte reactions (MLR) when the spleen is present even in a rudimentary form. Schneider (1983) points out that, in *Cyprinus carpio*, in fish of only 10 mm the spleen's structure is already well formed. Moreover, splenectomy has no effect on antibody responses against bovine serum albumin (BSA) in some teleosts (Ferren, 1967), although in others the spleen has been considered a major lymphoid organ (Yu et al., 1970). Antigen-binding cells and/or antibody-producing cells have been detected in rainbow trout spleen (Anderson, 1978; Chiller et al., 1969; Warr and Marchalonis, 1977; Pontius and Ambrosius, 1972), bluegill (Smith et al., 1967), perch (Pontius and Ambrosius, 1972) and the Mozambique mouth-brooder (Sailendri and Muthukkaruppan, 1975).

Antigen Binding

Electron microscopy reveals that antigen binds to lymphocytes, blast-like cells, macrophages and even cells which resemble eosinophils (Chiller et al., 1969). Moreover splenocytes of rainbow trout (Cuchens et al., 1976; Etlinger et al., 1976) can be stimulated by LPS, PPD and Con A, which suggests that the spleen is a source of T-like and B-like cells. Morphology of lymphocyte transformation revealed that Con A-induced blast cells are larger and possess a lighter staining nucleus than lymphocytes, have a higher cytoplasmic nuclear ratio and an increased amount of mitochondria and rough endoplasmic reticulum. Plasma cells occur infrequently. Blast cell morphology, after culture in the presence of LPS and PPD, is similar to that with Con A (Etlinger et al., 1978).

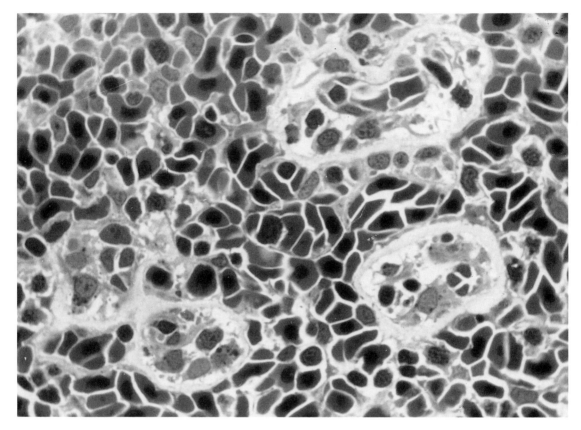

Figure 6.13 Ellipsoid in the spleen of the goldfish *Carassius auratus*. Phagocytic cells may be found in the wall (× 1260).

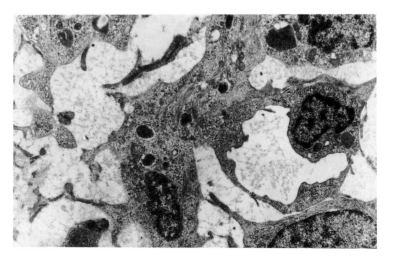

Figure 6.14 Processes of phagocytic cells showing numerous filaments and phagocytic vacuoles in the ellipsoidal walls of the spleen in *Carassius auratus* (× 5640).

Melanomacrophage Centers

General Features

The structure and function of melanomacrophage centers (MMCs) deserve special attention, since they are best developed in fish; this is not to discount, however, their presence in amphibian and even reptilian lymphoid organs (see description later). MMCs have been exhaustively investigated by Roberts and Agius and presented in several papers which describe their phylogeny, ontogeny and functional significance (Roberts, 1975, 1976; Agius, 1979, 1980, 1981a, b, 1983; Agius and Agbede, 1984). Changes in the MMCs after primary and secondary immunization have recently been analyzed in goldfish (Herraez and Zapata, 1986). Melanomacrophage centers are aggregations of closely packed macrophages which contain heterogeneous inclusions, the most frequent of which are melanin, hemosiderin and lipofucsin (Agius and Agbede, 1984). Lipofucsins are closely related to steroids which are possibly derived from the oxidation of polyunsaturated fatty acids (Agius and Agbede, 1984; Brown and George, 1985). Hemosiderin is one of the breakdown products of hemoglobin from senescent, degenerated erythrocytes. Fish which contain a high content of unsaturated fatty acid (Sargent, 1976) and relatively low levels of vitamin E (Tappel, 1975) are particularly prone to the formation of lipofucsin and melanin.

With respect to immunity, Edelstein (1971) has discussed the possible role of melanin pigments in defense mechanisms against disease and tissue damage in a wide range of living organisms. A particularly interesting suggestion is that melanin may be employed along with the peroxidase–peroxidase system to aid in the killing of bacteria, which is achieved by iodinating the bacterial cell walls. In this respect, melanin is known to produce hydrogen peroxide from the oxidation of NADH (van Woert and Palmer, 1969). This in turn can then be utilized in the bactericidal iodination system which occurs in polymorphonuclear leukocytes or neutrophils. Another characteristic of MMCs refers to their morphology and content, which can vary during different conditions: after bleeding (Grover, 1968; Yu et al., 1971), vitamin-deficient or rancid diets (Blazer and Wolke, 1983), starvation (Agius and Roberts, 1981; Agius, 1983; Agius and Agbede, 1984), senescence (Brown and George, 1985) and disease processes (Roberts, 1975).

In flatfish spleen, MMCs are often found in the axillary of an ellipsoidal branch and a fine fibrous membrane, continuous with that of ellipsoids, usually delimits the center. A few leukocytes and pyroninophilic cells are dispersed among the pigmented cells. A lymphocyte cuff surrounds the entire arterial system and its associated MMCs (Ellis, 1974; Ferguson, 1976; Roberts, 1975). In the flatfish kidney as well, the centers are bounded by a thin fibrous membrane which is surrounded by lymphoid tissue devoid of erythrocytes, through which thin-walled, narrow vessels have been observed (Ellis, 1974). In salmonids, the morphology of MMCs is less well-defined and the cells are distributed at random throughout the interstitial lymphohemopoietic tissue of the kidney, the white pulp of the spleen and the periportal areas of the liver (Roberts, 1975). The MMCs which occur in the spleen of *Carrasius auratus* are yellowish-brown clusters of phagocytic cells, the largest of which show an incomplete capsule and are associated with blood vessels (Figure 6.15). In the kidney, the MMCs are distributed randomly throughout the lymphohemopoietic tissue and they contain a part of the yellowish-brown melanin pigments which are more abundant in the pronephros than in the mesonephros (Figure 6.16).

Histochemistry

Histochemical analyses have demonstrated enormous heterogeneity in the content of MMCs of goldfish (Herraez and Zapata, 1986). Traces of lipids, neutral mucopolysaccharides and basic proteins have been found within them. Lipofucsin was demonstrated by the Schmorl's method but not by the more selective Nile blue reagent. Melanins were strongly positive in MMCs of the kidney but only slightly in those of the spleen. Perl's reaction was positive in all three organs—a bit of confirming evidence—at the ultrastructural level, for the presence of erythrocytic debris. Finally, acid phosphatase, but not alkaline phosphatase or endogenous peroxidase, is only slightly reactive in some of the MMCs. According to these histochemical results, the MMCs of *Carassius auratus* contain principally lipofucsin, crystalline inclusions which probably represent hematoidin

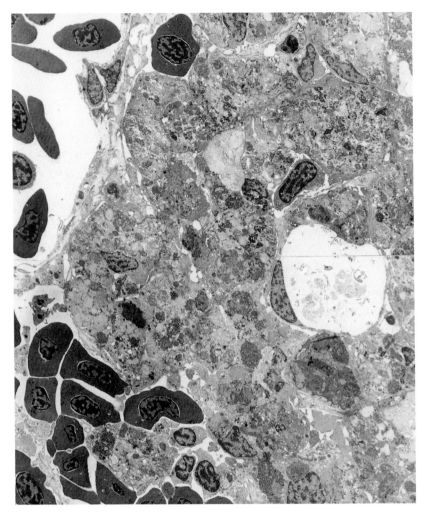

Figure 6.15 Melanomacrophage center in the spleen of the goldfish *Carassius auratus*. Note its relation with sinusoidal blood vessels and reticular cells (× 5500).

and/or hemosiderin, as well as fragments of erythrocytes and granulocytes (Figure 6.17). Some investigators consider that these cellular remains reveal a greater activity directed toward the destruction of erythrocytes (Graf and Schulns, 1979; Fulop and McMillan, 1984) whereas others (Agius and Agbede, 1984) consider lipofucsin to be a product that is derived from degraded mitochondria. The most widespread pigments, and in some conditions and/or species the most abundant, are melanins (Agius and Agbede, 1984). In any case, all authors have emphasized the heterogeneity of pigments in MMCs.

Evolution

All fish examined contain pigment cells, except for *Lampetra fluviatilis* (Agius, 1980). In contrast, Ardavin and Zapata (1987) found them in *Petromyzon marinus*—like *Lampetra*, another lamprey. There is an evolutionary pattern which occurs in these structures with respect to their distribution as well as their degree of organization. Thus, a progressive increase in the abundance of pigment cells and in their proclivity for the main lymphoid organs has been observed.

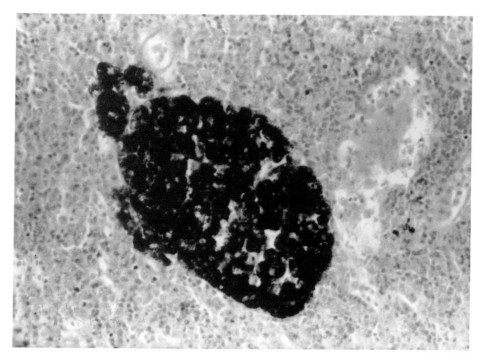

Figure 6.16 Melanomacrophage center showing abundant melanin pigment in the pronephros of the margate ($\times$ 600).

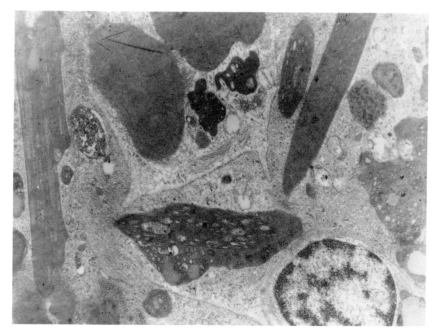

Figure 6.17 Melanomacrophage center containing numerous large crystalline inclusions after SRBC immunization ($\times$ 12 000).

MMCs seem to have evolved structurally from a random distribution of isolated pigment macrophages as in Agnatha and Chondrichthyes, to the characteristic, organized centers present in all Osteichthyes except salmonids (Agius, 1980). The change from liver of Agnatha, Chondrichthyes and primitive bony fishes to the spleen and kidney of the most evolved Osteichthyes seems to follow a pattern similar to that which parallels the evolution of lymphoid tissue. This represents a major advance in the evolution of lymphoreticular relationships (Agius, 1980). Thus, the increased complexity of the melanomacrophage centers is probably a concomitant event which accompanies a greater sophistication of the immune system. At least in *Salmo gairdneri*, *Scolophthalmus maximum* and *Tilapia zillii*, MMCs appear for the first time during ontogeny after the first feeding (Agius, 1981). Many other physiological processes of fish coincide with the first feeding but the causative effects of this phenomenon are unknown.

Function

How MMCs function has been presented in several hypotheses. MMCs have been related to age pigments (Roberts, 1975; Brown and George, 1985), to tissue breakdown (Agius, 1979; Agius and Roberts, 1981; Moccia *et al.*, 1984) and to defense mechanisms (Ellis *et al.*, 1976; Ferguson, 1976; Ellis, 1980; Secombes and Manning, 1980; Agius, 1981; Secombes *et al.*, 1982a; Fulop and McMillan, 1984; Lamers, 1985; Herraez and Zapata, 1986). These two later findings, i.e. tissue breakdown and defense mechanisms, deserve a more detailed description. A relationship between MMCs and iron metabolism has been suggested (Grover, 1968; Yu *et al.*, 1971; Agius, 1979; Graf and Schulns, 1979) and Grover (1968) and Yu *et al.* (1971) have found that the products of erythrocyte breakdown in fish MMCs can be reutilized during erythropoiesis. The amount of hemoglobin in fish spleen killed immediately after bleeding has been found to be equal to that observed in control fish; however, the numbers of MMCs decreased within 24–48 hours following bleeding. Agius (1979) concluded that under conditions of starvation and in diseased fish a markedly increased deposition of ferric ion occurred in splenic centers. Moreover, the induction of a fast and massive anemia induced by exposure to phenyl-hydrazine produced important changes in the MMCs of *Carassius auratus* (Herraez and Zapata, 1986). These MMCs accumulate huge amounts of altered erythrocytes and after 5 days they degenerate coincidentally with the appearance of erythroblasts, which then serve to recover the previously lost erythroid population. Involvement with erythrocyte development suggests a certain relationship between the need for iron during erythropoiesis and the disappearance of MMCs.

Finally, a role for splenic and kidney MMCs of teleosts in the trapping of antigenic and non-antigenic material has been established conclusively. The role of splenic ellipsoids and sinusoidal cells of the kidney as points for an initial trapping of material such as carbon has been found repeatedly by Lamers (1985) and by Herraez and Zapata (1986). From this location free macrophages migrate to the MMCs, where they apparently accumulate. Whether the carbon-laden macrophages move to pre-existing MMCs (Mori, 1980) or from new aggregates (Ellis *et al.*, 1976) is a matter of discussion, the results of which will probably depend on the amount of engulfed material and the number of MMCs present. In goldfish, carbon trapping as revealed by electron microscopy appears to be an intracellular process (Herraez and Zapata, 1986) although other workers have suggested an intra- and extracellular localization (Lamers, 1985). In contrast, the differences in carbon trapping by the kidney and spleen may be related to the route of injection, i.e. intraperitoneal or intramuscular (Herraez and Zapata, 1986).

In *Cyprinus carpio* and *Pleuronectes platessa*, soluble antigens have been detected by immuno-fluorescence in the splenic ellipsoidal sheaths which are associated with reticular fibers of the ellipsoidal walls (Ellis, 1980; Secombes and Manning, 1980; Secombes *et al.*, 1982a). Antigen trapping also appears to be related to Ig deposition in the same region, which suggests a trapping of extracellular antigen–antibody complexes. Moreover, after a second challenge with a soluble antigen such as HGG, clusters of pyroninophilic cells mainly in the kidney were found in *Cyprinus carpio* (Secombes and Manning, 1980; Secombes *et al.*, 1982b). After injecting a particulate antigen such as *Aeromonas salmonicida* or *Aeromonas hydrophila*, similar phenomena induced by non-antigenic, particulate material were observed, as revealed by fluorescence in macrophages of splenic ellipsoidal walls (Secombes and Manning, 1980, 1982). An extracellular deposition was, however, never found after SRBC immunization in goldfish (Herraez and Zapata, 1986).

Ultrastructural analyses have revealed that erythrocytes appeared first in the cytoplasm of macrophages in splenic ellipsoids (Figure 6.18) and in the endothelial cells of the kidney (Figure 6.19). These observations also suggest that macrophages in the spleen or phagocytic reticular cells in the kidney might serve to transport material such as *Aeromonas hydrophila*. Apparently, therefore, antigen processed by macrophages accumulates finally in the MMCs over long periods (Figure 6.20), which suggests a phylogenetic relationship to the germinal centers of higher vertebrates, despite their inherent morphological differences. In this sense, the quantitative variations which have occurred in the MMCs of spleen and kidney in goldfish seem to confirm the involvement of MMCs in antigenic trapping and processing (Herraez and Zapata, 1986).

Condition After Immunization

After primary immunization, significant differences between control and immunized fish have been observed in the number and size of splenic MMCs. Their numbers increased rapidly at 5 and 7 days, whereas the size of MMCs became prominent at 14 and 21 days. Following a secondary immunization, an increase in number but not in size of splenic MMCs was induced. Apparently the effects of immunization on pronephric MMCs were faster than those observed in the spleen. The pronephros showed the greatest quantitative modifications in MMCs, especially after secondary immunization. Events in the mesonephros as related to immunization, by contrast, were slower than those as related in the pronephros and spleen, which reveals only a few alterations after primary immunization at 5 and 7 days, which were still significant at 21 days. With respect to antibody titers and number and size of MMCs, there is apparently no correlation. Fish with the highest levels of circulating antibodies did not possess a correspondingly high

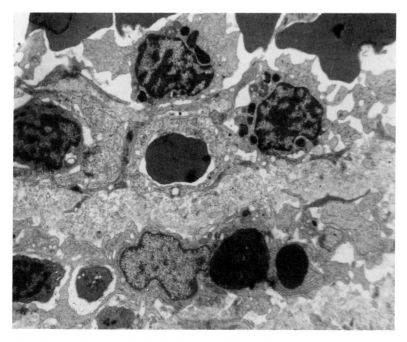

Figure 6.18 Phagocytic cells containing engulfed cell debris, possibly erythrocytes, appear in the walls of splenic ellipsoid of a goldfish, *Carassius auratus*, 5 days after primary immunization with sheep erythrocytes ($\times$ 5600).

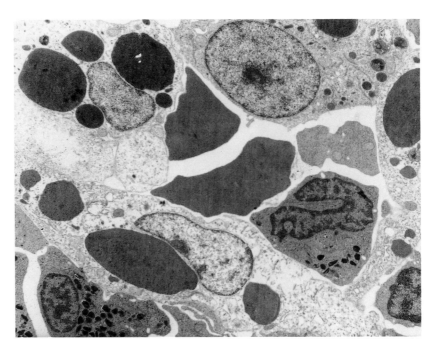

Figure 6.19 Sinusoidal lining cell contains engulfed erythrocytes in the pronephros of *Carassius auratus* after immunization with SRBC (× 5640).

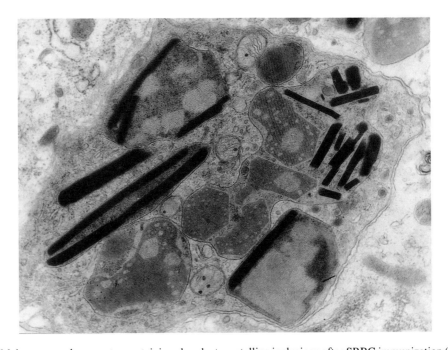

Figure 6.20 Melanomacrophage center containing abundant crystalline inclusions after SRBC immunization (× 10 500).

number of MMCs (Herraez and Zapata, 1986). In summary, MMCs probably represent a non-specific physiological system which is related to various processes, including those of the immune system.

AMPHIBIANS

Introduction

The spleen of amphibians represents an enigma. First, despite the key position occupied by amphibians in the phylogeny of immune responses and the recognized importance of the spleen in immunity, its structure has not been subject to intense scrutiny. Second, splenic morphology in amphibians shows remarkable differences in functional significance about which little is known. These differences are clear not only between the three principal groups of amphibians—the apodans, urodeles and anurans—but even, for example, among the various families of anurans. In any case, structural homologies probably exist between the spleen in apodans and urodeles but there are differences, on the contrary, between them and the anuran spleen. Resemblances and differences may reflect an evolutionary trend which is also evident in the immune reactions of this crucial group of ecto-thermic vertebrates (Cooper, 1976).

Apodans

In general, information on apodan immune responses (and for that matter any experimental work) is extremely restricted, which is also true for what is known concerning the microscopic organization of the spleen. In *Siphonopus indistinctus* and *Hypogeophis rostratus*, Weilacher (1933) reported that the spleen produced 'round cells', presumably lymphocytes, and it eliminated erythrocytes. Weilacher described further the white pulp as consisting of large, primary Malpighian corpuscles and smaller secondary cor-puscles. In *Nectrocaecilia cooperi* (formerly *Typhlonectes compressicauda*), the spleen is an elongated organ containing lymphoid and myeloid components (Garcia-Herrera and Cooper, 1968) whereas in *Ichthyophis kohtaoensis* it has been described as resembling the urodelan spleen (Zapata *et al.*, 1982) which consists mainly of red pulp and a few, small lymphoid aggregates (Figure 6.21). A clear

demarcation between both areas has not been observed. More recently, Welsch and Storch (1982) have published preliminary ultrastructural studies on the spleen of two other caecilians, *Ichthyophis paucisulcus* and *Afrocaecilia taitana*, confirming its primitive, simple organization. Despite these scattered bits, there is essentially no information on the role of the apodan spleen in immune responses.

Urodeles

General Features

The spleen of urodeles is an elongated organ, vascular-ized by multiple, intermediate branches of the major splenic arteries and veins (Cowden and Dyer, 1971). The parenchyma is not clearly separated into red and white pulp (Figure 6.22a) (Hartmann, 1926; Cowden and Dyer, 1971; Hightower and St Pierre, 1971), although in some genera such as *Megalobatrachus* and *Hynobius* (Nakajima, 1929a, b; Ohuye, 1932) and *Ambystoma mexicanum* (Ardavia and Zapata, in preparation) these regions are clearly recognizable after primary (Figure 6.22b) and secondary (Figure 6.22c) immunization. In any case, ultrastructural observations have revealed lymphoid cells, mainly small lymphocytes, which are distributed in cell cords that form the splenic red pulp (Figure 6.23). In parti-cular, the urodelan splenic red pulp consists of numerous cell cords which contain erythrocytes, thrombocytes, lymphocytes, granulocytes and macro-phages, supported in a meshwork of reticular cells and fibers arranged between sinusoidal blood vessels. Red pulp is a major site where erythropoiesis and thrombo-poiesis occur (Dawson, 1932; Tooze and Davies, 1967; Charlemagne, 1972b; Zapata *et al.*, 1979) and it is also a site where basophil precursors originate (Cowden, 1965).

Lymphoid follicles which constitute the white pulp of the spleen in urodeles are formed by aggregates of lymphoid cells, intermingled with mature erythrocytes and giant, pigment-containing phagocytic cells (Figure 6.24). These cells, quite similar to isolated melanomacrophages reported in fish, have been observed in the liver and spleen of numerous urodeles (Nakajima, 1929a, b; Zapata *et al.*, 1979) and their possible functional significance, which has been exten-sively discussed, does not deserve major attention in

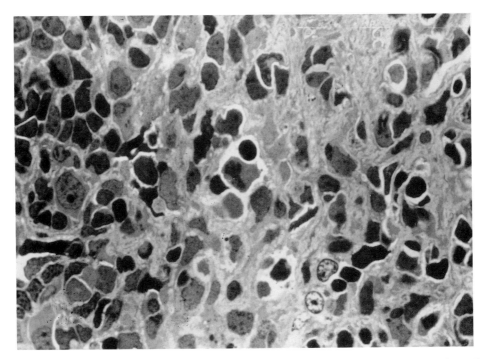

Figure 6.21 Spleen of the apodan *Nectrocaecilia cooperi*. Note the absence of clear lymphoid accumulations which form a white pulp (× 600).

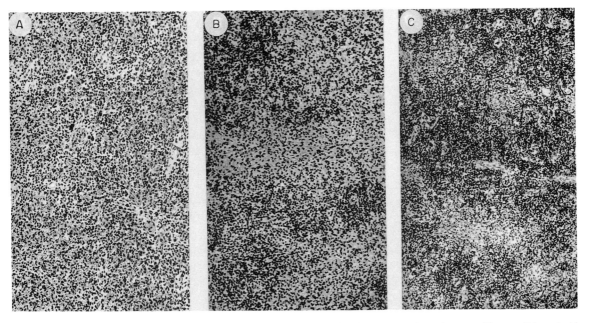

Figure 6.22 Spleen of *Pleurodeles waltlii* before and after immunization. In (a) there is no evidence of lymphoid accumulations which form white pulp, but lymphocytes increase after primary (b) and secondary immunization (c) (× 248).

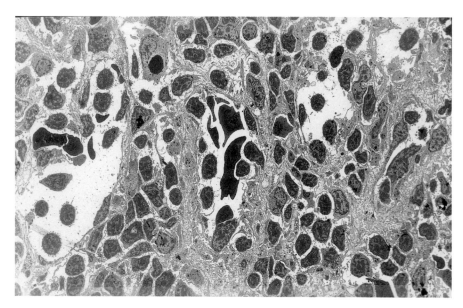

Figure 6.23 Numerous small lymphocytes occur in cell cords and sinusoids of splenic red pulp in the newt *Triturus alpestris* (× 2500).

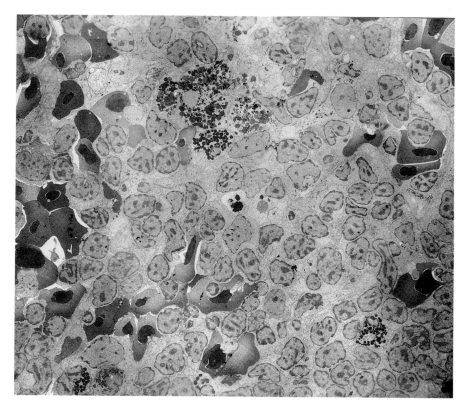

Figure 6.24 Panoramic survey of a lymphoid follicle in the spleen of *Ambystoma mexicanum*. A clear demarcation between white and red pulp is lacking and erythrocytes occur among lymphocytes and melanomacrophages (× 1100).

this context. The cytoplasm of these phagocytic cells contains numerous remains of various materials, some of which resemble engulfed cells, probably erythroid whereas others clearly represent melanin pigment (Figure 6.25). Large phagocytic cells can occur isolated, scattered at random throughout the cytoplasm, or inside the cytoplasmic granules, presumably as primary and/or secondary lysosomes.

Ontogeny

In *Triturus alpestris*, the embryonic spleen appears at week 7 of development as a mediodorsal enlargement of the mesenchymal epithelium in the stomach region (Tournefier, 1973). At week 8 the splenic primordium is only a cellular, sponge-like mass where no erythroblasts have been observed. However, at week 9, the spleen is essentially an erythropoietic organ surrounded by a connective tissue capsule. From week 10,

the young spleen is histologically similar to that in adults: loose red pulp which contains mainly erythroid cells can be distinguished from lymphoid areas where densely packed lymphocytes are grouped around splenic arteries.

Immune Reactions

Immune reactions are comparatively less strong in urodeles than in anurans. The splenic rosette-forming cell response seems slow to develop and is low in magnitude in *Pleurodeles waltlii* (Debons and Deparis, 1973). However, intraperitoneal, primary immunizations with SRBC have been associated with a notable increase in the amounts of lymphoid tissue (Figure 6.22b). No variations have been found, however, after intraoral or intracloacal immunization, an observation which seems to rule out the route as a major variable in determining strength of certain

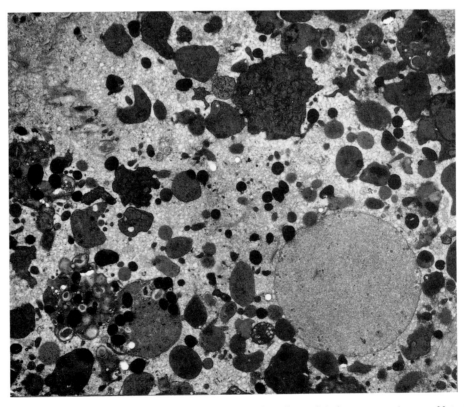

Figure 6.25 Detail of the cytoplasm of a melanomacrophage from the spleen of *Ambystoma mexicanum*. Note the pigment granules scattered at random in the cytoplasm or included in dense bodies ($\times$ 6100).

immune responses (Ardavin, 1981). A secondary challenge with the same antigen elicits a substantial growth of lymphoid tissue which forms densely stained lymphoid accumulations that are clearly demarcated from the red pulp (Figure 6.22c). Charlemagne (1983) described that a heavy-density spleen cell population which is sensitive to adult thymectomy, low-dose irradiation and hydrocortisone treatment may have a homeostatic suppressive function on the axolotl antibody synthesis. Ruben and Edwards (1979) using *Notophthalmus viridescens* reported the release of sensitized cells from the spleen after secondary challenge, a response which may serve to boost continued antibody synthesis elsewhere. Furthermore, levels of responses of urodele spleen cells to B-cell mitogens appear to be similar to those observed in anurans (Collins *et al.*, 1975). The responses to T-cell mitogens and those observed in mixed lymphocyte cultures are, however, significantly lower in urodeles than in anurans (Cohen and Collins, 1977), a finding which suggests to some comparative immunologists that an earlier evolution of B-cell reactivity occurred during urodele evolution. Recently, however, Suzuki and Cohen (1987) demonstrated that splenocytes derived from the newt *Notophthalmus viridescens* exhibit up to a 20-fold increase in [^{3}H]thymidine incorporation when cultured in a 4-day mitogen assay with phorbol 12-myristate (PMA). Furthermore, PMA potentiates a two-way mixed lymphocyte reaction. A preliminary report by these same authors suggests that the PMA effects on newt splenocytes are mediated through a receptor similar or identical to protein kinase C.

With respect to typical T-cell reactions, Tahan and Jurd (1979) were able to passively transfer hypersensitivity in *Ambystoma* by means of splenocytes. Likewise, autologous spleen cells can restore alloimmunity in Japanese newts, *Cynops pyrrhogaster*, after transfer to irradiated hosts (Murakawa, 1968). There is also other evidence that non-sensitized spleen cell populations, which include K-like cells, can effect cytotoxic killing of antibody-coated target cells (Jurd and Doritis, 1977). Despite these recognized capacities of splenic cells, splenectomy seems to have no marked effect on health and growth in general. Absence of the spleen does not affect allograft rejection (Cohen, 1971; Charlemagne, 1972a; Deparis and Flavin, 1973) either during first-set or second-set responses (Cohen and Horan, 1977).

Anurans

General Features

The anuran spleen is a reddish organ located dorsally in the body cavity. Blood supply occurs via branches of the mesenteric artery and splenic vein (Cooper, 1976). In all species studied so far, the spleen is surrounded by a connective tissue capsule, the outside of which is coated by peritoneum. The arrangements of various histological components, mainly the red and white pulp which comprise the splenic parenchyma, are, however, highly variable in different anuran species. With some exceptions the amount of splenic lymphoid tissue is apparently scarce, a condition which resembles the teleost spleen. Regarding phylogeny of the anuran spleen, Cooper and Wright (1976) completed a comparative analysis of splenic histology in several representative families. According to their observations, the trend from a primitive to a more advanced type of white pulp develops from a diffuse type to one which consists of a concentrated arrangement of lymphocytes.

Apart from its lymphoid condition, the spleen is also a major erythropoietic organ in adult anurans, while in larvae it destroys erythrocytes (Jordan and Speidel, 1923a, b; Jordan, 1938; Fey, 1962; Le Douarin, 1966; Maclean and Jurd, 1972; Carver and Meints, 1977). A clear distinction between red and white pulp is lacking in the primitive anuran *Ascaphus truei* (Cooper and Wright, 1976). In *Scaphoipus couchii*, of the family Pelobatidae, the spleen contains small groups of lymphocytes scattered throughout the parenchyma, whereas in *Bufo powerii* and *Rana pipiens* the white pulp is distinguishable, although a clear marginal zone has not been described (Cooper and Wright, 1976).

Ontogeny

Recently Nagata (1986a) used a monoclonal antibody which recognizes determinants (XT-1) expressed by most thymocytes and a subpopulation of thymus-dependent sIgM-negative lymphocytes (Nagata, 1985). He found that the percentage of XT-1-positive cells in the spleen at stage 50 of development was less than 2% but reached significant levels at stage 52 (6%) and increased to adult levels (approximately 30%) by stage 56.

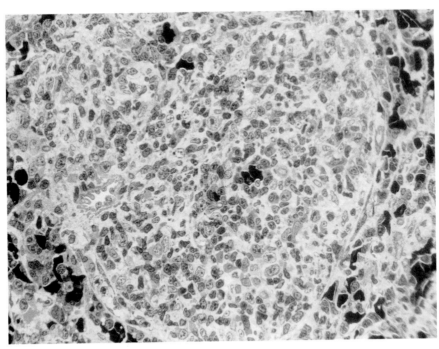

Figure 6.26 Lymphoid follicle in the spleen of the natterjack, *Bufo calamita*, which shows the distribution of lymphoid cells around an eccentric arteriole. Note the sharp demarcation between the white and red pulp due to the presence of a layer of flat reticular cells. Erythrocytes in the red pulp are black (× 425).

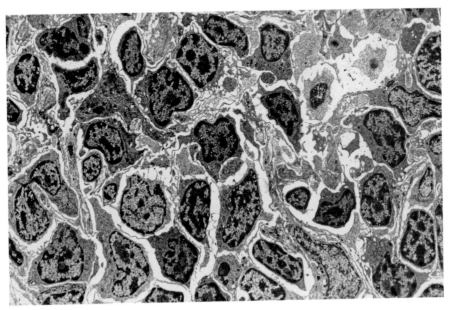

Figure 6.27 Distribution of lymphoid cells between reticular cells in a lymphoid follicle of the spleen in the natterjack, *Bufo calamita* (× 2200).

Spleen histogenesis has been studied in detail in *Xenopus laevis* (Manning and Horton, 1969) and *Rana pipiens* (Horton, 1971). In *Xenopus*, the spleen begins to be distinguished as a cell condensation in the dorsal mesogastrium (stage 46) which establishes a differentiation into red and white pulp at stage 48. Between stages 48 and 51 the organ continues to increase in size, with the white pulp becoming fully lymphoid. cIg sIg-positive lymphocytes appear at stage 49 and then the spleen commences its immunological function (Hadji-Azimi *et al.*, 1982). In *Rana pipiens* spleen histogenesis is similar.

White Pulp

The white pulp of *Xenopus laevis* is, in contrast to other anurans, highly elaborate, consisting of two more or less compact layers of lymphocytes which surround a central arteriole and a patent, marginal zone that separates the white pulp from the red pulp (Sterba, 1951; Manning, 1975). Curiously, this most distinctive organization occurs in a species which is relatively primitive when viewed according to the usual amphibian taxonomy. Thus, the presence of a complex white pulp may account for the lack of lymphomyeloid nodes in *Xenopus laevis* as is the case in the more advanced anurans, so that the spleen rests as the most important mass of lymphoid tissue (Turner, 1969). In agreement with this point, Barrutia *et al.* (1983) recently described a well-organized splenic white pulp in the natterjack, *Bufo calamita*, another anuran species devoid of lymphomyeloid nodes. Both animal models—*Xenopus laevis* and *Bufo calamita*—are undoubtedly the best ones for studying splenic histophysiology, at least with respect to distribution and function of lymphocytes.

The spleen of *Xenopus laevis*, which has been described so thoroughly by Sterba (1951), consists of several regions of white pulp that are sharply delimited first by a boundary layer. Second, there is a cuff of scattered lymphocytes, which extends irregularly into the red pulp, thus constituting a perifollicular zone (Turner and Manning, 1973). In *Bufo calamita* the spleen shows two clearly differentiated areas: the white pulp which is lymphoid and the red pulp which is composed of cell cords and sinusoids (Figure 6.26). These two areas are separated by a conspicuous marginal zone formed by flat reticular cells (Figure

6.27). The lymphoid follicles which surround eccentric arteries are composed of muscle walls (Figure 6.27) and reticular elements, macrophages, lymphoid cells and mature and developing plasma cells (Figure 6.27). By electron microscopy, Barrutia *et al.* (1983) found two kinds of splenic, supporting reticular elements in lymphoid follicles. One is an electron-dense, irregularly shaped cell which shows a nucleus that contains an abundant, condensed chromatin. The other cell is extremely large and ramified, possesses an electron-lucent nucleus, displaying prominent nucleoli and a cytoplasm which contains numerous dense mitochondria, abundant microfilaments and small, lysosome-like, dense bodies. These two reticular cell types correspond apparently to those described in human fetuses (Weiss and Chen, 1974) and rodent spleens (Galindo and Imaeda, 1962). Thus dark reticular cells reported as fibroblastic reticular cells by light microscopy might be related to the formation of a splenic supporting network. The other reticular cell type is similar to one found in rat spleens (Saito, 1977) and it represents a fibromuscular cell, i.e. an intermediate form between a smooth muscle cell and a fibroblast. We shall now pass to the red pulp first by traversing an intermediate marginal zone.

Red Pulp

A marginal zone is formed by expanded, electron-dense processes of reticular cells that constitute a continuous layer except for occasional gaps through which free cells move. The red pulp consists of a labyrinth of cell cords which contain free elements such as macrophages, lymphocytes, plasma cells and mature and developing erythroid cells. All of them are enmeshed in a network of reticular cells and fibers which are interrupted by blood sinuses (Barrutia *et al.*, 1983). The most remarkable component of the spleen in both *Xenopus laevis* and *Bufo calamita* is the presence of a giant, non-lymphoid cell which resembles the antigen-trapping dendritic cell of mammals. The structure, function and presence of these dendritic-like cells in other anurans will be discussed later in relation to trapping and processing of antigens in the spleen.

In the internal margins of splenic lymphoid follicles in *Bufo calamita*, presumptive, interdigitating cells have been described recently (Barrutia *et al.*, 1985b). Interdigitating cells, previously found in the thymus of

Rana sp. (Bigaj and Plytycz, 1984), are characterized mainly by numerous folds of their surface membrane, absence of organelles in the peripheral cytoplasm and, by contrast, concentration of organelles around the nucleus (Figure 6.28). In these cells, Barrutia *et al.* (1985b) found large, electron-dense, but no Birbeck granules, the significance of which is unknown. However, the expected function of interdigitating cells has already been discussed in the chapter on the thymus.

Existence and Distribution of Lymphocytic and Non-lymphoid Cells

We will consider now the existence and distribution of lymphocyte subpopulations in the spleen before discussing the structure and function of giant dendritic cells. Several comparative immunologists have postulated the existence of at least two lymphocyte subsets in anurans— views mainly derived from studies of the spleen in *Xenopus*. Supporting evidence is presented in the following summary:

1. Early larval thymectomy induces severe reduction but not elimination of splenic lymphocytes (Manning, 1971; Horton and Manning, 1974a; Tochinai, 1976a). Repopulation of splenic lymphocytes can be induced after implanting the thymus or injecting thymocytes (Tochinai *et al.*, 1976; Katagiri *et al.*, 1980; Kawahara *et al.*, 1980; Nagata, 1980).

2. In the spleen of *Xenopus*, Ig-positive and -negative lymphocytes occur (Jurd and Stevenson, 1976; Hadji-Azimi, 1977; Nagata and Katagiri, 1978).

Furthermore, Coosemans and Hadji-Azimi (1987) recently reported membrane-associated receptor for Ig on a large percentage of *Xenopus* splenocytes. Cells (28.4% and 5.3%) bore receptors for IgY and receptors for IgM respectively. All *Xenopus* splenic B-lymphocytes bearing sIg bind also antigen-complexed IgY, while a small percentage of splenocytes carry receptors for IgY alone on their surface. The identity of these latter cells and that of cells bearing receptors for IgM remains to be

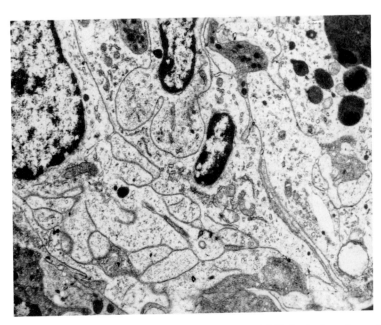

Figure 6.28 Presumptive interdigitating cells in the periphery of lymphoid follicles in the spleen of the natterjack, *Bufo calamita* (× 16 200).

established. Apparently, the membrane receptors detected on *Xenopus* splenocytes are homologous to the Fc receptor described in mammals.

The Ig-positive cells, not eliminated by early thymectomy, might be responsible for immune responses against thymus-independent antigens such as bacterial lipopolysaccharide or polyvinyl-pyrrolidone (Collie et al., 1975; Tochinai, 1976b).

3. Noticeable changes occur in splenic lymphocytes in response to different immunological conditions such as transplantation of allografts (Horton *et al.*, 1977) or antigenic stimulation (Tochinai, 1976a; Turner and Manning, 1973) (see later description).

Another parameter which characterizes different lymphocyte subpopulations is their localization in the spleen. There have been several approaches using *Xenopus laevis* but results which have attempted to answer the question are contradictory. First, the peri-follicular zone in the spleen of *Xenopus laevis* has been proposed as a thymus-dependent area, based upon the following results:

1. Severe depletion of lymphocytes after early thymectomy occurs in this splenic region (Manning, 1971; Horton and Manning, 1974a; Tochinai, 1976b).
2. The perifollicular zone shows increased incorporation of tritiated thymidine during skin allograft rejection (Horton *et al.*, 1977).
3. Histocompatible thymus (Tochinai *et al.*, 1976) or injected splenic or peripheral blood lymphocytes (Nagata and Tochinai, 1978) will repopulate this perifollicular region in thymectomized *Xenopus*.
4. Exposure to a carcinogen (*N*-methyl-*N*-nitro-sourea) depletes this region as well as the thymic cortex, but other splenic areas will recover (Balls *et al.*, 1980).

Thymic-dependent lymphocytes have also been associated with the red pulp, which is based upon the following results:

1. Manning (1971) found a notable reduction of lymphocytes in the splenic red pulp, while those of the white pulp were apparently normal in *Xenopus* after larval thymectomy.
2. Obara (1982) demonstrated that the localization

of transferred labeled donor cells in the spleen of hosts was dependent upon both the route of entry and time after transfer. Thus, grafted cells apparently migrated initially into the red pulp and later into the white pulp. According to Obara's interpretation, there was a preferential localization of thymocytes in the red pulp and splenocytes in the white pulp.

3. Lymphoid proliferation or formation of pyro-ninophilic cells occurs in white pulp in response to polyvinylpyrrolidone (Tochinai, 1976a) or HGG in adjuvant (Turner and Manning, 1973), particularly in the periphery of the white pulp, which suggests that it is involved significantly in humoral responses.

4. By immunohistochemical analysis, Nagata (1980) found that plasma cells specific for injected horseradish peroxidase do occur mostly in the white pulp.

5. Cells with Ig-positive surfaces were mostly arranged in the white pulp of *Xenopus laevis*, although their fluorescence was weak (Obara *et al.*, 1982). Cells with weak fluorescence appear occasionally, forming thin layers around the central arterioles of white pulp. In red pulp, positive cells show much weaker fluorescence and are confined to the area surrounding white pulp as single cells or as small clusters (Obara *et al.*, 1982).

Answers to the question of how various cell populations are distributed in splenic parenchyma have come from studies on carbon and antigen trapping. Carbon particles can be detected in red pulp shortly after injection (within 1–3 hours). In *Bufo marinus*, particles remain in the red pulp but do not enter the white pulp (Diener and Nossal, 1966), whereas in *Ascaphus truei* carbon-engulfing cells circumscribe the white pulp (Cooper and Wright, 1976). In *Xenopus laevis*, by contrast, the white pulp, although containing no carbon immediately following injections, does contain dense aggregates by 3–4 weeks. Likewise in *Bufo calamita* carbon deposits occur rapidly after injections, are scattered at random in the red pulp but are distributed later in the white pulp (Barrutia *et al.*, 1983).

In both locations, electron microscopy has revealed macrophages to be the unique cells which contain engulfed carbon. During larval life, free macrophages in the body cavities of *Xenopus laevis* trap intra-peritoneally injected particles as early as seven days.

Once other lymphoid organs have developed, carbon particles are removed, mainly by the spleen and liver of both larvae and adults (Turner, 1969), although some differences in this basic pattern occur in those anurans which possess lymphomyeloid organs. By contrast, Coleman and Phillips (1972) detected deposits in splenic macrophages and in Kupffer cells of the liver even three years after injecting colloidal thorium dioxide. This remarkable retention suggests an inability to effectively eliminate this substance.

Antigen trapping. In *Bufo marinus*, Diener and Marchalonis (1970) found extracellular trapping of ^{125}I-labeled *Salmonella adelaide*. Antigen was distributed randomly on dendritic cells in the jugular bodies and in the splenic red pulp but not in the white pulp where fluorescence accumulates (Horton and Manning, 1974b). According to these workers, this kind of antigen is trapped extracellularly in the form of antigen—antibody complexes. In contrast, the fluorescence pattern is different when particulate antigens such as formalin-killed *Aeromonas salmonicida* are used. In this instance, fluorescence occurs but it is distributed more randomly in the white pulp, with a conspicuous staining of the boundary layer (Secombes and Manning, 1980). In *Rana pipiens*, by contrast, no distinct antigen trapping occurs at any time in the spleen after injecting HGG in adjuvant since all of the antigen is retained in the jugular bodies (Manning, unpublished). Although there are variations in the exact site where antigen is trapped, the dendritic pattern of antigen localization seems to remain similar (Manning and Horton, 1982).

Vacuole formation and the XL-cell. Vacuole formation is another phenomenon which remains a distinct feature in the spleens of immunized anurans. It has been induced in *Xenopus* which have been previously injected with HGG in adjuvant (Manning and Turner, 1972) and in *Rana catesbeiana* larvae immunized with SRBC (Moticka *et al.*, 1973). According to one suggestion these vacuoles correspond to regions of phagocytic activity. In hyperimmunized anurans and when adjuvant is used, these areas become filled with pale staining histiocytic tissue (Turner *et al.*, 1974) and the so-called 'degenerating macrolymphocytes', first described by Sterba (1950), later by Manning (1971), and recently named XL-cells, constitute 3% of the cells

in the splenic white pulp of healthy juvenile *Xenopus laevis*. They are truly giant, mitotically active cells that trap foreign material on the surfaces of their cytoplasmic extensions (Baldwin and Cohen, 1981). XL-cells contain no demonstrable cytoplasmic Ig, fail to stain for non-specific esterase and do not phagocytose (Baldwin and Cohen, 1981).

By electron microscopy, they are large cells which contain few lysosomes with cytoplasmic extensions in contact with adjacent lymphocytes. Their hyperlobulated nuclei and prominent nucleoli resemble, according to these workers, Reed—Sternberg cells, a type of giant cell found in malignant and reactive lymphoid tissue, probably derived from dendritic cells (Baldwin and Cohen, 1981). Thus, Baldwin and Cohen (1981) have proposed that the XL-cells of *Xenopus laevis* are primitive dendritic cells because of their weak phagocytic capacity, failure to stain for non-specific esterase (neither in a diffuse pattern as macrophages nor in a punctate pattern typical of most lymphoid cells), failure to stain for cytoplasmic Ig and lack of interference by early larval thymectomy on their development (Manning, 1971).

Baldwin and Sminia (1982) demonstrated that isolated XL-cells are capable of trapping antigenic material on their cell projections and transporting it along their cell surfaces. Moreover, by immunofluorescence, bacteria (*Aeromonas*) have been found trapped on XL-cells in the spleen and on large cells in the bone marrow, liver, blood, gut, thymus and kidney. Anti-XL serum stained large cells and the endothelium of certain vessels with a similar pattern (Baldwin, 1983). In essence, Baldwin and his colleagues have proposed a model in which XL-cells, trapping and transporting antigens, may function as a bridge between T-cells, presumably in the marginal zone and B-cells in the white pulp follicle. Thus antigens and other materials would be extravasated into the red pulp to be processed by macrophages, trapped on the surface of XL-cells and then transported to the marginal zone of the white pulp. Once it is within the white pulp, antigenic material might be retained on the surface of XL-cells to be presented to neighboring lymphocytes which, under these conditions, are able to divide and transform into functionally active cells.

Giant cells, similar in many respects to XL-cells, have also been found in spleens of the natterjack, *Bufo calamita* (Barrutia *et al.*, 1983, 1985a). The main differences between both cell types concern their distribution throughout the spleen. While XL-cells occur exclusively in the white pulp of *Xenopus laevis*, giant cells in *Bufo calamita* appear in the red pulp mainly near the marginal zone (Figure 6.29) (Barrutia *et al.*, 1985a). Only sometimes can giant cells or their processes be observed in lymphoid follicles which constitute the white pulp of *Bufo calamita*, suggesting that they move freely through the marginal zone. The ultrastructure of giant cells in *Bufo calamita*, by contrast, resembles that of XL-cells. They are large cells, sometimes binucleated, with a prominent nucleolus and large amount of cytoplasm. XL-cells also contain abundant components, mainly several dictyosomes, electron-dense granules, and smooth and rough endoplasmic reticulum (Figure 6.30). Sometimes they form cell clusters, making contact with lymphocytes, developing and mature plasma cells (Barrutia *et al.*, 1983).

Likewise, in the spleen of another toad, *Bufo bufo*, giant cells similar to dendritic cells of *Bufo calamita* and *Xenopus laevis* occur in the red pulp. Their cell processes also make surface contact with neighboring lymphocytes (Figure 6.31). Giant, dendritic cells increase enormously in number in the red pulp of *Bufo calamita* ten days after a primary, intraperitoneal immunization with SRBC (Barrutia *et al.*, 1985a). They appear as very active, large ramified elements apparently capable of moving throughout the red pulp. The cytoplasm of some of them has been found to contain phagocytosed foreign particles, cytoplasmic dense bodies and cell debris. Barrutia and her colleagues also found increased numbers of circulating monocytes in blood sinusoids of red pulp in immunized natterjacks and other cells which show intermediate morphology between them and giant, dendritic cells. They concluded, finally, in contrast to the situation in *Xenopus*, that the giant cells of *Bufo calamita*, originating apparently from circulating monocytes may be able to process antigens in the red pulp and cooperate with lymphocytes. This suggests an evolutionary functional relationship between white pulp in its neighboring marginal zone.

To recapitulate, there are two basically different models that describe the distribution of lymphoid and non-lymphoid cells in the anuran spleen: one in *Xenopus laevis*, a member of the primitive family

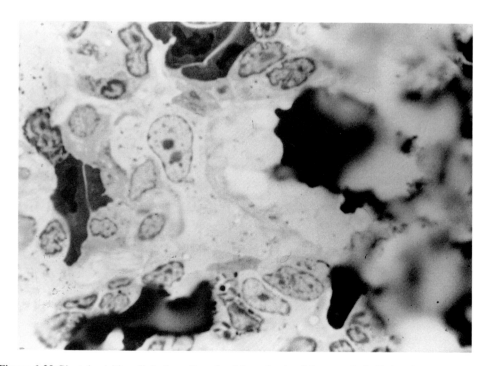

Figure 6.29 Giant dendritic cell in the cell cords of the red pulp of the natterjack, *Bufo calamita* ($\times$ 1200).

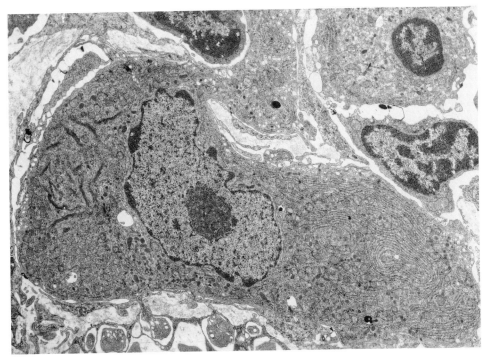

Figure 6.30 Giant dendritic cell of the spleen in *Bufo calamita*. Note small electron-dense granules, well-developed Golgi apparatus and arrangement of the endoplasmic reticulum (× 5500).

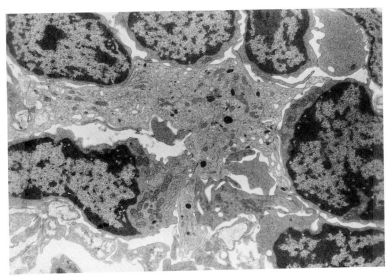

Figure 6.31 Process of a dendritic cell making contact with neighboring small lymphocytes suggesting a role in antigen processing. Spleen of *Bufo bufo* 15 days after primary immunization (× 6500).

Pipidae, the second in the more highly evolved natterjack, *Bufo calamita*. In *Xenopus*, lymphoid tissue which surrounds arterial blood vessels seems to be T-independent. Whether T-dependent tissue is distributed near the marginal zone, is located inside lymphoid follicles or forms a perifollicular layer in the immediately adjacent red pulp is a matter of discussion. In contrast, giant, non-lymphoid cells, probably dendritic ones, occur exclusively in lymphoid follicles. Their processes collect antigen–antibody complexes from throughout the marginal zone. These complexes have been previously processed by free macrophages which retain them on their surfaces, where they can collaborate with T- and B-lymphocytes. In *Bufo calamita*, although evidence is only morphological, results suggest a T-independent condition for lymphoid tissue which surrounds the arteries. As in *Xenopus*, T-lymphocytes probably occupy the outside region of lymphoid follicles just beneath the marginal zone, as suggested by the presence in this area of interdigitating cells. Giant cells, located exclusively in red pulp and throughout the marginal zone, phagocytose, process antigens and present them to lymphocytes in the white pulp. Whether they retain antigen–antibody complexes on their surfaces is an important point that has not been conclusively demonstrated.

Related to antigen trapping and processing and to immune capacities of anuran spleen are those morphological changes which affect it after immune stimulation. Despite the limited studies in a few species, clearly the spleen usually responds to antigen by producing increased numbers of large lymphocytes and blast cells, identified classically by light microscopy, as pyroninophilic cells (Diener and Nossal, 1966; Manning and Turner, 1972; Moticka *et al.*, 1973; Turner and Manning, 1973; Horton *et al.*, 1977) following enhanced responses during booster conditions (Diener and Nossal, 1966; Manning and Turner, 1972). However, in *Rana catesbeiana* pyroninophilia has been more evident in other lymphoid organs than in the spleen (Minagawa *et al.*, 1975). *Xenopus* injected with *Salmonella tennessee* failed to show pyroninophilic cells in any lymphoid loci despite the evident antibody production (Mitsuhashi *et al.*, 1971). According to Clothier and Balls (1973), when antigen is a live organism such as *Mycobacterium marinus* the initial splenic response in

Xenopus follows the usual pattern of proliferation and granulomata formation if large doses are administered.

In *Xenopus*, the proliferative responses and increased pyroninophilia peaked at approximately eight weeks after antigen administration, while the peak of serum antibodies occurred at week 8 (Turner and Manning, 1973). The pyroninophilia appeared first in sites where antigens are retained, but later, pyroninophilic cells have been observed in the perifollicular zone and throughout the red pulp. In *Bufo marinus*, after injecting BSA, pyroninophilic cells appear at the periphery of lymphoid areas and around blood vessels (Evans *et al.*, 1966). In immunized bullfrog (*Rana catesbeiana*) larvae, blast cells and lymphocytes increased in the red pulp while in the white pulp, which consists primarily of small lymphocytes, both areas became more extensive than in unstimulated controls (Baculi and Cooper, 1973).

Ultrastructural changes in the spleen of immunized anuran species have also been observed in *Xenopus laevis* (Obara *et al.*, 1982) and *Bufo calamita* (Barrutia *et al.*, 1985a). Increased numbers of lymphoblasts, mitotic figures, developing and mature plasma cells were the most remarkable features. In immunized *Xenopus*, the area around the central arteriole consists of small lymphocytes but there are also a small number of large cells with a well-developed rough endoplasmic reticulum (Obara *et al.*, 1982). Outside this area as well as in the red pulp, a number of plasma cells were found; they appeared to be more mature. In *Bufo calamita* increased numbers of lymphoid follicles, blast cells and mature plasma cells characterize this specific immune response (Barrutia *et al.*, 1985a). Numerous blast cells and medium lymphocytes occur in the red pulp near the marginal zone after primary immunization, a primitive feature reported in other anurans (Diener and Nossal, 1966; Manning and Turner, 1972; Moticka *et al.*, 1973; Turner and Manning, 1973). Increased numbers of mature plasma cells, some of them in the sinusoids, appeared also in the red pulp, a finding which agrees with observations of Borysenko (1976a, b) and Leceta (1984) in turtles.

Activities of Immune Cells

Conditions for Cell Culture

Anuran splenic cells produce antibodies which can be

detected by analyzing immunofluorescence patterns (Kent et al., 1964; Evans et al., 1966) and by enumerating plaque-forming cells (Moticka et al., 1973). In *Alytes obstetricans* Du Pasquier (1970) demonstrated specific PFC production in larval spleen when each tadpole only possessed less than one million lymphocytes. Furthermore, splenic cells could be stimulated by mitogen, showed mixed lymphocyte reactivity (Wright et al., 1978) and expressed delayed hypersensitivity reactions *in vitro*, as determined by macrophage migration inhibition tests (Ambrosius and Drossler, 1972; Rimmer and Gearing, 1980). The finding of stimulation by certain mitogens must, like all experimental results, be viewed critically. Proliferation of splenocytes from adult *Xenopus* cultured with commercial (Difco) lipopolysaccharide (LPS) from *S. abortus equii* largely (if not exclusively) appears to reflect a response to non-LPS contaminants in the commercial preparation (Bleicher et al., 1983). Thus whether the polyclonal activating property of commercial LPS is affected by LPS *per se* or results from a contaminant is unknown.

Monoclonal Antibodies and Cell Responses

In contrast, Bleicher and Cohen (1981), using a monoclonal antibody to *Xenopus* IgM to deplete surface IgM-positive lymphocytes from spleen cell suspensions, showed that responses of spleen cells to PHA, Con A and allogeneic cells are associated with sIgM-negative lymphocytes. Moreover, Nagata (1986b) has studied the role played by XT-1$^+$ and XT-1$^-$ cells in *in vitro* proliferative responses of *Xenopus* splenic cells. Early larval thymectomy depleted XT-1$^+$ lymphocytes in the spleen (Nagata, 1986a) and completely abrogated the *in vitro* splenic responses to PHA, Con A and allogeneic cells in MLC (Green and Cohen, 1979; Bleicher et al., 1983). Depletion of XT-1$^+$ lymphocytes by cell affinity chromatography on a protein A-Sepharose column produces still 3–6% XT-1$^+$ lymphocytes in the non-adherent spleen cell fraction and only partially eliminates the proliferative response (Nagata, 1986b). Although this small proportion of XT-1$^+$ cells could be responsible for generating considerable levels of PHA, Con A and MLC responses, it seems more likely that XT-1$^-$ splenic cells are reactive under those conditions. Results from costimulation experiments suggest either that Con A

reactive cells are XT-1$^-$ or that there is an interaction between XT-1$^+$ and XT-1$^-$ cells that enhances cell proliferation during normal Con A responses. In any case Nagata's results support the view that there is a difference in cell types required for PHA/MLC and Con A responses by *Xenopus* spleen cells.

Behavior of Alloreactive Cells

Alloreactive cells demonstrated by transfer and autoradiographic studies (Horton et al., 1977) as well as graft-versus-host reactive cells have been found in the anuran spleen (Clark and Newth, 1972; Brown et al., 1975). Other workers, however, failed to restore the capacity for allograft rejection in irradiated larvae after autologous spleen cell transfers (Brown and Cooper, 1976). Furthermore, spleen and thymic implants in larval *Xenopus* can suppress the timing of initiation and intensity of allograft rejection. The spleen is more effective than the thymus, which suggests the presence of suppressor lymphocytes in both organs (Ruben et al., 1972). Suppressor activity in *Xenopus* is antigen dependent and partially antigen specific but not MHC restricted (Ruben et al., 1983), while helper function is genetically restricted by the MHC (Bernard et al., 1981). Despite all these capacities, splenectomy in general has no marked effects on anuran immunological responses. Thus splenectomy does not affect allograft rejection (Brown and Cooper, 1976) and antibody production usually remains efficient (Turner, 1973) except against high antigenic doses in *Xenopus* (Collie and Turner, 1975) or in *Rana catesbeiana* larvae, where a reduction was found (Brown and Cooper, 1976).

T-Cell Growth Factor

T-cell growth factor (TCGF)-like stimulatory molecules associated with a 20–40-kD fraction have been obtained from serum-free supernatants from PHA-stimulated cultures of adult *Xenopus* splenocytes (Cohen et al., 1987). These supernatants induce proliferation of adult splenic and thymic T-lymphoblasts, costimulate (with PHA) adult thymocytes and support the continued growth of alloreactive T-cell lines (Watkins, 1985; Watkins and Cohen, 1985). According to previous results, larval spleens but not thymuses in *Xenopus* had significant numbers of

TCGF-producing cells (Rollins-Smith *et al.*, 1984). Moreover, Langeberg *et al.* (1987b) have characterized subpopulations of *Xenopus* splenocytes which bind an anti-human IL-2 receptor antibody (anti-Tac) and recombinant DNA-produced IL-2 (rIL-2). According to their protocol, a PHA/IL-2-sensitive splenocyte population is removed by injecting *N*-methyl-*N*-nitrosourea (NMU), a drug which removes the thymic cortex and other lymphocytes throughout the body and requires helper and cytotoxic cell functions. Many of the remaining NMU-insensitive cells are Tac positive but fail to bind rIL-2. In contrast, splenocytes with constitutive IL-2 receptor can be found by panning in both the sIg$^-$ and sIg$^+$ populations (Langeberg *et al.*, 1987a).

Both populations can bind the ligand with equal efficiency. Nevertheless our colleagues suggest that the predominant PHA-activatable rIL-2-binding cell populations are T-cells involved in helper and cytotoxic function (Langeberg *et al.*, 1987b). Previous work by the same group indicates that the IL-2 receptor on *Xenopus* splenocytes is not identical to its mammalian homologue (Langeberg *et al.*, 1987a). Furthermore *Xenopus* cells contain constitutive receptors. This fact could be related, according to these workers, to a special requirement of these ectotherms to respond to a myriad of pathogens present in both aqueous and terrestrial environments, although they could have been characteristic of ancestral forms which utilized similar autologous immune mediators and their relevant receptors (Langeberg *et al.*, 1987a).

REPTILES

Histology and Ontogeny—Light Microscopy

The spleen of reptiles shows important histological changes when compared to its condition in other more primitive vertebrates. These include increasing compartmentalization in some families, which suggests some specialization in the reptilian immune system, although germinal centers are apparently not evident. Anatomical and histological studies on reptilian spleens have revealed substantial variation from species to species relative to size, shape, anatomical location and histological organization. The spleen in general is a large heavily encapsulated lymphoid organ

associated with the systemic blood circulation (Krause, 1921; Murata, 1959; Evans *et al.*, 1965; Schubart, 1966; Marchalonis *et al.*, 1969; Miller, 1969; Tischendorf, 1969; Borysenko and Cooper, 1972; Wetherall and Turner, 1972; Kanakambika and Muthukkarruppan, 1973; Borysenko, 1975, 1976a; Hussein *et al.*, 1978a, b, 1979a, b; Pitchappan, 1980; Zapata *et al.*, 1981a; Kroese and van Rooijen, 1982; Kroese *et al.*, 1985; Leceta and Zapata, 1985). However, there are differences that may be due in part to seasonal variations which affect reptilian lymphoid organs (Muthukkaruppan *et al.*, 1982; Leceta and Zapata, 1985, see also Chapter 9). In fact, seasonal changes are emerging as a seemingly general characteristic of all vertebrate immune systems. This phenomenon alone brings the immune and neuroendocrine systems in close functional collaboration.

Ontogenesis has been analyzed histologically in two lizards, *Calotes versicolor* (Pitchappan and Muthukkaruppan, 1977a) and *Chalcides ocellatus* (El Deeb *et al.*, 1985), and in a turtle, *Chelydra serpentina* (Borysenko, 1978). Splenic histogenesis commences with a thickening of the dorsal mesogastrium, where a closely aggregated mass of mesenchymal elements occurs. Later this mass is well vascularized and contains blood sinuses which appear as separate cavities in the mesenchyme. During early phases of development, the spleen, before becoming lymphopoietic, contains a large number of granulocytes arranged between a syncytial network of mesenchymal cells. During subsequent stages, splenic lymphopoietic activity increases, producing as a result large, medium and small lymphocytes which finally form the first lymphoid aggregates which serve as precursors to organized white pulp. Because of this level of development, the first plasma cells in *Chelydra serpentina* appear around the time of hatching (Borysenko, 1978).

In some reptilian species, the spleen is composed primarily of white pulp, whereas in others both the red and white pulp are well developed (Murata, 1959; Evans *et al.*, 1965; Marchalonis *et al.*, 1969; Wetherall and Turner, 1972; Kanakambika and Muthukkaruppan, 1973; Borysenko, 1976a; Zapata *et al.*, 1981a; Kroese and van Rooijen, 1982). In several lizards, the white pulp is not well demarcated and the red pulp consists of narrow strands of blood sinuses between confluent areas of white pulp. The spleens of the lizard *Calotes versicolor* (Pitchappan

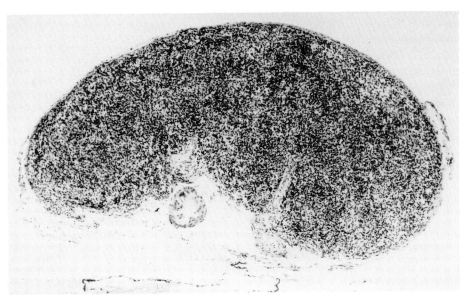

Figure 6.32 Spleen of *Lacerta hispanica*. Lymphoid aggregates are densely stained and scattered throughout the parenchyma (× 60).

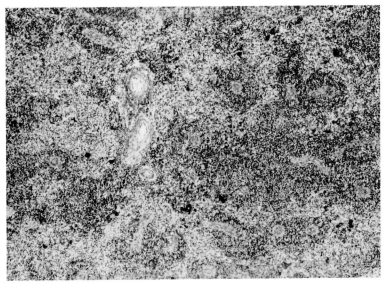

Figure 6.33 Spleen of the turtle *Mauremys caspica*. Note large lymphoid aggregates which form the white pulp (× 100).

and Muthukkaruppan, 1977a) and the snake *Phyton reticulatus* (Kroese *et al.*, 1985) contain trabeculae composed of dense connective tissue which divides the splenic parenchyma into a few lobes.

A similar arrangement of lymphoid tissue occurs in the spleens of chelonians (Murata, 1959, in *Amyda japonica* and *Clemmys japonica*; Borysenko and Cooper, 1972; Borysenko, 1976a, in *Chelydra serpentina*; Zapata *et al.*, 1981a, in *Mauremys caspica*). It shows a definitive demarcation into a red and white pulp. The white pulp consists of two types of lymphoid tissue called the periarteriolar lymphoid sheath (PALS) and the ellipsoids, the so-called peri-ellipsoidal lymphoid sheath (PELS) (Figure 6.32, 6.33). Both PALS and PELS occur and form two distinct compartments. This compartmentalization is also reflected in how reticular fibers, the supporting framework, are distributed. In *Chrysemys scripta elegans* reticular fibers are found throughout PALS but are absent in PELS (Kroese and van Rooijen, 1982), while in *Mauremys caspica* PALS contains a regular reticular network (Figure 6.34) and PELS comprises an inner region devoid of reticular fibers and an outer

one with reticular fibers arranged circumferentially (Figure 6.35) (see also Zapata *et al.*, 1981a).

The splenic white pulp is organized differently in other reptilian orders. In Squamata and in the Tautara, white pulp is located only around a central arteriole (Murata, 1959; Marchalonis *et al.*, 1969; Wetherall and Turner, 1972; Kanakambika and Muthukkaruppan, 1973; Hussein *et al.*, 1978a, b, 1979a, b). A central arteriole is, however, not found in the snake *Elaphe quadrivirgata* (Murata, 1959). In *Python reticulatus*, the white pulp consists of lymphoid tissue arranged around a kind of 'central arteriole', although these vessels are often difficult to see. Smaller branches of central arterioles are extended towards the periphery to open into the sinusoids of red pulp. Thus ellipsoids could be absent in the spleen of lizards and snakes (Murata, 1959; Tischendorf, 1967), although sheathed capillaries have been reported in spleens of the lizard *Uromastyx aegyptia* (Hussein *et al.*, 1978b); they were not encircled by lymphocytes as in chelonians. Furthermore, Weiss (1972) found a similar organization to that described in chelonian spleens in an unidentified lizard. In contrast, ellipsoids

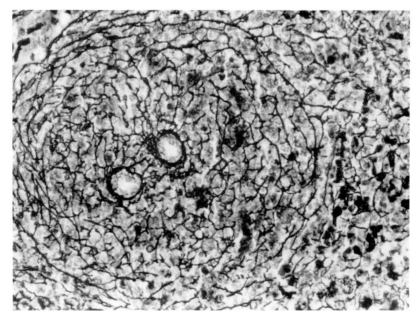

Figure 6.34 Arrangement of reticular fibers demonstrated by silver impregnation in periarteriolar lymphoid sheaths (PALS) in white pulp of the turtle *Mauremys caspica* (× 125).

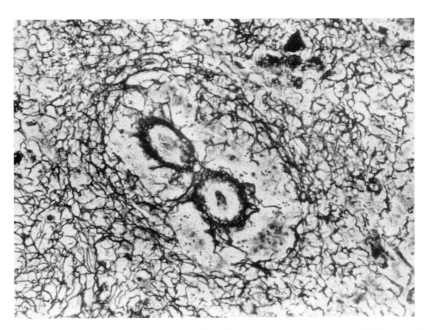

Figure 6.35 Arrangement of reticular fibers demonstrated by silver impregnation in the periellipsoidal lymphoid sheaths (PELS) in white pulp from the turtle *Mauremys caspica*. Note an inner area devoid of fibers and an outer region rich in fibers (× 240).

have not been observed in spleens of the turtles *Lessemys punctatus* and *Chelydra serpentina*, although reticular cells enclose a central arteriole which is surrounded by lymphoid cells. This could represent true ellipsoids with their corresponding lymphoid sheath. In conclusion, these results suggest an evolutionary trend for the histological structure of the spleen in reptiles. It culminates in chelonians, where some compartmentalization of the white pulp occurs.

Lymphoid components in the spleen of *Mauremys caspica*, as revealed by electron microscopy, consist mainly of lymphocytes and plasma cells which appear to be associated with various non-lymphoid cells. These include interdigitating cells, dendritic cells and macrophages which are probably involved in antigen trapping and processing. Stromal support is provided by a network of reticular cells and fibers (Figure 6.35). The specific arrangements of all these components vary in distinct splenic areas. In PALS small lymphocytes, lymphoblasts and interdigitating cells predominate (Figure 6.36). Ultrastructural characteristics of the splenic IDCS agree with those described earlier for

the IDCS in the turtle thymus but in the spleen they frequently contain engulfed intracytoplasmic material that has been phagocytosed, which suggests some phagocytic capacity. In PELS, ultrastructural analysis confirms the existence of two— an inner and an outer zone— as demonstrated by silver impregnation. In the inner zone of PELS small and medium lymphocytes are associated with large dendritic cells whose morphology resembles that of antigen-presenting cells found in peripheral lymphoid organs of higher vertebrates (Figure 6.37).

The outer zone, by contrast, contains less lymphoid tissue but reticular cells and macrophages abound (Figure 6.38). Between both zones of PELS there is a discontinuous layer formed by flat reticular cell processes (Figure 6.38). A similar layer of reticular cells interposed between the arteriole and the lymphocyte sheath and the marginal zone has been reported in lizards (Pitchappan and Muthukkaruppan, 1977a). A layer of reticular cells which also constitutes a limit between the splenic red and white pulp has been observed in various reptiles, which suggests a phylo-

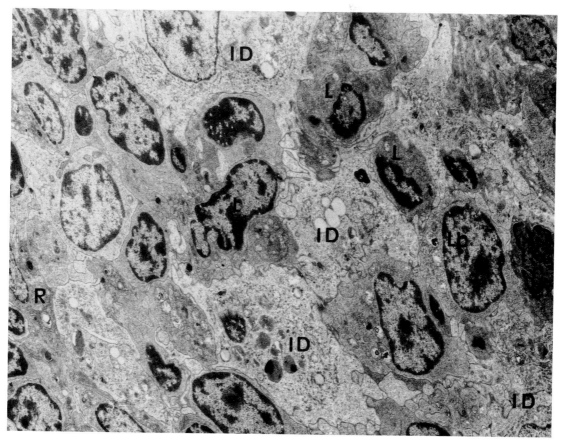

Figure 6.36 Ultrastructure of PALS in the spleen *Mauremys caspica*. Note the presence of mature interdigitating cells (ID) between small lymphocytes (L), lymphoblasts (Lb) and reticular cells (R) ($\times$ 5510).

genetic relationship with the mammalian marginal zone (Kroese and van Rooijen, 1982; Zapata *et al.*, 1981a; Muthukkaruppan *et al.*, 1982). In this area, as revealed by our images, phagocytic cells have been found (Kanakambika and Muthukkaruppan, 1973 in *Calotes versicolor*; Borysenko, 1975 in *Chelydra serpentina*; Kroese and van Rooijen, 1983 in *Chrysemys scripta elegans*). The increasing compartmentalization of the reptilian spleen as revealed at both the histological and cytological levels raises the question of whether the separated compartments have their own specialized functions in the immune response. Some available data on the specific distribution of lymphocyte subpopulations in distinct areas and the mechanism of antigen trapping support this hypothesis.

Activities of Immune Cells

Ig-positive Cells

Apparently 50% of reptilian splenocytes are sIgM-positive cells, as demonstrated by immunofluorescence using anti-IgM heteroserum (Kawaguchi *et al.*, 1980 in *Elaphe quadrivirgata*; Muthukkaruppan *et al.*, 1982; Natarajan and Muthukkaruppan, 1985 in *Calotes versicolor*; Mead and Borysenko, 1984a, b in *Chelydra serpentina*). A small number of lymphocytes also express sIgM and sIgY simultaneously since IgY is the second Ig class in reptiles (Natarajan and Muthukkaruppan, 1985). Fiebig and Ambrosius (1976) have identified it immunochemically on the surfaces of tortoise splenocytes. There is another approach to identifying Ig cells. A heterologous anti-

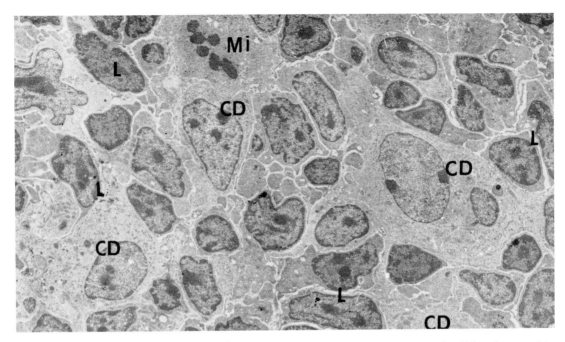

Figure 6.37 Cell component of the inner area of PELS in the spleen of *Mauremys caspica*. Small lymphocytes (L) and lymphoblasts, some in mitosis (Mi), appear scattered between large dendritic cells (CD) (× 3800).

serum has been raised in rabbits against *Chalcides ocellatus* thymocytes absorbed with lizard erythrocytes, kidney and liver cells. In the presence of guinea-pig complement, this antibody will selectively kill 50% of splenic cells (El Ridi and Kandil, 1981). Turning to the condition during development, in this same species El Deeb (1983) found that approximately 80–90% of embryonic splenocytes showed surface membrane components recognized by a heterologous antiserum which reacted with both embryonic and adult thymocytes. These cells appear early in the embryonic spleen and their proportions remained almost constant until birth. Moreover 40–50% of splenic lymphocytes were cIg and sIg positive and they decreased in number as embryos grew (El Deeb, 1983).

Preliminary observations suggest that splenic PALS of reptiles consists predominantly of T-cells, whereas in PELS B-lymphocytes are more abundant. In the lizard *Calotes versicolor*, adult thymectomy or treatment with rabbit anti-*Calotes* thymocyte serum results in severe depletion of the white pulp. During lymphoid regeneration the juxta-arteriolar region is repopulated by medium and then small lymphocytes (Pitchappan and Muthukkaruppan, 1977a). Staining of cryostat sections of the spleen of *Mauremys caspica* with an anti-IgM heteroserum by indirect immunohistochemical methods demonstrated high numbers of Ig-positive cells in the inner zone of PELS and others scattered at random throughout the outer zone. Ig-positive lymphocytes were, however, totally absent from the PALS, although some cytoplasmic Ig-positive, presumably plasma cells were found scattered throughout (Leceta and Zapata, unpublished). In *Chelydra serpentina*, adults after thymic involution exhibit some lymphoid cell depletion in the juxta-arteriolar region, whereas in juveniles there is a continuous sheath of lymphoid cells from the arteriole to the marginal zone (Borysenko and Cooper, 1972). Moreover, in humoral responses, lymphoblast and plasma cell development in the spleen basically occur in the outer lymphocyte sheath which extends into the red pulp (Borysenko, 1976a).

Strong primary responses have been observed after

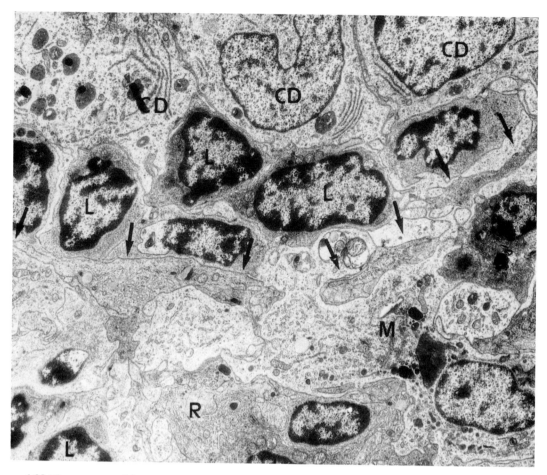

Figure 6.38 Ultrastructure of the outer area of PELS in the spleen of *Mauremys caspica*. Small lymphocytes (L) occur together with dendritic cells (CD) near a marginal zone formed by flattened processes of reticular cells (R). Note a macrophage (M) migrating through a gap in the marginal zone (× 7000).

stimulating lizards with SRBC (Kanakambika and Muthukkaruppan, 1972a) and turtles with keyhole limpet hemocyanin (KLH) (Borysenko 1976a, b). After antigenic stimulation a marked increase in lymphoblasts which differentiate into plasma cells occurs in white pulp of *Chelydra serpentina* (Borysenko, 1976b). Following an apparent migration of cells from the white to the red pulp, plasma cells, in various stages of development, appear in the red pulp cords and sinuses. A large number of immature macrophages and monocytes have also been observed in immunized spleens (Borysenko, 1976b). Although in both of these cases further antigenic challenge elicited no new

proliferative responses, the situation is different in *Mauremys caspica* following a second challenge three months after a primary immunization with SRBC. This elicited a greater increase in splenic lymphoid tissues mainly ten days after immunization (Zapata *et al.*, 1981b). Furthermore this greater increase was affecting mostly PELS (Leceta and Zapata, 1986). Some of this variability may be due to other factors. Evidently most reptiles when challenged with potent antigens and maintained in optimal conditions produce good secondary responses (Lerch *et al.*, 1967; Ambrosius *et al.*, 1970; Wetherall and Turner, 1972; Wright and Shapiro, 1973; Muthukkaruppan *et al.*, 1982).

Non-lymphoid Dendritic Cells

Trapping of immune complexes by non-lymphoid dendritic cells has been observed in spleens of *Chrysemys scripta elegans* (Kroese and van Rooijen, 1983) and *Phyton reticulatus* (Kroese *et al.*, 1985) using peroxidase – antiperoxidase complexes. Dendritic cells seem to retain the immune complexes on their external surfaces but some have been found within the cytoplasm by electron microscopy. From a morphological viewpoint, the dendritic cells of reptilian spleens closely resemble mammalian follicular cells (Chen *et al.*, 1978). These cells extend their processes between the surrounding lymphocytes; their nucleus is large, often lobulated and the cytoplasm contains no phagolysosomes. In *Mauremys caspica* dendritic cells form cell clusters with neighboring lymphocytes (Zapata *et al.*, 1981b). Dendritic cells have little phagocytic capacity (Kroese and van Rooijen, 1983; Kroese *et al.*, 1985; Leceta and Zapata, unpublished observations), are weakly positive for acid phosphatase but negative for non-specific esterase and ATPase (Kroese *et al.*, 1985).

These data confirm the antigen-trapping capacity of vertebrate spleens, which include those of fish, amphibians and reptiles where germinal centers are absent. However, during evolution, splenic morphology has changed considerably. It shows increased levels of compartmentalization in the white pulp, a development which seems to correlate well with the appearance of a more delimited 'antigen-trapping compartment'. Thus, Kroese and van Rooijen (1983) have demonstrated that trapping of peroxidase – antiperoxidase immune complexes is restricted exclusively to the PELS of *Chrysemys scripta elegans*. In PELS of *Mauremys caspica* there are cells identifiable ultrastructurally as dendritic. In the snake *Python reticulatus*, where histologically distinct areas are found, antigen-trapping dendritic cells, although present throughout the white pulp, are more prominent at the outer border (Kroese *et al.*, 1985). The condition is different in mammals, where follicular dendritic cells are involved in generating germinal centers (Klaus *et al.*, 1980). In ectothermic vertebrates germinal centers are lacking despite the existence of dendritic cells which trap immune complexes. Whether this condition creates a less efficient immune response particularly with respect to eliciting anamnestic responses is unknown.

Function of the Spleen in Immune Responses

General Considerations

Reptiles show humoral and cell-mediated immune responses but the role played by the various lymphoid organs, mainly the spleen, in each response is unclear and may be species specific (Muthukkaruppan *et al.*, 1982). Reptiles respond to a variety of antigens, including proteins (Evans, 1963; Ambrosius and Lehmann, 1965; Grey, 1966; Lerch *et al.*, 1967; Lykakis, 1968), bacteria (Evans, 1963; Maung, 1963) and heterologous erythrocytes (Rothe and Ambrosius, 1968). Kinetics of antibody responses have been investigated in spleens of several lizards and snakes (Muthukkaruppan *et al.*, 1982). There is a wide range of variability which depends on the nature of antigen, dose, route of injection, temperature, type of assays used to detect responses, species as well as reproductive and seasonal cycles (Cohen, 1971). As an example utilizing the Jerne plaque assay, antibody-forming cells have been identified in the spleen of chelonians (Rothe and Ambrosius, 1968; Sidky and Auerbach, 1968; Kassin and Pevenitskii, 1969) and lizards (Kanakambika and Muthukkaruppan, 1972a; Subramonia Pillai, 1977).

Cell-mediated Immune Responses

Spleen cells are capable of typical cell-mediated immune responses such as mixed lymphocyte reactions and graft-versus-host reactions. Vigorous proliferation in random one- and two-way MLC combinations has been observed using spleen cells derived from various reptilian groups (Cuchens and Clem, 1979 in *Alligator mississippiensis*; Saad and El Ridi, 1984 in *Chalcides ocellatus*; Farag and El Ridi, 1985 in *Spalerosophis diadema*). In addition, Farag and El Ridi (1985) have emphasized that whereas macrophages of the stimulator cell genotype are of little importance, macrophages autologous to the responding cells apparently play a major role in mixed lymphocyte reactions of snakes, probably as accessory cells. Lymphoproliferative responses to allogeneic cells can occur in reptiles, a finding which is also supported by the results of graft-versus-host reaction experiments in turtles and lizards (Borysenko and Tulipan, 1973; Badir *et al.*, 1981; El Ghareeb *et al.*, 1983; Saad and El Ridi, 1984).

Splenic lymphocytes undergo strong proliferative responses after mitogenic stimulation (Cuchens and Clem, 1979 in *Alligator mississippiensis*; Farag and El Ridi, 1986 in *Psammophis sibilans*; Saad *et al.*, 1987 in *Chalcides ocellatus*; El Ridi *et al.*, 1987 in *Spalerosophis diadema*). Recently a soluble lymphokine has been found in conditioned medium derived from snake splenocytes which had been activated previously by Con A (El Ridi *et al.*, 1987a). Apparently this IL2-like molecule of *Spalerosophis diadema* does not differ significantly from IL-2 of other vertebrates with respect to either charge heterogeneity or biological and biochemical properties. Thus, it possesses a molecular weight of approximately 15 000. The 39 − 42-kD form observed following Sephadex G-100 chromatography is apparently an aggregate, possibly a trimer. Finally isoelectric focusing of snake conditioned medium revealed the presence of two major IL-2 active forms of pI in ranges of 5.5 − 5.8 and 6.4 − 6.8, respectively (El Ridi *et al.*, 1987).

Splenectomy

Cell-mediated responses. The role of the spleen in the reptilian immune system has been analyzed employing the classical experimental approach of adult splenectomy. Splenectomy in *Calotes versicolor* did not impair skin allograft rejection or migration inhibition responses by peritoneal exudate cells using several doses of SRBC (Muthukkaruppan *et al.*, 1976a; Jayaraman and Muthukkaruppan, 1977, 1978a, b). In *Chalcides ocellatus*, however, adult splenectomy induced a significant prolongation of allograft survival time (El Masri, 1979).

Antibody production. A complete abrogation of antibody production has been reported in *Calotes versicolor* after immunization with SRBC or BSA administered five to seven days post-splenectomy, which suggests that the spleen is the major locus for generating antibody-producing cells in this species (Kanakambika and Muthukkaruppan, 1972b; Muthukkaruppan *et al.*, 1976b). Splenectomy does not prevent antibody production. Antigenic stimulation of splenectomized lizards with rat erythrocytes or HSA resulted in a strong antibody response with no significant differences in serum antibody titers between splenectomized, sham and non-operated controls (El Masri, 1979 in *Chalcides ocellatus*; Hussein *et al.*,

1979c in *Scincus scincus*). According to these results, immunological tasks are apparently shared in lizards between the spleen and other lymphoid organs. Some comparative immunologists have stressed the importance of gut-associated lymphoid tissue (GALT) because it is well developed in *Chalcides ocellatus* (Hussein *et al.*, 1978a) and *Scincus scincus* (Hussein *et al.*, 1979b), while others suggest an important role for bone marrow (Leceta and Zapata, 1986).

BIRDS

Introduction

Little attention has been paid to the structure and function of the avian spleen despite the known structural dichotomy between the T- and B-cell system of birds, exemplified morphologically by the thymus and bursa of Fabricius. We must remember that general studies of the vertebrate immune system have been driven by this discovery. Although the available data are restricted mainly to the chicken, there is some information that has been derived from analyzing aspects of lymphoid organs of, among others, the pigeon, the cowbird, the spotless starling, the weaver birds and the pied flycatcher.

Anatomy and Vascularization

The avian spleen is a reddish, ellipsoidal organ located on the right angle of the proventriculum. In the New Hampshire chicken strain, accessory spleens occur in one-third of the birds (Glick and Sato, 1964). They are located cranial, adjacent or caudal to the main spleen, and following splenectomy the cranial accessory spleen hypertrophies (Glick, 1970). The chicken spleen grows rapidly during the first six weeks after hatching, with maximum spleen-to-body weight ratio attained by ten weeks of age (Norton and Wolfe, 1949; Wolfe *et al.*, 1962).

The spleen is encapsulated by connective tissue below the mesothelial layer. Fibroblasts, some smooth muscle cells and abundant thick and thinner collagenous fibers form the capsule's connective tissue. Collagenous fibers within the inner layers of the capsule continue with the reticulum of the splenic parenchyma and with the reticular fibers which limit the subcapsular blood sinuses. Although some authors have pointed out that the avian spleen cannot undergo rhythmic changes in volume or that it stores blood, physiological (Fange and Nilsson, 1985) and experimental evidence (Herradon, 1987) demonstrates volume changes which involve the splenic capsule. On the other hand, a lack of trabeculae has been reported in some birds (Kaupp, 1918; Bradley, 1938; Ewart and McMillan, 1970), whereas in others their presence is well documented (Hartmann, 1930; Lucas *et al.*, 1954).

The vascularization of the avian spleen is extremely complex but its pattern probably governs the distribution of lymphoid tissue within the splenic parenchyma. This may explain in part the important differences which have been found between the avian and mammalian spleen. In any case unanswered questions on splenic vasculature in birds arise as a result of the organization and functional significance of the so-called Schweigger — Seidel sheaths or ellipsoids and their nature, i.e. open or closed. Detailed descriptions concerning the vascularization of avian spleen, with special emphasis on the ellipsoidal organization, have been reported extensively by light microscopy (Billroth, 1857; Muller, 1865; Whiting, 1897; Greschick, 1915; Klemperer, 1938; Ewart and McMillan, 1970; Hoshi, 1972; Dustin, 1975; Fange and Silverin, 1985) and recently its ultrastructure has been analyzed (Hoshi and Mori, 1975; Miyamoto *et al.*, 1980; Olah and Glick, 1982).

The avian spleen is supplied by several ramifications of the coeliac artery called primary arteries, which gain entrance into it through the hilum. New ramifications from the primary arteries give off secondary and then tertiary arteries. Gradually the number of muscle layers and the amount of connective tissue which surrounds the blood vessels diminishes. The tertiary arteries give off five or six central (terminal) arterioles, the walls of which contain no more than one or two layers of smooth muscle cells in the tunica media. The wall of the central arteriole undergoes an abrupt change and forms the penicilliform capillaries, in which the muscle layer is lacking, and the cuboidal endothelial cells appear to be surrounded by a thick fibrous connective tissue layer (Figure 6.39).

In the penicilliform capillary we can distinguish three regions (Diagram 6.1). The proximal one is the shortest and is devoid of a muscle layer. The mid-

portion is larger and can bifurcate three or four times. It is characterized by a change in the morphology of endothelial cells, which become higher and sometimes bulge into the lumen. A thick layer of connective tissue fibers with fenestrations (which will be commented upon later) surrounds the endothelium in this portion, which represents the so-called ellipsoid. In this region, unmyelinated nerve fibers have been described in the chicken (Olah and Glick, 1982). The distal or terminal portion lined by gradually flattening endothelial cells branches many times before entering the red pulp. The penicilliform capillaries surround circumferentially the central artery from which they are derived. Therefore the ellipsoids are limited by the lymphoid tissue which surrounds the central artery, by other ellipsoids and by the red pulp, whose sinusoids are partially interspersed among the ellipsoids and the periarterial lymphoid sheath (PALS) (Diagram 6.2).

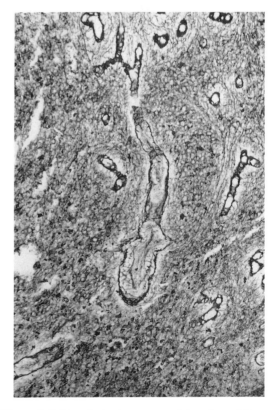

Figure 6.39 Vascularization pattern of the spleen of *Sturnus unicolor.* Central artery undergoes abrupt changes and forms penicilliform capillaries (silver impregnation) (× 212).

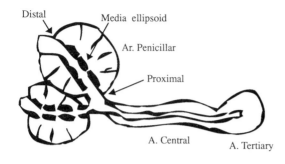

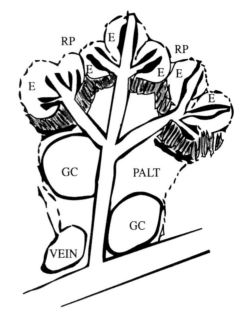

Diagrams 6.1, 6.2 Patterns of circulation in the red and white pulp.

The red pulp sinusoids are lined by flat endothelial cells surrounded by a thin layer of reticular fibers. According to their location, sinusoids join with either the subcapsular veins or artery-associated veins. Finally the subcapsular veins form radial veins which in turn join in to form a unique central vein leaving from the spleen through the hilar zone. This description corresponds to the vascular pattern in the spleen of the spotless starling, *Sturnus unicolor*, and for other avian species (Ewart and McMillan, 1970): the cowbird (Miyamoto *et al.*, 1980), chickens (Olah and Glick, 1982) and the pied flycatcher (Fange and Silverin, 1985).

In chickens, 11-day embryonic spleens contain sinusoidal blood vessels and a few developing arteries (Herradon, 1987). Incipient ellipsoids become evident at day 15 of incubation and on days 17 and 19 the vascular pattern of the embryonic spleen shows adult characteristics. Nerve endings occur in addition in the arteriolar walls of 17–19-day embryonic spleens (Herradon, 1987).

The functions of ellipsoids remain poorly understood, although they have been mainly related to mechanical or filtering processes. In mammals, they are absent in rodents, difficult to observe in humans and well delimited in the spleens of cats and dogs

(Dustin, 1975; Hatoe, 1978). The presence of cytoplasmic filaments in the endothelial cells of the ellipsoids in mammalian spleens suggests a sphincteric function which regulates blood flow into the splenic sinuses (Weiss, 1972; Dustin, 1975; Small and Sobieszek, 1977; Hatoe, 1978; Blue and Weiss, 1981a, b). Other authors who support this view have pointed out that ellipsoids serve also as a filtration apparatus (Solnitzky, 1937; Blanstein, 1963; Dustin, 1975; Ferguson, 1976; Hatoe, 1978; Graf and Schlons, 1979; Blue and Weiss, 1981a).

The localized thickening of macrophages in ellipsoidal walls (see later) and the aforementioned incomplete basement membrane around the capillaries may enable the ellipsoid to serve as a first filter for arterial blood. A similar proposal was claimed to exist in the avian spleen by Miyamoto *et al.* (1980). Moreover, intravascularly injected tracers (dyes, carbon, bacteria, parasites) promptly leave the circulation in these animals which have ellipsoids and only a very small amount of them passes into the red pulp (Blue and Weiss, 1981a). Later in this chapter we will review the proposed filtering function of the ellipsoidal blood vessel in relation to the mechanisms that govern antigen trapping and processing in the avian spleen. Finally, evidence for both an open (Fukuta *et al.*,

1969; Payne, 1971) and closed (Greschik, 1915; Fukuta et al., 1976) circulation in the avian spleen is now available. Apparently, however, both situations occur simultaneously (Ewart and McMillan, 1970; Miyamoto et al., 1980). Thus it appears that some ellipsoids empty into the reticular meshwork of the red pulp (open) while others may open directly into sinusoids (closed).

Histology—Cell Components

In the avian spleen, two easily distinguishable areas—the white and the red pulp—are present. The white pulp consists of collections of various-sized lymphocytes, plasma cells and accessory non-lymphoid cells associated with different portions of the vascular channels. This association characterizes distinct compartments: a periarteriolar (PALS) and perivenous lymphoid sheath which in addition contains germinal centers and a periellipsoidal lymphoid sheath (PELS) (Diagram 6.2; Figure 6.40). PALS occupies the areas around the central arteries up to the middle portion of the penicilliform capillaries. The perivenous lymphoid tissue occurs discontinuously along the course of the large veins in the red pulp, usually as nodular masses of lymphoid tissue. In fully developed chicken spleens, the perivenous lymphoid tissue is often continuous with or appears to be an extended portion of the PALS (Hoshi, 1972). Actually both PALS and perivenous lymphoid sheaths are morphologically similar, i.e. they are essentially T-dependent lymphoid areas (see later). PELS occurs in a less defined region around connective tissue walls of ellipsoids as two or three cell layers of mainly medium-sized lymphocytes, plasma cells and macrophages.

Periarteriolar and Perivenous Lymphoid Tissue

By electron microscopy the splenic PALS and perivenous lymphoid tissue consist of densely packed lymphoid elements including large, medium and small lymphocytes, scattered plasma cells and macrophages arranged in a meshwork of both electron-dense and -lucent reticular cells (Figure 6.41). Mitoses are frequent in large, pale lymphocytes and the limits with PELS are difficult to see. Fibrocyte-like reticular cells constitute the main supporting elements in PALS

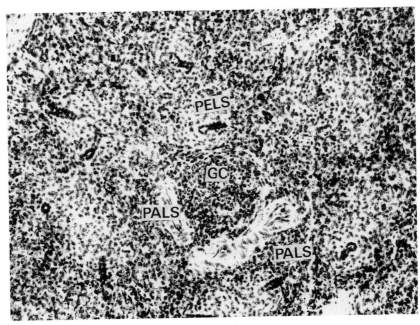

Figure 6.40 Distribution of lymphoid tissue in the spleen of *Sturnus unicolor*. Note the PELS, PALS and germinal centers (× 120).

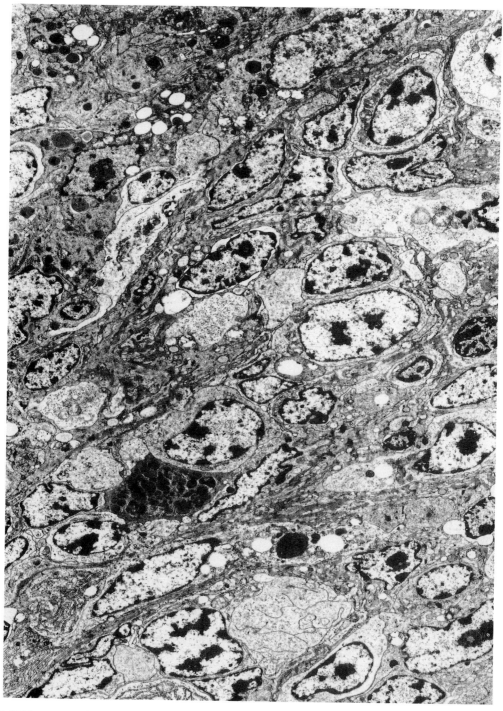

Figure 6.41 Ultrastructural organization of PALS. Note the distribution of lymphoid cells arranged in a reticular meshwork around the central artery. Pale and dark reticular cells constitute the supporting stroma of the parenchyma (× 6400).

(Figure 6.42). They are electron-lucent cells with a round or irregular nucleus which contains a few clumps of condensed chromatin arranged peripherally, with a pale cytoplasm where ribosomes and profiles of rough endoplasmic reticulum occur (Figure 6.42). The irregular processes of reticular cells frequently embrace areas of ground substance which contain reticular fibers.

Germinal Centers

Germinal centers have been found in PALS of avian spleen in association with tertiary arteries (Ewart and McMillan, 1970; Fange and Silverin, 1985), especially close to the bifurcating angle of these arteries within lymphoid tissue (Hoshi, 1972) (Diagram 6.2). They are delimited by a capsular tissue formed by reticular cells and fibers demonstrable by silver-staining methods (Ewart and McMillan, 1970;

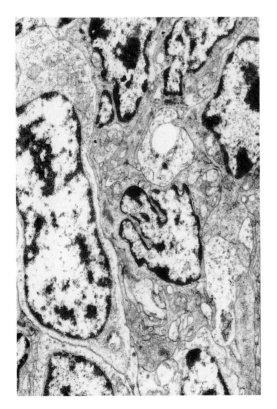

Figure 6.42 Pale reticular cell of the supporting stroma of PALS. Note its association with reticular fibers (× 10000).

Hoshi, 1972; Fange and Silverin, 1985) and confirmed ultrastructurally (Figure 6.43). It is remarkable that no vascular channels occur in them as in mammals (Hoshi, 1972; Olah and Glick, 1982), although Fange and Silverin (1985) claimed that in the spleen of *Ficedula hypolevca* they are penetrated by one to four small arteries and capillaries. On the contrary, small vessels appear which surround the germinal centers in the spleen of *Sturnus unicolor* (Figure 6.43) and in the cowbird spleen (Ewart and McMillan, 1970).

The connective tissue capsule which surrounds the germinal centers is formed by flat fibrocyte-like reticular cells which are continuous with the walls of an accompanying vessel (Figure 6.43). The supporting stroma of the germinal centers consists of reticular cells whose ultrastructure resembles that described for reticular cells of PALS, although association with reticular fibers is not easy to observe (Figure 6.44). Medium and large lymphocytes, some mature and developing plasma cells are the most abundant lymphoid components in the germinal centers of the spleen in *Sturnus unicolor* (Figure 6.44). Small lymphocytes are, however, few and a dark corona, as in mammalian germinal centers, is lacking in those of *Sturnus unicolor*, but it has been observed by light microscopy in *Ficedula hypolevca* (Fange and Silverin, 1985). Large macrophages occur also, with most showing abundant engulfed material equivalent to the tangible body macrophages of the mammalian germinal centers (Figure 6.44). Other non-lymphoid elements of germinal centers will be described later.

Germinal centers appear in the chicken spleen for the first time at about 4−5 weeks of age (Thorbecke *et al.*, 1957; Cooper *et al.*, 1965; Fukuta *et al.*, 1979). Fukuta *et al.* (1980) observed the formation of primary germinal centers in chicken spleen cells which arrive from PELS. This agrees with the migration of antigen-bearing cells which has been observed in chicken spleens immunized with human serum albumin (White *et al.*, 1970). After intravenous injections of SRBC in 21-day-old chickens, the antigen was trapped rapidly in the ellipsoids. The number of cells in the PALS was gradually depleted, leaving large pyroninophilic cells in the periphery of PALS four hours after injection; they then increased in number and migrated centrally toward PALS. On the fourth day they had accumulated in the vicinity of the central arteries, where they formed nodular structures. Morphologically mature

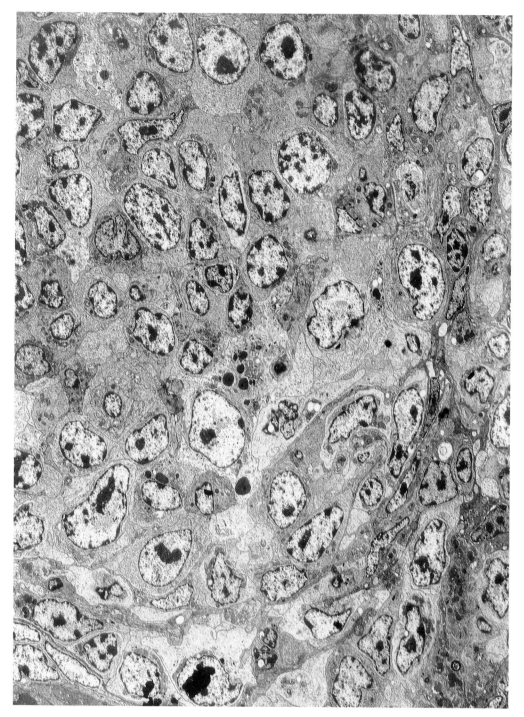

Figure 6.43 Encapsulated germinal centers in PALS of *Sturnus unicolor*. Note the absence of vascularization inside the germinal center. No dark lymphocytic corona occurs in the germinal center but lymphoblasts, plasma cells and tingible body macrophages are frequent (× 2800).

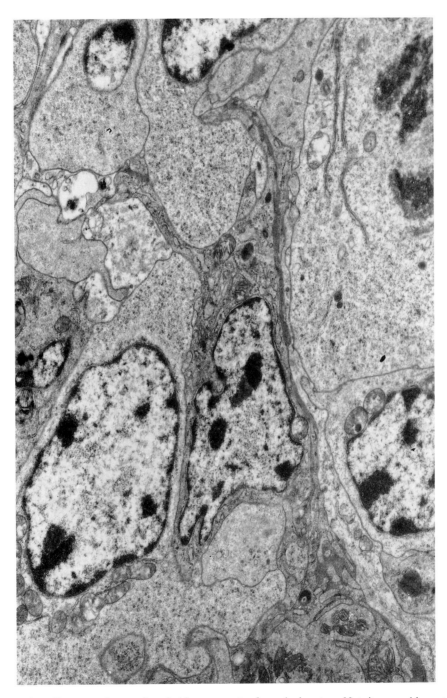

Figure 6.44 Reticular cells arranged among lymphoid components of germinal centers. Note its resemblance to the reticular cells of PALS but no association with reticular fibers was found ($\times$ 8250).

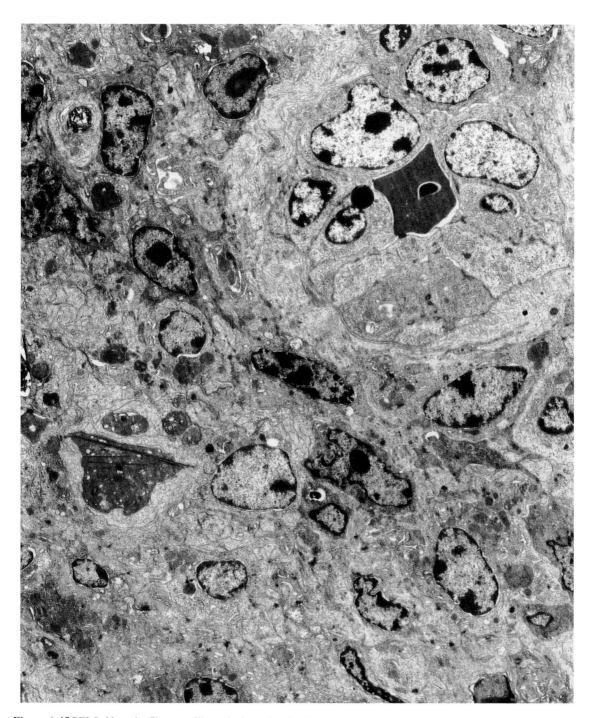

Figure 6.45 PELS. Note the fibrocyte-like reticular cell delimiting PELS and the presence of a few lymphoid components and crystalline inclusions containing macrophages ($\times$ 6000).

germinal centers encapsulated by connective tissue were found on the sixth day, became numerous on the eighth day but then decreased gradually. These same authors found decreased numbers of germinal centers after secondary immunization but these results require further confirmation (Fukuta *et al.*, 1979). We will review the antigen-trapping mechanism later, and the role different cell types play in this process and in the generation of germinal centers.

Ellipsoids— Periellipsoidal Lymphoid Sheaths

Different workers have commented on the presence of blast-like cells (Hoshi, 1972) or pyroninophilic cells (Fange and Silverin, 1985) in PELS of avian spleens. It is, however, important to distinguish between cells associated with ellipsoidal walls and lymphoid tissue which outlines the ellipsoids, the so-called PELS (see Diagram 6.2; Figure 6.45). Unfortunately authors who describe the avian spleen by light microscopy only refer to the cell content of PELS. However, recent electron microscopic analyses have revealed quite interesting non-lymphoid cells in the ellipsoidal walls (Olah and Glick, 1982).

In *Sturnus unicolor* the ellipsoidal sheaths are formed by a meshwork of reticular cells and reticular fibers arranged in the ground substance similar to those described in the PALS. Within spaces of the meshwork there are free cells which include mainly macro-phages, cells morphologically resembling those referred to as ellipsoid-associated cells (EAC) described in chicken spleens (Olah and Glick, 1982) and bursa of Fabricius (Olah and Glick, 1978; Olah *et al.*, 1979) and lymphoid cells (Figure 6.45). The spaces between closely neighboring ellipsoids (see Diagram 6.2) are occupied mainly by cells which become impregnated by techniques which use silver. At the electron microscopic level they appear as groups of flat reticular cells which delimit the ellipsoids laterally. Apparently ellipsoids are not fully encircled by PELS. Instead there is a close direct relationship between ellipsoids and red pulp, whereas a lymphoid tissue which represents the PELS is interposed between the ellipsoidal walls and PALS (Diagram 6.2).

The splenic PELS consists of macrophages, mature and developing plasma cells and large lymphocytes (Figure 6.45). Macrophages occur in these areas and

are completely filled by engulfed, globular debris of unknown significance, especially in some seasons of the year (Figure 6.46). Seasonal variations in lym-phoid organs of *Sturnus unicolor* have been previously reported (Fonfria *et al.*, 1983). Macrophages contain crystalline bars and bodies which result from the destruction of engulfed erythrocytes (Figure 6.45). In contrast, Olah and Glick (1982) did not observe many macrophages in and around chicken ellipsoids.

Cells which resemble ellipsoid-associated cells (EAC) occur in several locations in the splenic white pulp of *Sturnus unicolor*, in the ellipsoidal walls (Figure 6.47), PELS, PALS and germinal centers. A similar distribution occurs for chicken EACs (Olah and Glick, 1982; Olah *et al.*, 1984) and von Rautenfeld and Budras (1980) detected them in the avian germinal centers of the intestinal tonsils of *Gallus* and various other birds. The ultrastructure of EACs in *Sturnus unicolor* differs slightly in various locations. A point also reported by these other authors, for example in the ellipsoidal walls, is that they show short, thick cell processes (Figure 6.47) which resemble the ultrastruc-ture of cells that trap immune complexes in chicken ellipsoids (Eikelenboom *et al.*, 1983). The cytoplasm contains a moderate amount of electron-dense, large granules and an incipient Golgi complex. In contrast, EACs in PELS and germinal centers are more irregular, with long cell processes intermingled with neighboring lymphoid elements (Figures 6.48, 6.49). In addition, the number of cytoplasmic granules has increased, mainly in those cells which comprise PELS. On the other hand EAC-resembling cells have been demonstrated ultrastructurally in the outer zone of the ellipsoidal sheaths of 17−19-day embryonic spleens of chickens (Herrodon, 1987).

Finally, typical interdigitating cells occur in both PALS and PELS (Figures 6.50, 6.51). The presence of IDCs in the PALS of avian spleen agrees with numer-ous reports assuming a T-dependence for this area (see later description). However, it is remarkable to find them in a T-independent area such as PELS. In hamsters, presumptive pro-interdigitating cells have been identified and found migrating throughout the splenic marginal zone (de Cardenas, 1987), a region proposed to be related to avian PELS by some authors. From our information, the presence of interdigitating cells in avian spleen has not been observed but they have been described in the thymus (Kendall and

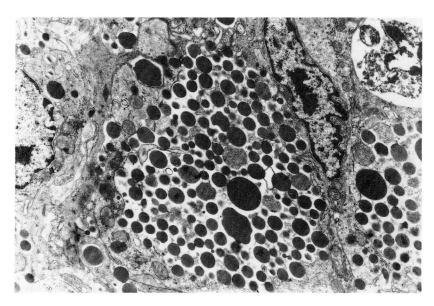

Figure 6.46 Macrophage in the border of PELS containing globular material which fully occupies its cytoplasm (× 1200).

Frazier, 1979; Fonfria *et al.*, 1982). The ultrastructural analysis of splenic interdigitating cells of *Sturnus unicolor* demonstrates numerous folds on the surface membrane, scarcity of cytoplasmic membranous organelles and phagocytic capacity exemplified by engulfed cell debris. This last feature has been reported also for interdigitating cells in turtles (Leceta *et al.*, 1984). The importance of these non-lymphoid cells in trapping antigenic and non-antigenic material in the avian spleen emerges from the repeatedly mentioned role of avian ellipsoids in this process. This is especially due to the extensive studies on the origin and functional significance of chicken EACs (Olah and Glick, 1982; Olah *et al.*, 1984, 1985; Glick and Olah, 1987).

Antigen-trapping Mechanisms

Immune complexes are segregated in the chicken ellipsoidal sheaths, taken up by non-lymphoid cells, reported as macrophages in the peripheral regions of the sheaths (White *et al.*, 1970). These cells migrate with the immune complexes through the white pulp and are subsequently found as dendritic cells within the germinal centers (White *et al.*, 1970). Similar results were found by Eikelenboom *et al.* (1983), who defined acid phosphatase-positive dendritic cells which contained considerable numbers of primary lysosomes but not phagolysosomes. They resemble mammalian follicular dendritic cells which are engaged in trapping chicken immune complexes. The authors also suggested a possible relationship between these cells and the marginal metallophils located at the inner border of the marginal zone (Snook, 1964; Streefkerk and Veerman, 1971; Eikelenboom, 1978a, b). Such a relationship has been pointed out by other authors (Olah and Glick, 1982; Fange and Silverin, 1985).

Eikelenboom *et al.* (1983) observed, nevertheless, some differences in the antigen-trapping process between mammals and birds. In chickens, the cell processes of trapping cells are shorter and thicker and the cells are dispersed throughout the germinal center, while in mammals these cells are mainly located in a special area of the germinal center, the so-called cap region at the border of the germinal center and another region, the corona. As mentioned earlier, a corona is lacking in the germinal centers in spleens of most birds.

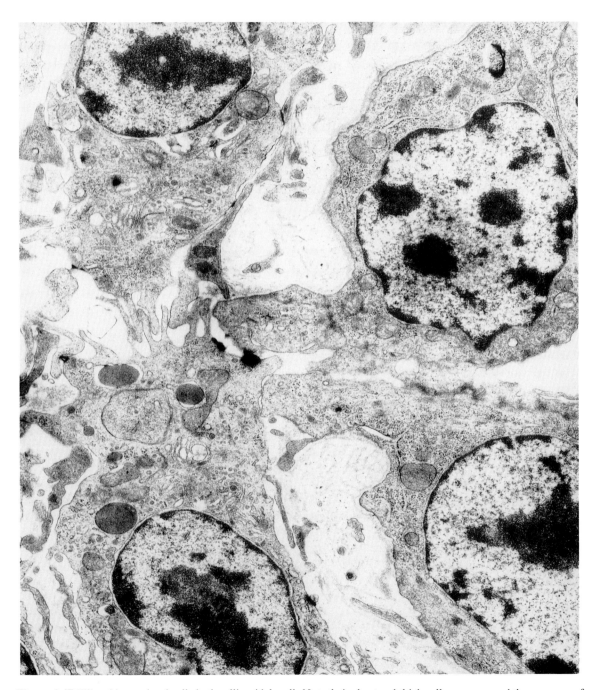

Figure 6.47 Ellipsoid-associated cells in the ellipsoidal wall. Note their short and thick cell processes and the presence of electron-dense, medium cytoplasmic granules (× 21 850).

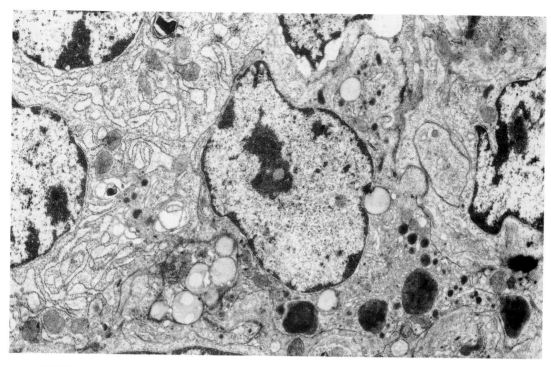

Figure 6.48 EAC in the PELS of *Sturnus unicolor*. Note increased cell processes and number of cytoplasmic granules (× 11 660).

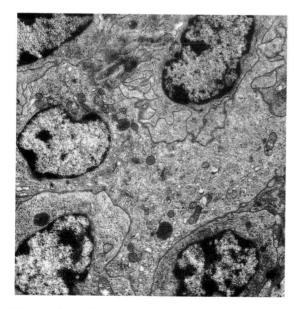

Figure 6.49 EAC in a germinal center of *Sturnus unicolor* (× 9600).

An important point of discussion is concerned with the mechanisms governing antigen distribution from the ellipsoids to germinal centers. Several authors found that immune complexes and deposits of carbon show, unlike in mammals, an identical pattern shortly after intravenous injection, but the distribution patterns differ some days later (White, 1969; Olah and Glick, 1982; Eikelenboom *et al.*, 1983; Olah *et al.*, 1984). Eikelenboom *et al.* (1983) consider that both immune complexes and non-antigenic particles are segregated on the periphery of ellipsoidal sheaths by a non-specific process. From here redistribution of both compounds may occur by simple diffusion. White suggested, however, that non-lymphoid cells in the periphery of ellipsoidal sheaths pick up immune complexes and migrate toward the follicles when they become follicular dendritic cells. Olah *et al.* (1984) identified these cells as EACs which do not discriminate between inert and immunogenetic substances and may enter the systemic circulation serving as antigenic messengers.

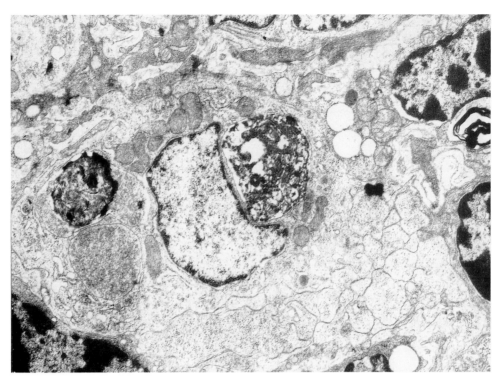

Figure 6.50 Mature interdigitating cell in PALS. Note the surface folds and the engulfed material in the cytoplasm (×
15 625).

According to their view EACs which are easily
detached from the ellipsoidal surface by carbon (Olah
and Glick, 1982), carrageen (Olah *et al.*, 1981) and
antigens (Olah *et al.*, 1984) after antigenic and non-
antigenic stimulation leave ellipsoidal walls to migrate
to red pulp, appearing later in the systemic circulation
as monocytes (Olah *et al.*, 1984), to the splenic PALS
and then to germinal centers (Olah and Glick, 1982). It
is not known whether the EACs migrate directly (without leaving the spleen) to PALS or whether they return
from the circulation.

Recently, it was proposed that the mesenchyme
which surrounds the embryonic bursa of Fabricius on
days 11–14 of incubation contains precursors for
secretory (dendritic EA) cells of both bursa and spleen
(Glick and Olah, 1987). This group had reported

previously that bursectomy impaired the capacity for
carbon binding of splenic EACs and restricted their
migration, suggesting furthermore that the decreased
numbers of germinal centers found in bursectomized
irradiated chickens (Cooper *et al.*, 1966) could be due
to an impaired functional capacity of EACs (Olah
et al., 1985). The results in the spleen of *Sturnus
unicolor* introduce a new dimension to these problems
since apparently cells with an assumed role in antigen-
trapping and processing, such as macrophages, EACs
and interdigitating cells, occur in ellipsoidal walls, but
also in red pulp, PELS, PALS and germinal centers.
Further experiments must be focused on the antigenic
and non-antigen trapping capacities of various non-
lymphoid cell populations in the spleen of *Sturnus
unicolor*.

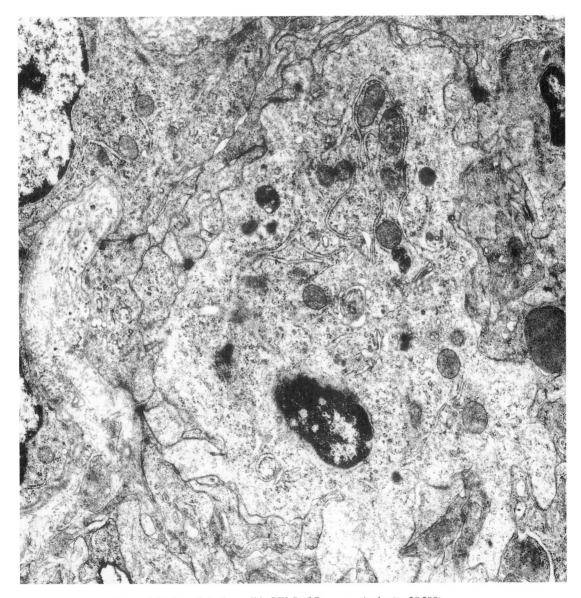

Figure 6.51 Interdigitating cell in PELS of *Sturnus unicolor* (× 20 500).

Ontogeny

The embryonic avian spleen is essentially a granulo-poietic organ since white pulp does not appear until after hatching (Lucas and Jamroz, 1961; De Lanney and Ebert, 1962; Mori and Hoshi, 1971; Hoshi, 1972; Sorell and Weiss, 1982; Boyd and Ward, 1984; Herradon, 1987). The splenic stroma is established from the seventh day of incubation, when reticular cells without associated reticular fibers appear (Fukuta and Mochizuchi, 1982). From the ninth day onward the intercellular spaces become occupied by a fine material which aggregates later and exhibits the characteristics of mature reticular fibers. A first delimitation into red and white pulp has been demonstrated in 18-day-old embryos (Boyd and Ward, 1984). Around the first day after hatching small lymphocytic aggregates occur around small arteries and veins (Hoshi, 1972; Boyd and Ward, 1984). There is a gradual increase in lymphoid elements which become nodular accumulations by day 10. They then resemble adult PALS and perivenous lymphoid sheaths (Hoshi, 1972).

Development of PELS begins when medium-sized lymphoid cells appear at the margins of ellipsoids at 2–3 days of age. Within a week these cells increase in number and become arranged in a single cell layer at the periphery of each ellipsoid. By the end of the second week two events occur: the development of PELS is basically accomplished, and immature, non-encapsulated germinal centers appear mainly on day 10 (Hoshi, 1972). Plasma cells, scattered at random throughout the splenic parenchyma, have been reported from days 5 or 6 (Hoshi, 1972). This documented increase in splenic lymphocytes following hatching is probably a consequence of their having been stimulated by external antigen to migrate (Kincade and Cooper, 1971; Back and Linna, 1973; Glaister, 1973; Milne *et al.*, 1975).

The ontogeny of bursa-dependent lymphoid tissue in chickens has been analyzed by using rabbit antisera specific for B-lymphocyte subpopulations and two components of the bursal microenvironment (Boyd and Ward, 1984). These investigators defined a chicken B-lymphocyte antigen (CBLA) which is expressed on 7% of 12-day-old embryonic spleen cells. These cells increased around hatching and represented 30% of the spleen in 3-week-old chickens.

Around hatching CBLA-positive cells were apparently localized in primitive PELS and also later in germinal centers. The time just after hatching represents a crucial period for two events: first, Ig-positive cells increase in the spleen, reaching adult levels by 3 weeks of age and appearing as CBLA-positive cells; second, by anti-IgG serum cells which appear in the splenic B-dependent areas. The development of a cell population defined by the so-called mature B-lymphocyte antigen (CMBLA) closely paralleled the appearance of IgG-positive cells. Day 18 embryonic and 1-day-old spleens had low levels of fetal-associated antigen (CEAA)-bearing cells but older ages were negative. Finally the fetal spleen specific antigen (CFSA) stained approximately 20% of 12- and 15-day embryo spleno-cytes, decreasing gradually until hatching when no fluorescence was observed.

Distribution of Lymphoid Populations

The histological compartmentalization in the avian spleen also has a counterpart when we consider the specific distribution of T- and B-lymphoid subpopulations, although finer aspects of this condition still remain to be clarified. Based upon morphological, immunohistochemical and autoradiographic studies in the chicken spleen, plasma cells and PELS are bursa dependent whereas PALS and the perivenous lymphoid tissue are regarded as thymus dependent (Isakovic and Jankovic, 1964; Jankovic and Isakovic, 1964; Cooper *et al.*, 1965, 1969; Weber and Weidanz, 1969; Nagy, 1970; Hoshi, 1972; Hoffman-Fezer *et al.*, 1977). In ducks, cyclophosphamide treatment (Hashimoto and Sugimura, 1976; Sugimura and Hashimoto, 1976) or bursectomy and irradiation (Sugimura and Hashimoto, 1980) depleted PELS, which confirms their bursal dependence. In contrast, germinal center formation seems to be mainly bursa dependent although interaction with the T-cell system is required (Toivanen and Toivanen, 1977).

Romppanen and Sorvari (1981) demonstrated a decrease in the lymphoid components of PALS in bursectomized chickens by morphometrical analysis. This discrepancy has been explained by the authors as due to a different sensitivity of morphometrical methods when compared to semi-quantitative techniques used by other workers. This difference is not without some support since, in fact, a few B-cells have also been observed in PALS (Krueff *et al.*, 1977; Hoffman-Fezer *et al.*, 1977), and thymectomized chickens do not show complete disappearance of PALS (Jankovic and Isakovic, 1964; Cooper *et al.*, 1965). Furthermore germinal centers are also located in the PALS. Finally, an indirect effect of the bursa through the thymus cannot be completely discarded since lymphoid traffic from the bursa to the thymus and then to the spleen has been reported (Woods and Linna, 1965; Hemmingsson and Linna, 1972). All these data, although difficult to compare with the situation in mammals, undoubtedly demonstrate a high level of efficiency and compartmentalization in immune functions of the avian spleen.

FINAL COMMENT

The spleen is a lymphoreticular organ which has unique morphological and functional features. It arises from a mesenchymal proliferation in the dorsal mesentery or mesogastrium. In the adult, one of its main functions is its imposition in the path of circulating blood, thus making it a very special filter. As a consequence of its anatomical position throughout the evolutionary scale, the spleen has the added responsibility of acting as a major component housing cells necessary in the immune response.

REFERENCES

Agius C (1979). The role of melano-macrophage centres in iron storage in normal and diseased fish. *J Fish Dis* **2**: 337–343.

Agius C (1980). Phylogenetic development of melano-macrophage centres in fish. *J Zool (Lond)* **191**: 11–31.

Agius C (1981a). The effects of splenectomy and subsequent starvation on the storage of haemosiderin by melano-macrophages of rainbow trout *Salmo gairdneri* Richardson. *J Fish Biol* **8**: 41–44.

Agius C (1981b). Preliminary studies on the ontogeny of the melano-macrophages of teleost haemopoietic tissues and age-related changes. *Dev Comp Immunol* **5**: 597–606.

Agius C (1983). On the failure to detect haemosiderin in the melano-macrophages of the dogfish *Scylorhinus caniculia* L. after prolonged starvation. *Experientia* **39**: 64–66.

Agius C and Agbede SA (1984). An electron microscopical study on the genesis of lipofucsin, melanin and haemosiderin in haemopoietic tissues of fish. *J Fish Biol* **24**: 471–488.

Agius C and Roberts RJ (1981). Effects of starvation on the melano-macrophage centres of fish. *J Fish Biol* **19**: 161–169.

Ambrosius HJ and Drossler K (1972). Spezifische zellvermittelte immunitat bei Froschlurchen. I. Quantitative nachweistechnick mit dem Makrophagen-Migrations-Hemmtest fur peritoneal exsudat zellen und Milzstucken. *Acta Biol Med Ger* **29**: 437–440.

Ambrosius HJ and Lehmann R (1965). Beitrage zur immunobiologie poikilothermer wirbeltiere. II. Immunologische untersuchungen an schildkroten *Testudo hermanni*. *Z Immunol Forsch Exp Ther* **128**: 81–104.

Ambrosius HJ, Hammerling R, Richter R and Schimke R (1970). Immunoglobulins and the dynamics of antibody formation in poikilothermic vertebrates (Pisces, Urodela, Reptilia). In Sterzl J and Riha I (Eds), *Developmental Aspects of Antibody Formation and Structure*. Vol II. Academic Press: New York. pp 727–744.

Anderson DP (1974). *Fish Immunology*. TFH Publ: Neptune.

Anderson DP (1978). Passive hemolytic plaque assay as a means for detecting antibody producing cells in rainbow trout immunized with the O-antigen of enteric redmouth bacteria. Doctoral thesis, University of Maryland.

Ardavin CF (1981). Tejido linfoide asociado al tubo digestivo en el anfibio urodelo *Pleurodeles waltlii*. Efecto de la immunizacion primaria y secundaria. MSc thesis, Faculty of Biology, Complutense University, Madrid.

Ardavin CF and Zapata A (1987). Ultrastructure and changes during metamorphosis of the lympho-hemopoietic tissue of the larval anadromous sea lamprey *Petromyzon marinus*. *Dev Comp Immunol* **11**: 79–94.

Bach R, Chen PK and Chapman GB (1978). Changes in the spleen of the catfish *Cetalurus punctatus* Rafinesque induced by infection with *Aeromonas hydrophila*. *J Fish Dis* **1**: 205–217.

Back R and Linna TJ (1973). Influence of antigenic stimulation on lymphoid cell traffic in the chicken. I. Increased homing of thymus-derived cells to the bone marrow after antigenic stimulation. *Arch Allergy Appl Immunol* **43**: 657–670.

Baculi BS and Cooper EL (1973). Lymphoid changes during antibody synthesis in larval *Rana catesbeiana*. *J Exp Zool* **183**: 185–192.

Badir N, Afifi A and El Ridi R (1981). Cell-mediated immunity in the gecko *Tarentola annularis*. *Folia Biol* **27**: 28–39.

Baldwin III WM (1983). Antigen trapping cells in *Xenopus laevis*: tissue distribution. *Dev Comp Immunol* **7**: 709–710.

Baldwin III WM and Cohen N (1981). A giant cell with dendritic cell properties in spleens of the anuran amphibian *Xenopus laevis*. *Dev Comp Immunol* **5**: 461–474.

Baldwin III WM and Sminia T (1982). Antigen trapping cells: advantages of phylogenetic studies. *Dev Comp Immunol* Suppl **2**: 59–67.

Balls M, Clothier R, Hodgson R and Berridge D (1980).

Effects of *N*-methyl-*N*-nitrosourea and cyclosporin A on the lymphocytes and immune responses of *Xenopus laevis* and other amphibians. In Horton JD (Ed), *Development and Differentiation of Vertebrate Lymphocytes*. Elsevier/North-Holland: Amsterdam. pp 183–184.

Barrutia MSG, Leceta J, Fonfria J, Garrido E and Zapata A (1983). Non-lymphoid cells of the anuran spleen: an ultrastructural study in the natterjack *Bufo calamita*. *Am J Anat* **167**: 83–94.

Barrutia MSG, Villena A, Gomariz RP, Rasquin B and Zapata A (1985a). Ultrastructural changes in the spleen of the natterjack *Bufo calamita* after antigenic stimulation. *Cell Tissue Res* **239**: 435–441.

Barrutia MSG, Villena A, Rasquin B. Gomariz RP and Zapata A (1985b). Presence of presumptive interdigitating cells in the spleen of the natterjack *Bufo calamita*. *Experientia* **41**: 1393–1394.

Bernard CCA, Bordmann G, Blomberg B and Du Pasquier L (1981). Genetic control of T helper function in the clawed toad *Xenopus laevis*. *Eur J Immunol* **11**: 151–155.

Bigaj J and Plytycz B (1984). Cytoarchitecture of the thymus gland of the adult frog *Rana temporaria*. *Folia Histochem Cytobiol* **22**: 63–70.

Bigaj J and Plytycz B (1987). Interdigitating cells in the thymus of the frog *Rana temporaria*. *Folia Histochem Cytobiol* **24**: 65–68.

Billroth T (1857). Beitrage zur vergleichenden histologie der milz. *Mueller's Arch* **88**: 88–108.

Blaustein A (1963). *The Spleen*. McGraw-Hill: New York.

Blazer VS and Wolke RE (1983). Ceroid deposition, retinal degeneration and renal calcium oxalate crystals in cultured clownfish *Amphiprion ocellaris*. *J Fish Dis* **6**: 365–376.

Bleicher PA and Cohen N (1981). Monoclonal anti-IgM can separate T cell from B cell proliferative responses in the frog *Xenopus laevis*. *J Immunol* **127**: 1549–1555.

Bleicher PA, Rollins-Smith LA, Jacobs D and Cohen N (1983). Mitogenic responses of frog lymphocytes to crude and purified preparations of bacterial lipopolysaccharide (LPS). *Dev Comp Immunol* **7**: 483–496.

Blue J and Weiss L (1981a). Periarterial macrophage sheaths (ellipsoids) in cat spleen. An electron microscope study. *Am J Anat* **161**: 115–134.

Blue J and Weiss L (1981b). Vascular pathways in non-sinusal red pulp. An electron microscope study of the cat spleen. *Am J Anat* **161**: 135–168.

Borysenko M (1975). Cellular aspects of humoral immune responsiveness in *Chelydra*. *Adv Exp Med Biol* **64**: 277–291.

Borysenko M (1976a). Changes in spleen histology in response to antigenic stimulation in the snapping turtle *Chelydra serpentina*. *J Morph* **149**: 223–241.

Borysenko M (1976b). Ultrastructural analysis of normal and immunized spleen of the snapping turtle *Chelydra serpentina*. *J Morph* **149**: 243–264.

Borysenko M (1978). Lymphoid tissues and cellular components of the reptilian immune system. In Gershwin ME

and Cooper EL (Eds), *Animal Models of Comparative and Developmental Aspects of Immunity and Disease*. Pergamon Press: New York. pp 63–79.

Borysenko M and Cooper EL (1972). Lymphoid tissue in the snapping turtle *Chelydra serpentina*. *J Morph* **138**: 487–498.

Borysenko M and Tulipan P (1973). The graft-versus-host reaction in the snapping turtle *Chelydra serpentina*. *Transplantation* **16**: 496–504.

Boyd RL and Ward HA (1984). Lymphoid antigenic determinants of the chicken: ontogeny of bursa-dependent lymphoid tissue. *Dev Comp Immunol* **8**: 149–168.

Bradley OC (1938). *The Structure of the Fowl*. Oliver & Boyd: Edinburgh and London.

Brown BA and Cooper EL (1976). Immunological dichotomy in the larval bullfrog spleen. *Immunology* **30**: 299–305.

Brown BA, Wright RK and Cooper EL (1975). Lymphoid organs and amphibian immunity. In Hildemann WH and Benedict AA (Eds), *Immunologic Phylogeny*. Plenum Press: New York. pp 267–275.

Brown CL and George CJ (1985). Age dependent accumulation of macrophage aggregates in the yellow perch *Perca fluviatilis* (Mitchell). *J Fish Dis* **8**: 135–138.

Carver FJ and Meints RH (1977). Studies on the development of frog hemopoietic tissue *in vitro*. 1. Spleen culture assay of an erythropoietic factor in anemic frog blood. *J Exp Zool* **201**: 37–46.

Charlemagne J (1972a). Les reactions immunitaires chez les amphibiens urodeles. I. Resultats acquis et possibilites experimentales. In *Phylogenic and Ontogenic Study of the Immune Response and its Contribution to the Immunological Theory*. Colloque INSERM, Ministry of Public Health, Paris. pp 89–95.

Charlemagne J (1972b). Aspects morphologiques de la differenciation des elements sanguins chez l'axolotl *Ambystoma mexicanum* Shaw. *Z Zellforsch Mikrosk Anat* **123**: 224–239.

Charlemagne J (1983). Effects of immunization, adult thymectomy and irradiation on axolotl spleen lymphocytes: Discontinuous Ficoll density gradients analysis. *Dev Comp Immunol* **7**: 385–390.

Chen LL, Adams JC and Steinman RM (1978). Anatomy of germinal centers in mouse spleen with special reference to follicular dendritic cells. *J Cell Biol* **77**: 148–164.

Chiller JM, Hodkins HO, Chambers VC and Weiser RS (1969). Antibody response in rainbow trout *Salmo gairdneri*. I. Immunocompetent cells in the spleen and anterior kidney. *J Immunol* **102**: 1193–1201.

Clark JC and Newth DR (1972). Immunological activity of transplanted spleens in *Xenopus laevis*. *Experientia* **28**: 951–953.

Clothier RH and Balls M (1973). Mycobacteria and lymphoreticular tumours in *Xenopus laevis*, the South African clawed toad. I. Isolation, characterization and pathogenicity for *Xenopus* of *M. marinum* isolated from lymphoreticular tumour cells. *Oncology* **28**: 445–457.

Cohen N (1971). Amphibian transplantation reactions: A review. *Am Zool* **11**: 193−205.

Cohen N and Collins NH (1977). Major and minor histocompatibility systems of ectothermic vertebrates. In Gotze D (Ed), *The Major Histocompatibility System in Man and Animals*. Springer-Verlag: Berlin. pp 313−337.

Cohen N and Horan M (1977). Lack of correlation between the rapidity of newt allograft rejection and the frequency and magnitude of stimulation in the mixed lymphocyte culture reaction. In Solomon JB and Horton JD (Eds), *Developmental Immunobiology*. Elsevier/North-Holland: Amsterdam. pp 259−266.

Cohen N, Watkins D and Parsons SV (1987). Interleukins and T-cell ontogeny in *Xenopus laevis*. In Cooper EL, Langlet C and Bierne J (Eds), *Developmental and Comparative Immunology*. Alan R Liss: New York. pp 53−68.

Coleman R and Phillips AD (1972). Longterm retention of colloidal thorium dioxide in the liver and spleen of *Xenopus laevis* (Daudin). *Experientia* **28**: 1326−1327.

Collie MH and Turner RJ (1975). Influence of antigen dose on antibody production of intact and splenectomised *Xenopus laevis. J Exp Zool* **192**: 173−179.

Collie MH, Turner RJ and Manning MJ (1975). Antibody production to lipopolysaccharide in thymectomized *Xenopus. Eur J Immunol* **5**: 426−427.

Collins NH, Manickavel V and Cohen N (1975). *In vitro* responses of urodele lymphoid cells. Mitogenic and mixed lymphocyte culture reactivities. In Hildemann WH and Benedict AA (Eds), *Immunologic Phylogeny*. Plenum Press: New York. pp 305−314.

Cooper EL (1976). Immunity mechanism. In Lofts B (Ed), *Physiology of the Amphibia*. Vol 3. Academic Press: New York. pp 163−272.

Cooper EL and Wright RK (1976). The anuran amphibian spleen. An evolutionary model for terrestrial vertebrates. In Battisto JR and Streilen JW (Eds), *Immuno-Aspects of the Spleen*. Elsevier/North-Holland: Amsterdam. pp 47−60.

Cooper MD, Peterson RDA and Good RA. (1965). Delineation of the thymic and bursal lymphoid systems in the chicken. *Nature* **205**: 143−146.

Cooper MD, Schwartz ML and Good RA (1966). Restoration of gamma globulin production in agammaglobulinemic chickens. *Science* **151**: 471−473.

Cooper MD, Cain WA, Van Alten PJ and Good RA (1969). Development and function of the immunoglobulin producing system. I. Effect of bursectomy at different stages of development on germinal centers, plasma cells, immunoglobulins and antibody production. *Int Arch Allergy* **35**: 242−252.

Coosemans V and Hadji-Azimi I (1987). *Xenopus laevis* splenocyte receptors for immunoglobulins (Abstract). *Dev Comp Immunol* **11**: 447.

Cowden RR (1965). Quantitative and qualitative cytochemical studies on the *Amphiuma* basophil leukocyte. *Z Zellforsch* **67**: 219−233.

Cowden RR and Dyer RF (1971). Lymphopoietic tissue and plasma cells in amphibians. *Am Zool* **11**: 183−192.

Cuchens MA and Clem LW (1979). Phylogeny of lymphocyte heterogeneity. III. Mitogenic responses of reptilian lymphocytes. *Dev Comp Immunol* **3**: 287−297.

Cuchens M, McLean E and Clem LW (1976). Lymphocyte heterogeneity in fish and reptiles. In Wright RK and Cooper EL (Eds), *Phylogeny of Thymus and Bone Marrow—Bursa Cells*. Elsevier/North-Holland Biomedical Press: Amsterdam. pp 205−213.

Dawson AB (1932). Hemopoietic loci in *Necturus maculosus. Anat Rec* **52**: 367−379.

De Cardenas L (1987). Desarrollo postnatal del bazo del hamster *Mesocricetus auratus*. Masters thesis, Faculty of Biology, Complutense University, Madrid.

De Lanney LE and Ebert JD (1962). On the chick spleen: origin, patterns of normal development and their experimental modification. *Contrib Embryol* **255**: 59−89.

Debons MC and Deparis P (1973). Mise en evidence des immunocytes par immunocytoadherence chez l'amphibien Urodele *Pleurodeles waltlii* Michah. après immunisation par les globules rouges de mouton. *CR Soc Biol* **167**: 568−572.

Deparis P and Flavin M (1973). Les effects de la splenectomie precoce chez l'amphibien urodele *Pleurodeles waltlii* Michah. *J Physiol (Paris)* **66**: 19.

Dicks (1965).

Diener E and Marchalonis JJ (1970). Cellular and humoral aspects of the primary immune response of the toad *Bufo marinus. Immunology* **10**: 535−542.

Diener E and Nossal GJV (1966). Phylogenetic studies on the immune response. Localization of antigens and immune response in toad *Bufo marinus. Immunology* **10**: 535−542.

Dragotoiu-Untu C (1970). Sistemul reticulo-histocitar di splina de Tinca. *St Si Cerc Biol Seria Zool Bucuresti* **22**: 337−340.

Du Pasquier L (1970). Ontogeny of the immune response in animals having less than one million lymphocytes: the larvae of the toad *Alytes obstetricans. Immunology* **19**: 353−362.

Dustin P (1934). Recherches sur les organes hematopoietiques du *Protopterus dolloi. Archs Biol* **45**: 1−26.

Dustin P (1939). Les housses spleniques de Schweigger-Seidel. Etude d'histologie et d'histophysiologie comparees. *Archs Biol* **49**: 1−99.

Dustin P (1975). Ultrastructure and function of the ellipsoids of the spleen. Their relationship with fat metabolism and red blood cells. *Haematologica* **60**: 136−154.

Edelstein LM (1971) Melanin: a unique biopolymer. In Ioachim HL (Ed), *Pathobiology Annual*. Vol 1. Butterworth: London. pp 309−324.

Eikelenboom P (1978a). Dendritic cells in the rat spleen follicles. A combined immuno- and enzyme histochemical study. *Cell Tissue Res* **190**: 79−87.

Eikelenboom P (1978b). Characterization of non-lymphoid cells in the white pulp of the mouse spleen: an *in vivo* and *in vitro* study. *Cell Tissue Res* **195**: 445−460.

Eikelenboom P, Kroese FGM and van Rooijen N (1983). Immune complex trapping cells in the spleen of the chicken. Enzyme histochemical and ultrastructural aspects. *Cell Tissue Res* **231**: 377−386.

Eikelenboom P, Dijkstra CD, Boorsma DM and van Rooijen N (1985). Characterization of lymphoid and nonlymphoid cells in the white pulp of the spleen using immunohisto-peroxidase techniques and enzyme-histochemistry. *Experientia* **41**: 209−215.

El Deeb S (1983). Ontogeny of the immune system of the lizard *Chalcides ocellatus*. PhD thesis, Faculty of Sciences, Cairo University.

El Deeb S, Zada S and El Ridi R (1985). Ontogeny of hemopoietic and lymphopoietic tissues in the lizard *Chalcides ocellatus* (Reptilia, Sauna, Scincidae). *J Morph* **185**: 241−253.

El Ghareeb A, Wahby AF, El Ridi R and Badir N (1983). Cellular and humoral immune response of the GALT-less lizard *Agama stellio*. *Dev Comp Immunol* **7**: 719−720.

El Masri M (1979). Role of thymus and spleen in immune response of the lizard *Chalcides ocellatus*. MSc thesis, Faculty of Sciences, Cairo University.

El Ridi R and Kandil O (1981). Membrane markers of reptilian lymphocytes. *Dev Comp Immunol* **5** (Suppl 1): 143−150.

El Ridi R, Wahby AF, Saad AH and Soliman MA-W (1987). Concanavalin responsiveness and interleukin-2 production in the snake *Spalerosophis diadema*. *Immunobiology* **174**: 177−189.

Ellis AE (1974). Aspects of the lymphoid and reticulo-endothelial system in the plaice *Pleuronectes platessa* L. PhD thesis, University of Aberdeen.

Ellis AE (1977). Ontogeny of the immune response in *Salmo salar*. Histogenesis of the lymphoid organs and appearance of membrane immunoglobulin and mixed leukocyte reactivity. In Solomon JB and Horton JD (Eds), *Developmental Immunobiology*. Elsevier/North-Holland Biomedical Press: Amsterdam. pp 225−231.

Ellis AE (1980). Antigen trapping in the spleen and kidney of the plaice *Pleuronectes platessa*. *J Fish Dis* **3**: 413−426.

Ellis AE and de Sousa M (1974). Phylogeny of the lymphoid system. I. A study of the plaice *Pleuronectes platessa*. *Eur J Immunol* **4**: 338−343.

Ellis AE, Munroe ALS and Roberts RJ (1976). Defense mechanisms in fish. I. A study of the phagocytic system and the fate of intraperitoneally injected particulate material in the plaice *Pleuronectes platessa* L. *J Fish Biol* **8**: 67−78.

Engle Jr RL, Woods KR and Pert JH (1958). Studies on the phylogenesis of gamma globulins and plasma cells (Abstract). *J Clin Invest* **37**: 892.

Etlinger HM, Hodgins HO and Chiller JM (1976). Evolution of the lymphoid system. I. Evidence for lymphocyte heterogeneity in rainbow trout revealed by the organ distribution of mitogenic responses. *J Immunol* **116**: 1547−1553.

Etlinger HM, Hodgins HO and Chiller JM (1978). Evolution of the lymphoid system. III. Morphological and functional consequences of mitogenic stimulation of rainbow trout lymphocytes. *Dev Comp Immunol* **2**: 263−276.

Evans EE (1963). Comparative immunology. Antibody response in *Dipsosaurus dorsalis* at different temperatures. *Proc Soc Exp Biol Med* **112**: 531−533.

Evans EE, Kent SP, Attleberger MH, Siebert C, Bryant RE and Booth B (1965). Antibody synthesis in poikilothermic vertebrates. *Ann NY Acad Sci* **126**: 629−646.

Evans EE, Kent SP, Bryant RE and Moyer M (1966). Antibody formation and immunological memory in the marine toad. In Smith RT, Good RA and Miescher PA (Eds), *Phylogeny and Immunity*. University of Florida Press: Gainesville. pp 218−226.

Ewart D and McMillan D (1970). The spleen of the cowbird. *J Morph* **130**: 187−206.

Fange R (1984). Lymphomyeloid tissues in fishes. *Vidensk Meddr Dansk Naturh Foren* **145**: 143−162.

Fange R and Mattison A (1981). The lymphomyeloid (hemopoietic) system of the Atlantic nurse shark *Ginglymostoma cirratum*. *Biol Bull* **160**: 240−249.

Fange R and Nilsson S (1985). The fish spleen: structure and function. *Experientia* **41**: 152−158.

Fange R and Silverin B (1985). Variation of lymphoid activity in the spleen of a migratory bird, the pied flycatcher *Ficedula hypolevca*: Aves Passeriformes. *J Morph* **184**: 33−40.

Farag MA and El Ridi R (1985). Mixed leucocyte reaction (MLR) in the snake *Psammophis sibilans*. *Immunology* **55**: 173−181.

Farag MA and El Ridi R (1986). Proliferative responses of snake lymphocytes to concanavalin A. *Dev Comp Immunol* **10**: 561−569.

Farr AG and de Bruyn PP (1975). The mode of lymphocyte migration through postcapillary venule endothelium in lymph node. *Am J Anat* **143**: 59−92.

Ferguson HW (1976). The relationship between ellipsoids and melano-macrophage centres in the spleen of turbot *Scophthalmus maximus*. *J Comp Pathol* **86**: 377−380.

Ferren FA (1967). Role of the spleen in the immune response of teleosts and elasmobranchs. *J Florida Med Assoc* **54**: 434−437.

Fey F (1962). Haematologische Untersuchungen an *Xenopus laevis* Daudin. I. Die morphologie des blutes mit einigen vergleichenden betrachtungen bei *Rana esculenta* und *Rana temporaria*. *Morphol Jahrb* **103**: 9.

Fey F (1965). Hematologische Untersuchungen der blut-bildenden Gewebe niederer Wirbeltiere. *Folia Haemat* **84**: 122−146.

Fiebig H and Ambrosius H (1976). Cell surface immunoglobulin of lymphocytes in lower vertebrates. In Wright RK and Cooper EL (Eds), *Phylogeny of Thymus and Bone Marrow— Bursa Cells*. Elsevier/North-Holland Biomedical Press: Amsterdam. pp 195−203.

Fonfria J, Barrutia MG, Villena A and Zapata A (1982). Ultrastructural study of interdigitating cells in the thymus of the spotless starling *Sturnus unicolor*. *Cell Tissue Res* **225**: 687–691.

Fonfria J, Barrutia MG, Garrido E, Ardavin CF and Zapata A (1983). Erythropoiesis in the thymus of the spotless starling *Sturnus unicolor*. *Cell Tissue Res* **222**: 445–455.

Fukuta K and Mochizuki K (1982). Formation of the reticular fibers in the developing spleen of the chick embryo. *Arch Histol Jap* **45**: 181–189.

Fukuta K, Nishida T and Mochizuki K (1976). Electron microscopy of the splenic circulation in the chicken. *Jap J Vet Sci* **38**: 241–254.

Fukuta K, Nishida T and Yasuda M (1969). Comparative and topographical anatomy of the fowl. LXIII. Structure and distribution of the fine blood vascular system in the spleen. *Jap J Vet Sci* **31**: 303–311.

Fukuta K, Nishida T and Mochizuki K (1979). Temporal decrease of germinal centers during the secondary immune response in the chicken spleen. *Jap J Vet Sci* **41**: 555–559.

Fukuta K, Nishida T and Mochizuki K (1980). Primary formation of germinal centers in the chick spleen after injection with sheep red blood cells. *Arch Histol Jap* **43**: 331–339.

Fulop GMI and McMillan D (1984). Phagocytosis in the spleen of the sunfish *Lepomis* sp. *J Morphol* **179**: 175–195.

Galindo B and Imaeda T (1962). Electron microscope study of the white pulp of the mouse spleen. *Anat Rec* **143**: 399–415.

Garcia-Herrera F and Cooper EL (1968). Organos linfoides del anfibio apoda *Typhlonectes compressicauda*. *Acta Med* **4**: 157–160.

Glaister JR (1973). Factors affecting the lymphoid cells in the small intestinal epithelium of the mouse. *Int Arch Allergy Appl Immunol* **45**: 719–730.

Glick B (1970). Hypertrophy of accessory spleens in splenectomized chickens. *Folia Biol (Prague)* **16**: 74–76.

Glick B and Olah I (1987). Contribution of a specialized dendritic cell, the secretory cell, to the microenvironment of the bursa of Fabricius. In Weber WT and Ewert DL (Eds), *Avian Immunology*. Alan R Liss: New York. pp 53–66.

Glick B and Sato K (1964). Accessory spleens in the chicken. *Poultry Sci* **43**: 1610–1612.

Good RA, Finstad B, Pollara B and Gabrielsen AE (1966). Morphologic studies on the evolution of the lymphoid tissues among the lower vertebrates. In Smith RT, Miescher PA and Good RA (Eds), *Phylogeny of Immunity*. University of Florida Press: Gainesville. pp 149–170.

Grace MF and Manning MJ (1980). Histogenesis of the lymphoid organs in rainbow trout *Salmo gairdneri*. *Dev Comp Immunol* **4**: 255–264.

Graf R and Schluns J (1979). Ultrastructural and histochemical investigation of the terminal capillaries of the spleen of the carp *Cyprinus carpio* L. *Cell Tissue Res* **196**: 289–306.

Green (Donnelly) N and Cohen N (1979). Phylogeny of immunocompetent cells. III. Mitogen response characteristics of lymphocyte subpopulations from normal and thymectomized frogs *Xenopus laevis*. *Cell Immunol* **48**: 59–70.

Greschick E (1915). Uber den bau der milz einiger vogel mit besonderer berucksichtigung der Schweigner–Scidelschen kapillarhulsen. *Aguila* **22**: 133–159.

Grey HM (1966). Structure and kinetics of formation of antibody in the turtle. In Smith RT, Miescher PA and Good RA (Eds), *Phylogeny of Immunity*. University of Florida Press: Gainesville. pp 227–233.

Grover JH (1968). Hemosiderins in bluegill spleens. *Trans Am Fish Soc* **97**: 48–50.

Hadji-Azimi I (1977). Distribution of immunoglobulin determinants on the surface of *Xenopus laevis* splenic lymphocytes. *J Exp Zool* **201**: 115–126.

Hadji-Azimi I, Schwager J and Thiebaud C (1982). B lymphocyte differentiation in *Xenopus laevis* larvae. *Dev Biol* **90**: 253–258.

Haider G (1966). Beitrag zur Kenntnis der mikroskopischen anatomie der Milz einiger Teleostier. *Zool Anz* **177**: 348–367.

Hartmann A (1926). Uber den feineren bau der milz bei urodelen amphibien (Axolotl). *Z Anat Entwickl Gesch* **80**: 454–491.

Hartmann A (1930). Die milz. *Handb mikr Anat Mollendorff*. Vol 6, pt 1: 416.

Hartwig H and Hartwig HG (1985). Structural characteristics of the mammalian spleen indicating storage and release of red blood cells. Aspects of evolutionary and environmental demands. *Experientia* **41**: 159–163.

Hashimoto Y and Sugimura M (1976). Effects of early cyclophosphamide treatment on lymphoid organs and its immune response in ducks. *Poultry Sci* **55**: 1441–1449.

Hatoe T (1978). Electron microscope studies on the ellipsoid of the cat spleen with special reference to the filaments in the endothelial cell. *Arch Histol Jap* **41**: 177–186.

Hemmeter J (1926). The special histology of the spleen of *Alopias vulpes*, its relation to hemolysis and hemopoiesis. *Z Zellforsch* **3**: 329–348.

Hemmingsson EJ and Linna TJ (1972). Ontogenic studies on lymphoid cell traffic in the chicken. I. Cell migration from the bursa of Fabricius. *Int Arch Allergy Appl Immunol* **42**: 693–710.

Herradon PG (1987). Relaciones entre el sistema neuroendocrino y el sistema inmune durante la ontogenia. Efecto de la decapitacion temprana sobre el desarrollo de los organos linfoides del embrion de pollo *Gallus gallus*. PhD thesis, University of Leon (Spain).

Herraez MP and Zapata A (1986). Structure and function of the melano-macrophage centres of the goldfish *Carassius auratus*. *Vet Immunol Immunopathol* **12**: 117–126.

Hightower JA and St Pierre RL (1971). Hemopoietic tissue in the adult newt *Notophthalmus viridescens*. *J Morph* **135**: 299–308.

Hoefsmit ECM, Kamperdijk EWA, Beelen RHJ, Hendriks HR and Balfour BM (1980). Lymph node macrophages. In

Carr I and Daems WT (Eds), *The Reticuloendothelial System. A Comprehensive Treatise*. Vol I. Plenum: New York. pp 417–468.

Hoffman-Fezer G, Rodt H, Gotze D and Thierfelder S (1977). Anatomical distribution of T and B lymphocytes identified by immunohistochemistry in the chicken spleen. *Int Arch Allergy Appl Immunol* **55**: 86–95.

Horton JD and Manning MJ (1974a). Lymphoid organ development in *Xenopus* thymectomized at eight days of age. *J Morph* **143**: 385–396.

Horton JD and Manning MJ (1974b). Effect of early thymectomy on the cellular changes occurring in the spleen of the clawed toad *Xenopus laevis* homologous with mammalian M(19s) and G(7s) immunoglobulins. *Immunology* **26**: 797–807.

Horton JD, Horton TL and Rimmer JJ (1977). Splenic involvement in amphibian transplantation immunity. *Transplantation* **24**: 247–255.

Horton JJ (1971). Ontogeny of the immune system in amphibians. *Am Zool* **11**: 219–228.

Hoshi H (1972). On the nature of the periellipsoidal lymphoid tissue of chick spleen. *Tohoku J Exp Med* **106**: 285–305.

Hoshi H and Mori T (1975). A light and electron microscopic study on the Schweigger–Seidel ellipsoid and periellipsoidal lymphoid tissue of the chicken spleen. *10th Int Congress of Anatomy*, Tokyo.

Hussein MF, Badir N, El Ridi R and Akef M (1978a). Differential effect of seasonal variation on lymphoid tissue of the lizard *Chalcides ocellatus*. *Dev Comp Immunol* **2**: 297–310.

Hussein MF, Badir N, El Ridi R and Akef M (1978b). Effect of seasonal variation on lymphoid tissues of the lizards *Mabuya quinquetaeniata* Licht and *Uromastyx aegyptia* Forsk. *Dev Comp Immunol* **2**: 469–478.

Hussein MF, Badir N, El Ridi R and Akef M (1979a). Lymphoid tissue of the snake *Spalerosophis diadema* in different seasons. *Dev Comp Immunol* **3**: 77–88.

Hussein MF, Badir N, El Ridi R and El Deeb S (1979b). Effect of seasonal variations on immune system of the lizard *Scincus scincus*. *J Exp Zool* **209**: 91–96.

Hussein MF, Badir N, El Ridi R and El Deeb S (1979c). Effect of splenectomy on the humoral immune response in the lizard *Scincus scincus*. *Experientia* **35**: 869–870.

Isakovic K and Jankovic BD (1964). Role of the thymus and the bursa of Fabricius in immune reactions in chickens. II. Cellular changes in the lymphoid tissues of thymectomized, bursectomized and normal chickens in the course of first antibody response. *Int Arch Allergy* **24**: 296–310.

Jankovic BD and Isakovic K (1964). Role of the thymus and the bursa of Fabricius in immune reactions in chickens. I. Changes in lymphoid tissues of chickens surgically thymectomized at hatching. *Int Arch Allergy* **24**: 278–295.

Jayaraman S and Muthukkaruppan VR (1977). *In vitro* correlation of transplantation immunity: spleen cell migration inhibition in the lizard *Calotes versicolor*. *Dev Comp Immunol* **1**: 133–144.

Jayaraman S and Muthukkaruppan VR (1978a). Influence of route and dose of antigen on the migration inhibition and plaque-forming cell responses to sheep erythrocytes in the lizard *Calotes versicolor*. *Immunology* **34**: 241–246.

Jayaraman S and Muthukkaruppan VR (1978b). Detection of cell mediated immunity to sheep erythrocytes by the capillary migration inhibition technique in the lizard *Calotes versicolor*. *Immunology* **34**: 231–240.

Jordan HE (1938). Comparative hematology. In Downey H (Ed), *Handbook of Hematology*. Harper: New York. pp 704–862.

Jordan HE and Speidel CC (1923a). An experimental study of the spleen of the frog, *Rana pipiens*. *Anat Rec* **25**: 136–137.

Jordan HE and Speidel CC (1923b). Blood cell formation and distribution in relation to the mechanism of thyroid accelerated metamorphosis in the larval frog. *J Exp Med* **38**: 529–541.

Jordan HE and Speidel CC (1930). Blood formation in cyclostomes. *Am J Anat* **46**: 355–391.

Jordan HE and Speidel CC (1931). Blood formation in the African lungfish under normal conditions and under conditions of prolonged estivation and recovery. *J Morphol Physiol* **51**: 319–371.

Jurd RD and Doritis A (1977). Antibody-dependent cellular cytotoxicity in poikilotherms. *Dev Comp Immunol* **1**: 341–352.

Jurd RD and Stevenson GT (1976). Surface immunoglobulins on *Xenopus laevis* lymphocytes. *Comp Biochem Physiol* **A53**: 381–387.

Kanakambika P and Muthukkaruppan VR (1972a). The immune response to sheep erythrocytes in the lizard *Calotes versicolor*. *J Immunol* **109**: 415–419.

Kanakambika P and Muthukkaruppan VR (1972b). Effects of splenectomy in the lizard *Calotes versicolor*. *Experientia* **28**: 1225–1226.

Kanakambika P and Muthukkaruppan VR (1973). Lymphoid differentiation and organization of the spleen in the lizard *Calotes versicolor*. *Proc Ind Acad Sci B* **78**: 37–44.

Kanesada A (1956). A phylogenetic survey of hemocytopoietic tissues in submammalian vertebrates. *Bull Yamaguchi Med School* **4**: 1–22.

Kassin LF and Pevitskii LA (1969). Detection of antibody forming cells in turtle spleens by means of a modified method of local hemolysis in gel. *Bull Exp Biol Med* **67**: 70–74.

Katagiri C, Kawahara H, Nagata S and Tochinai S (1980). The mode of participation of T-cells in immune reactions as studied by transfer of triploid lymphocytes into early-thymectomized diploid *Xenopus*. In Horton JD (Ed), *Development and Differentiation of Vertebrate Lymphocytes*. Elsevier/North-Holland: Amsterdam. pp 163–171.

Kaupp BF (1918). *The Anatomy of the Domestic Fowl*. Saunders: Philadelphia.

Kawaguchi S, Hiruki T, Harada T and Morikawa S (1980). Frequencies of cell-surface or cytoplasmic IgM-bearing cells in the spleen, thymus and peripheral blood of the snake *Elaphe quadrivirgata. Dev Comp Immunol* **4**: 559–564.

Kawahara H, Nagata S and Katagiri C (1980). Role of injected thymocytes in reconstituting cellular and humoral immune responses in early thymectomized *Xenopus*: use of triploid markers. *Dev Comp Immunol* **4**: 679–690.

Kendall MD and Frazier JA (1979). Ultrastructural studies on erythropoiesis in the avian thymus. I. Description of cell types. *Cell Tissue Res* **199**: 37–61.

Kent SP, Evans EE and Attleberger MH (1964). Comparative immunology: lymph nodes in the amphibian *Bufo marinus. Proc Soc Exp Biol Med* **116**: 456–459.

Kincade PW and Cooper MD (1971). Development and distribution of immunoglobulin containing cells in the chicken. An immunofluorescent analysis using purified antibodies to mu, gamma and light chains. *J Immunol* **106**: 371–382.

Klaus GGB, Humphrey JH, Kunkl A and Dongworth DW (1980). The follicular dendritic cell: its role in antigen presentation in the generation of immunological memory. *Immunol Rev* **53**: 3–28.

Klemperer P (1938). The spleen. In Downey H (Ed), *Handbook of Hematology*. Vol III. Hafner: New York. pp 1591–1754.

Krause R (1921). *Mikroskopische Anatomie der Wirbeltiere*. Walter de Gruyter: Berlin.

Kroese FG and Van Rooijan N (1982). The architecture of the spleen of the red-eared slider *Chrysemys scripta elegans* (Reptilia: Testudines). *J Morph* **173**: 279–284.

Kroese FG and Van Rooijen N (1983). Antigen trapping in the spleen of the turtle *Chrysemys scripta elegans. Immunology* **49**: 61–68.

Kroese FG, Leceta J, Dopp EA, Herraez MP, Nieuwenhuis P and Zapata A (1985). Dendritic immune complex trapping cells in the spleen of the snake *Python reticulatus. Dev Comp Immunol* **9**: 641–652.

Krueff de RH, Durkin HG, Gilmour DG and Thorbecke GJ (1977). Migratory patterns of B lymphocytes. II. Fate of cells from central lymphoid organs in the chicken. *Cell Immunol* **16**: 301–314.

Lamers CHJ (1985). The reaction of the immune system of fish to vaccination. PhD thesis, University of Wageningen (Netherlands).

Langeberg L, Ruben LN, Clothier RH and Shiigi S (1987a). The characterization of the toad splenocytes which bind mouse anti-human IL-2 receptor antibody. *Immunol Letters* **16**: 43–48.

Langeberg L, Ruben LN, Malley A, Shiigi S and Beadling C (1987b). Toad splenocytes bind human IL-2 and anti-human IL-2 receptor antibody specifically. *Immunol Letters* **14**: 103–110.

Le Douarin N (1966). L'hematopoiese dans les formes embryonnaires et jeunes des vertebres. *Annee Biol* **5**: 105–171.

Leceta J (1984). Cambios estacionales en el sistema inmune de *Mauremys caspica*. Papel regulador del sistema neuro-endocrino. PhD thesis, Complutense University, Madrid.

Leceta J and Zapata A (1985). Seasonal changes in the thymus and spleen of the turtle *Mauremys caspica*. A morphometrical, light microscopical study. *Dev Comp Immunol* **9**: 653–668.

Leceta J, Villena A, Rasquin B, Fonfria J and Zapata A (1984). Interdigitating cells in the thymus of the turtle *Mauremys caspica*. Possible relationships to macrophages. *Cell Tissue Res* **239**: 381–385.

Lerch EG, Huggins SE and Bartel AH (1967). Comparative immunology. Active immunization of young alligators with hemocyanin. *Proc Soc Exp Biol Med* **124**: 448–451.

Lucas AM and Jamroz C (1961). Atlas of avian hematology. *Agriculture Monograph 25*, US Department of Agriculture Superintendent of Documents, Washington, DC. p 58.

Lucas AM, Denengton EM, Cottral GE and Burnester BR (1954). Production of so-called normal lymphoid foci following inoculation with lymphoid tumor filtrate. *Poultry Sci* **33**: 562–582.

Lykakis JJ (1968). Immunoglobulin production in the European pond tortoise *Emys orbicularis* immunized with serum protein antigens. *Immunology* **14**: 799–808.

Maas MG and Bootsma R (1982). Uptake of bacterial antigens in the spleen of carp *Cyprinus carpio* L. *Dev Comp Immunol Suppl* **2**: 47–52.

Maclean N and Jurd RD (1972). The control of haemoglobin synthesis. *Biol Rev* **47**: 393–437.

Manning MJ (1971). The effect of early thymectomy on histogenesis of the lymphoid organs in *Xenopus laevis*. *J Embryol Exp Morphol* **26**: 219–229.

Manning MJ (1975). The phylogeny of thymic dependence. *Am Zool* **15**: 63–71.

Manning MJ and Horton JD (1969). Histogenesis of lymphoid organs in larvae of the South African clawed toad *Xenopus laevis* (Daudin). *J Embryol Exp Morphol* **22**: 265–277.

Manning MJ and Horton JD (1982). RES structure and function of the amphibia. In Cohen N and Sigel MM (Eds), *The Reticuloendothelial System. A Comprehensive Treatise*. Vol 3. *Phylogeny and Ontogeny*. Plenum Press: New York. pp 423–459.

Manning MJ and Turner RJ (1972). Some responses of the clawed toad *Xenopus laevis* to soluble antigens administered in adjuvant. *Comp Biochem Physiol* **42A**: 737–747.

Marchalonis JJ, Ealey EHM and Diener E (1969). Immune response of the tuatara *Sphenodon punctatum*. *Aus J Exp Biol Med Sci* **47**: 367–380.

Mattisson A and Fange R (1982). The cellular structure of the Leydig organ in the shark *Etmopterus spinax* L. *Biol Bull* **162**: 182–194.

Maung HT (1963). Immunity in the tortoise *Testudo iberica*. *J Pathol Bacteriol* **85**: 51–66.

Maximow A (1923). Untersuchungen uber Blut and Bindegewebe. X. Uber die Blutbildung bei den selachiern in erwachzenen und embryonalen Zustanden. *Arch Mikrosk Anat* **97**: 623–717.

Mead KF and Borysenko M (1984a). Surface immunoglobulin on granular and agranular leukocytes in the thymus and spleen of the snapping turtle *Chelydra serpentina*. *Dev Comp Immunol* **8**: 109 – 120.

Mead KF and Borysenko M (1984b). Turtle lymphocyte surface antigens in *Chelydra serpentina* as characterized by rabbit anti-turtle thymocyte sera. *Dev Comp Immunol* **8**: 351 – 358.

Miller JJ (1969). Studies of the phylogeny and ontogeny of the specialized lymphatic tissue venules. *Lab Invest* **21**: 484 – 490.

Millot J, Anthony J and Robineau D (1978). *Anatomie de Latimeria chalumnae*. III. Editions de Centre National de la Recherche Scientifique: Paris. pp 133 – 134.

Milne RW, Bienenstodk J and Perey DY (1975). The influence of antigenic stimulation on the ontogeny of lymphoid aggregates and immunoglobulin-containing cells in mouse bronchial and intestinal mucosa. *J Ret Soc* **17**: 361 – 369.

Minagawa Y, Ohnishi K and Murakawa S (1975). Structure and immunological function of lymphomyeloid organs in the bull frog *Rana catesbeiana*. In Hildemann WH and Benedict AA (Eds), *Immunologic Phylogeny*. Plenum Press: New York. pp 257 – 266.

Mitsuhashi S, Kurashige S, Mishima S, Yamaguchi N. and Fukai K (1971). Antibody production without reactive proliferation of pyroninophilic cells in the rainbow trout and African clawed toad. *Tohoku J Exp Med* **103**: 7 – 10.

Miyamoto H, Seguchi H and Ogawa K (1980). Electron microscopic studies of the Schweigger – Seidel sheath in hen spleen with special reference to the existence of 'closed' microcirculation. *J Electron Microsc* **29**: 158 – 172.

Moccia RD, Hung SSO, Slinger SJ and Ferguson HW (1984). Effect of oxidized fish oil, vitamin E and ethoxyquin on histopathology and haematology of rainbow trout *Salmo gairdneri* Richardson. *J Fish Dis* **7**: 269 – 282.

Mori M (1980). Studies on the phagocytic system in goldfish. I. Phagocytosis of intraperitoneally injected carbon particles. *Fish Pathol* **15**: 25 ff.

Mori T and Hoshi H (1971). The periellipsoidal lymphoid tissue in chick spleen: A bursa-dependent area of the white pulp. *Tohoku J Exp Med* **104**: 201 – 202.

Morrow WJW (1978). The immune response of the dogfish *Scyliorhinus canicula* L. PhD thesis, Plymouth Polytechnic (UK).

Moticka EJ, Brown BA and Cooper EL (1973). Immunoglobulin synthesis in bullfrog larvae. *J Immunol* **110**: 855 – 861.

Muller W (1865). *Uber den feineren Bau der Milz*. Leipzig, Heidelberg.

Murakawa S (1968). Studies in the transplantation immunity in the Japanese newt *Cynops pyrrhogaster*. *SABCO J* **4**: 17 – 32.

Murata H (1959). Comparative studies of the spleen in submammalian vertebrates. II. Minute structure of the spleen, with special reference to the periarterial lymphoid sheath. *Bull Yamaguchi Med School* **6**: 83 – 105.

Muthukkaruppan VR, Pillai PS and Jayaraman S (1976a). Immune functions of the spleen in the lizard *Calotes versicolor*. In Battisto JR and Streilein JW (Eds), *Immunodynamics of Spleen*. Elsevier/North-Holland Biomedical Press: Amsterdam. pp 61 – 73.

Muthukkaruppan VR, Pitchappan RM and Ramila G (1976b). Thymic dependence and regulation of the immune response to sheep erythrocytes in the lizard. In Wright RK and Cooper EL (Eds), *Phylogeny of Thymus and Bone Marrow—Bursa Cells*. Elsevier/North-Holland Biomedical Press: Amsterdam. pp 185 – 193.

Muthukkaruppan VR, Borysenko M and El Ridi R (1982). RES structure and function of the reptilia. In Cohen N and Sigel MM (Eds), *The Reticuloendothelial System. A Comprehensive Treatise*. Vol 3. *Phylogeny and Ontogeny*. Plenum Press: New York. pp 461 – 508.

Nagata S (1980). Restoration of antibody forming capacity in early thymectomized *Xenopus* by injecting thymocytes. *Dev Comp Immunol* **4**: 553 – 558.

Nagata S (1985). A cell surface marker of thymus-dependent lymphocytes in *Xenopus laevis* is identifiable by mouse monoclonal antibody. *Eur J Immunol* **15**: 837 – 841.

Nagata S (1986a). Development of T lymphocytes in *Xenopus laevis*: appearance of the antigen recognized by anti-thymocyte mouse monoclonal antibody. *Dev Biol* **114**: 389 – 394.

Nagata S (1986b). A T-cell specific surface marker in *Xenopus laevis* that is identified by a mouse monoclonal antibody. *Proceedings of the 6th International Congress of Immunology*, Toronto. p 63.

Nagata S and Katagiri C (1978). Lymphocyte surface immunoglobulin in *Xenopus laevis*. Light and electron microscopic demonstration by immunoperoxidase method. *Dev Comp Immunol* **2**: 277 – 286.

Nagata S and Tochinai S (1978). Isolated lymphocytes can restore allograft rejection capacity of early-thymectomized *Xenopus*. *Dev Comp Immunol* **2**: 637 – 645.

Nagy ZA (1970). Histological study of the topographic separation of thymus-type and bursa-type lymphocytes and plasma cell series in chicken spleen. *Zbl Veterinaermed (A)* **17**: 422 – 429.

Nakajima A (1929a). Uber die morphogenese der Milz von *Megalobatrachus japonicus*. *Folia Anat Jap* **7**: 93 – 112.

Nakajima A (1929b). Zur morphologie und entwicklungsgeschichte der Milz von *Hynobius fuscus*. *Folia Anat Jap* **7**: 305 – 323.

Natarajan K and Muthukkaruppan VR (1985). Distribution and ontogeny of B cells in the garden lizard *Calotes versicolor*. *Dev Comp Immunol* **9**: 301 – 310.

Nielsen MH, Jensen H, Braendstru O and Wenderlin O (1974). Macrophage lymphocyte clusters in the immune response to soluble protein antigen *in vitro*. II. Ultrastructure of cluster formed during the early response. *J Exp Med* **140**: 1260 – 1272.

Nilsson S (1983). *Autonomic Nerve Function in the Vertebrates*. Springer-Verlag: Berlin. p 253.

Norton S and Wolfe HR (1949). The growth of the spleen in

the chicken. *Anat Rec* **105**: 83 – 93.

Obara N (1982). Autoradiographic study on the distribution of thymus-derived and thymus-independent lymphocytes in the spleen of *Xenopus laevis*. *Dev Comp Immunol* **5**: 95 – 104.

Obara N, Tochinai S and Katagiri CH (1982). Splenic white pulp as a thymus independent area in the African clawed toad *Xenopus laevis*. *Cell Tissue Res* **226**: 327 – 335.

Ohuye T (1932). Hemocytopoietic effect of splenectomy in the newt. *Sci Rep Tohoku Imp Univ Sendai* **7**: 49 – 63.

Olah I and Glick B (1978). Secretory cells in the medulla of bursa of Fabricius. *Experientia* **34**: 1642 – 1643.

Olah I and Glick B (1982). Splenic white pulp and associated vascular channels in chicken spleen. *Am J Anat* **165**: 445 – 480.

Olah I, Glick B, McCorkle F and Stinson R (1979). Light and electron microscope structure of secretory cells in the medulla of bursal follicles on normal and cyclophosphamide treated chickens. *Dev Comp Immunol* **3**: 101 – 115.

Olah I, Yamamoto Y and Glick B (1981). Effect of carrageenan on the ellipsoid-associated antigen trapping cells of the spleen (Abstract). *Poultry Sci* **60**: 1705.

Olah I, Glick B and Taylor Jr RL (1984). Effect of soluble antigen on the ellipsoid-associated cells of the chicken's spleen. *J Leuk Biol* **35**: 501 – 510.

Olah I, Glick B and Taylor Jr RL (1985). Effect of surgical bursectomy on the ellipsoid, ellipsoid-associated cells and periellipsoid region of the chicken's spleen. *J Leuk Biol* **38**: 450 – 469.

Parrott DMV, de Sousa MAB and East J (1966). Thymus dependent area in the lymphoid organs of neonatally thymectomized mice. *J Exp Med* **123**: 191 – 204.

Payne L (1971). The lymphoid system. In Bell DJ and Freeman BM (Eds), *Physiology and Biochemistry of the Domestic Fowl*. Vol II. Academic Press: London. pp 985 – 1037.

Phisalix C (1885). Recherches sur l'anatomie et la physiologie de la rate chez les ichthyopsides. *Arch Zool Gen Exp* **3**: 369 – 464.

Pierce C and Benacerraf B (1969). Immune response in vitro: independence of 'activated' lymphoid cells. *Science* **186**: 1002 – 1004.

Pitchappan RM (1980). On the phylogeny of the splenic structure and function. *Dev Comp Immunol* **4**: 395 – 416.

Pitchappan RM and Muthukaruppan VR (1977a). Analysis of the development of the lizard *Calotes versicolor*. II. Histogenesis of the thymus. *Dev Comp Immunol* **1**: 217 – 231.

Pitchappan RM and Muthukkaruppan VR (1977b). Thymus-dependent lymphoid regions in the spleen of the lizard *Calotes versicolor*. *J Exp Zool* **199**: 177 – 188.

Pontius H and Ambrosius H (1972). Beitrage zur immunbiologie poikilothermer wirbeltiere. IX. Untersuchungen zur zellularen Grundlage humoraler immunoreaktionen der knochenfishe an beispiel des flussbarsches *Perca fluviatilis* L. *Acta Biol Med Ger* **29**: 319 – 339.

Pulsford A, Fange R and Morrow WJW (1982). Cell types and interactions in the spleen of the dogfish *Scyliorhinus canicula* L. An electron microscopic study. *J Fish Biol* **21**: 649 – 662.

Rafn S and Wingstrand KG (1981). Structure of intestine, pancreas and spleen of the Australian lungfish *Neoceratodus forsteri* (Krefft). *Zool Scripta* **10**: 223 – 239.

Rasquin P (1951). Effects of carp pituitary and mammalian ACTH on the endocrine and lymphoid system of the teleost *Astyana mexicanus*. *J Exp Zool* **117**: 317 – 334.

Rimmer JJ and Gearing AJH (1980). Antigen specific migration inhibition of peritoneal exudate cells in an anuran *Rana temporaria*. In Horton JD (Ed), *Development and Differentiation of Vertebrate Lymphocytes*. Elsevier/North-Holland: Amsterdam. pp 195 – 200.

Roberts RJ (1975). Melanin-containing cells of teleost fish and their relation to disease. In Ribelin WE and Migali G (Eds), *The Pathology of Fishes*. University of Wisconsin Press: Madison. pp 339 – 428.

Roberts RJ (1976). Experimental pathogenesis of lymphocytes in the plaice *Pleuronectes platessa* L. In Page LA (Ed), *Wildlife Diseases*. Plenum Press: New York. pp 431 – 441.

Rollins-Smith LA, Parsons SCV and Cohen N (1984). During ontogeny of *Xenopus*, PHA and Con A responsiveness of splenocytes precedes that of thymocytes. *Immunology* **52**: 491 – 500.

Romppanen T and Sorvari TE (1981). A morphometrical study of chicken spleen with special reference to the bursa dependence of the white pulp. *Int Arch Allergy Appl Immunol* **65**: 349 – 358.

Rothe F and Ambrosius H (1968). Beitrage zur immunobiologie poikilothermer wirbeltiere. V. Die proliferation antikorper bildender Zellen bei Schildkoten. *Acta Biol Med Ger* **21**: 525 – 536.

Ruben LN and Edwards BF (1979). The phylogeny of the emergence of 'T – B' collaboration on humoral immunity. In Cohen N and Marchalonis JJ (Eds), *Contemporary Topics in Immunobiology*. Vol 9. Plenum Press: New York. pp 55 – 89.

Ruben LN, Stevens JM and Kidder GM (1972). Suppression of the allograft response by implants of mature lymphoid tissues in larval *Xenopus laevis*. *J Morphol* **138**: 457 – 466.

Ruben LN, Buenafe A and Seivert D (1983). Some characteristics of thymus suppression of antibody production *in vitro* in *Xenopus laevis*, the South African clawed toad. *Thymus* **5**: 13 – 18.

Saad A-H and El Ridi R (1984). Mixed leukocyte reaction, graft-versus-host reaction and skin allograft rejection in the lizard *Chalcides ocellatus*. *Immunobiology* **166**: 484 – 493.

Saad A-H, El Ridi R, El Deeb S and Soliman MA-W (1987). Corticosteroids and immune system in the lizard *Chalcides ocellatus*. In Cooper EL, Langlet C and Bierne J (Eds), *Developmental and Comparative Immunology*.

Alan R Liss: New York. pp 129 – 140.

Sailendri K and Muthukkaruppan VR (1975). Morphology of lymphoid organs in a cichlid teleost *Tilapia mossambica* (Peters). *J Morph* **147**: 109 – 122.

Saito H (1977). Fine structure of the reticular cells in the rat spleen, with special reference to their fibromuscular features. *Arch Histol Jap* **40**: 333 – 345.

Saito H (1984). The development of the spleen in the Australian lungfish *Neoceratodus forsteri* Krefft, with special reference to its relationship to the 'gastro'-enteric vasculature. *Am J Anat* **169**: 337 – 360.

Sargent JR (1976). The structure, metabolism and function of lipids in marine organisms. In Malius DC and Sargent JR (Eds), *Biochemical and Biophysical Perspectives on Marine Biology*. Vol 3. Academic Press: London. pp 150 – 212.

Schneider B (1983). Ontogeny of fish lymphoid organs. *Dev Comp Immmunol* **7**: 739 – 740.

Schubart H (1966). Hemosiderin in the spleen and RES of the liver of various vertebrates. *Z Mikrosk Anat Forschung* **75**: 428 – 437.

Secombes CJ and Manning MJ (1980). Comparative studies on the immune system of fishes and amphibians. I. Antigen localization in the carp *Cyprinus carpio*. *J Fish Dis* **3**: 399 – 412.

Secombes CJ and Manning MJ (1982). Histological changes in lymphoid organs of carp following injection of soluble or particulate antigens. *Dev Comp Immunol* Suppl **2**: 53 – 58.

Secombes CJ, Manning MJ and Ellis AE (1982a). Localization of the immune complexes and heat-aggregated immunoglobulin in the carp *Cyprinus carpio* L. *Immunology* **47**: 101 – 105.

Secombes CJ, Manning MJ and Ellis AE (1982b). The effect of primary and secondary immunization on the lymphoid tissues of carp *Cyprinus carpio* L. *J Exp Zool* **220**: 277 – 287.

Sidky YA and Auerbach R (1968). Tissue culture analysis of immunological capacity of snapping turtles. *J Exp Zool* **167**: 187 – 196.

Smith AM, Potter M and Merchant EB (1967). Antibody-forming cells in the pronephros of the teleost *Lepomis macrochirus*. *J Immunol* **99**: 876 – 882.

Snook T (1964). Studies on the perifollicular region of the rat's spleen. *Anat Rec* **148**: 149 – 160.

Solnitzky S (1937). The Schweigger – Seidel sheath (ellipsoid) of the spleen. *Anat Rec* **69**: 55 – 75.

Sorell JM and Weiss L (1982). Development of the embryonic chick phagocytic system: intraembryonic erythrophagocytosis induced by phenyl-hydrazine. *J Morph* **171**: 183 – 194.

Sterba G (1950). Uber die morphologischen und histo-genetischen Thymus-probleme bei *Xenopus laevis* Daudin nebst einigen Bermerkungen uber die morphologie der Kaulquappen. *Abh Sachs Akad Wiss Leipzig Math Naturwiss KL44*: 1 – 54.

Sterba G (1951). Untersuchungen an der Milz des Krallenfrosches *Xenopus laevis*. *Morph Jb* **90**: 221 – 248.

Streefkerk JG and Veerman AJP (1971). Histochemistry and electron microscopy of follicle lining reticular cells in the rat spleen. *Z Zellforsch* **115**: 524 – 542.

Subramonia Pillai P (1977). Studies on the role of antigen-binding cells in the immune response to sheep erythrocytes in the lizard *Calotes versicolor*. PhD thesis, Madurai University, Tamilnadu (India).

Sugimura M and Hashimoto Y (1976). Cellular changes in the bursa of Fabricus and spleen of cyclophosphamide-treated ducks. *RES* **19**: 201 – 210.

Sugimura M and Hashimoto Y (1980). Quantitative histological studies on the spleen of ducks after neonatal thymectomy and bursectomy. *J Anat* **131**: 441 – 452.

Suzuki CK and Cohen N (1987). Phorbol ester stimulates *in vitro* proliferation of lymphocytes from the newt *Notophthalmus viridiscens* (Abstract). *Dev Comp Immunol* **11**: 452.

Tahan AM and Jurd RD (1979). Delayed hypersensitivity in *Ambystoma mexicanum*. *Dev Comp Immunol* **3**: 299 – 306.

Tahan AM and Jurd RD (1981). Antigen trapping in *Ambystoma mexicanum*: role of secondary lymphoid organs. *Dev Comp Immunol* **5**: 291 – 300.

Tait J (1927). A review of the structure and function of the spleen. *Br Med J* **2**: 291 – 294.

Tamura E and Honma Y (1970). Histological changes in the organs and tissues of the gobiid fishes throughout the life-span. III. Hemopoietic organs in the ice-goby *Leucopsariun petersi* Hilgendorf. *Bull Jap Soc Sci Fish* **36**: 661 – 669.

Tappel AL (1975). Lipid peroxidation and fluorescent molecular damage to membranes. In Troup BF and Arstila AV (Eds), *Pathobiology of Cell Membranes*. Vol I. Academic Press: London. pp 145 – 170.

Tatner MF (1985). The migration of labelled thymocytes to the peripheral lymphoid organs in the rainbow trout. *Salmo gairdneri* Richardson. *Dev Comp Immunol* **9**: 85 – 92.

Tatner MF and Manning MJ (1983). Growth of the lymphoid organs in rainbow trout *Salmo gairdneri* from one to fifteen months of age. *J Zool London* **199**: 503 – 520.

Thorbecke GJ, Gordon HA, Wostman B, Wagner M and Reyneirs JA (1957). Lymphoid tissue and serum gamma globulin in young germfree chickens. *J Infect Dis* **101**: 237 – 251.

Tischendorf F (1969). Die Milz. In Bargmann W (Ed), *Handbuch der Mikroskopischen Anatomie des Menschen*. Vol VI/6. Springer-Verlag: Berlin.

Tischendorf F (1985). On the evolution of spleen. *Experientia* **41**: 145 – 152.

Tochinai S (1976a). Lymphoid changes in *Xenopus laevis* following thymectomy at the initial stage of its histogenesis. *J Fac Sci Hokkaido Univ Ser VI Zool* **19**: 803 – 811.

Tochinai S (1976b). Demonstration of thymus-independent immune system in *Xenopus laevis*. *Immunology* **31**: 125–128.

Tochinai S, Nagata S and Katagiri C (1976). Restoration of immune responsiveness in early thymectomized *Xenopus* by implantation of histocompatible adult thymus. *Eur J Immunol* **6**: 711–714.

Toivanen A and Toivanen P (1977). Histocompatibility requirements for cellular cooperation in the chicken: generation of germinal centers. *J Immunol* **118**: 431–436.

Tomonaga S, Kobayashi K and Kajii T (1984). Two populations of immunoglobulin-forming cells in the skate *Raja kanojei*: their distribution and characterization. *Dev Comp Immunol* **8**: 803–812.

Tooze J and Davies HG (1967). Light and electron microscopic studies on the spleen of the newt *Triturus cristatus*: the fine structure of the erythropoietic cells. *J Cell Sci* **2**: 617–640.

Tournefier A (1973). Developpement des organes lymphoides chez l'amphibien urodele *Triturus alpestris* Laur: tolerance des allogreffes apres la thymectomie larvaire. *J Embryol Exp Morphol* **29**: 383–396.

Turner RJ (1969). The functional development of the reticuloendothelial system in the toad *Xenopus laevis* (Daudin). *J Exp Zool* **170**: 467–480.

Turner RJ (1973). Response of the toad *Xenopus laevis* to circulating antigens. II. Responses after splenectomy. *J Exp Zool* **183**: 35–46.

Turner RJ and Manning MJ (1973). Response of the toad *Xenopus laevis* to circulating antigens. I. Cellular changes in the spleen. *J Exp Zool* **183**: 21–34.

Turner RJ, Nguyen-Dang T and Manning MJ (1974). Effects of *Corynebacterium parvum* and Freund's adjuvants on amphibian antibody responses. *J Ret Soc* **16**: 232–238.

van Woert MH and Palmer SH (1969). Inhibition of the growth of mouse melanoma by chlorpromazine. *Cancer Res* **29**: 1925–1955.

Veerman AJP and van Ewijk W (1975). White pulp compartments in the spleen of rats and mice: a light and electron microscopic study of lymphoid and non-lymphoid cell types in T- and B-areas. *Cell Tissue Res* **156**: 417–441.

von Rautenfeld DB and Bubras K-D (1980). A comparative study on the bursa (Fabricii) and tonsilla caecalis in birds. *Folia Morphol (Praha)* **28**: 168–170.

Walvig F (1958). Blood and parenchymal cells in the spleen of the ice fish *Chaenocephalus aceratus* (Lonnberg). *Nytt Magasin Zool* **6**: 111–120.

Warr GW and Marchalonis JJ (1977). Lymphocyte surface immunoglobulin of the goldfish differs from its serum counterpart. *Dev Comp Immunol* **1**: 15–22.

Watkins D (1985). T-cell function in *Xenopus*: Studies on T-cell ontogeny and cytotoxicity using an IL-2 like growth factor. PhD thesis, University of Rochester, New York.

Watkins D and Cohen N (1985). The phylogeny of interleukin-2. *Dev Comp Immunol* **9**: 819–824.

Weber WT and Weidanz WP (1969). Prolonged bursal lymphocyte depletion and suppression of antibody formation following irradiation of the bursa of Fabricius. *J Immunol* **103**: 537–543.

Weilacher S (1933). Die Milz der gymnophionen. Beitrag zur kenntnis der gymnophione Nr. XVII. *Morphol Zb* **72**: 469–498.

Weiss L (1972). Spleen. In *The Cells and Tissues of the Immune System*. Prentice-Hall: Englewood Cliffs, New Jersey.

Weiss L and Chen LT (1974). The differentiation of white pulp and red pulp in the spleen of human fetuses (72–145 mm crown–rump length). *Am J Anat* **141**: 393–414.

Weiss L, Powell R and Schiffman FJ (1985). Terminating arterial vessels in red pulp of human spleen: a transmission electron mircoscopic study. *Experientia* **41**: 233–242.

Welsch U and Storch V (1982). Light and electron microscopical observations on the caecilian spleen. A contribution to the evolution of lymphatic organs. *Dev Comp Immunol* **6**: 293–302.

Wetherall JD and Turner KJ (1972). Immune response of the lizard *Tiliqua rugosa*. *Aust J Exp Biol Med Sci* **50**: 79–95.

White RG (1969). Recognition mechanisms in the chicken spleen. *Antibiot Chemother* **15**: 24–39.

White RG, French VI and Stark JM (1970). A study of the localization of a protein antigen in the chicken spleen and its relation to the formation of germinal centres. *J Med Microbiol* **3**: 65–83.

Whiting AJ (1897). On the comparative histology and physiology of the spleen. *Trans R Soc Edinb* **38**: 253–316.

Wislocki GB (1917). The action of vital dyes in teleost. *Anat Rec* **12**: 415–427.

Wolfe HR, Sheridan SA, Bilstad NM and Johnson MA (1962). The growth of lymphoidal organs and the testes of chickens. *Anat Rec* **142**: 485–493.

Woods R and Linna J (1965). The transport of cells from the bursa of Fabricius to the spleen and thymus. *Acta Pathol Microbiol Scand* **64**: 470–476.

Wright RK and Shapiro HC (1973). Primary and secondary immune response of the desert iguana *Dipsosaurus dorsalis*. *Herpetologica* **29**:275–280.

Wright RK, Eipert EF and Cooper EL (1978). Regulatory role of temperature on the development of ectothermic vertebrate lymphocyte populations. In Gershwin ME and Cooper EL (Eds), *Animal Models of Comparative and Developmental Aspects of Immunity and Disease*. Pergamon Press: New York. pp 80–92.

Yamada H (1951). The blood vascular system of the postbranchial alimentary canal in the lamprey (in Japanese). *Okayama Igakukai Zasstii* **63**: 1–51.

Yoffey JM (1929). A contribution to the study of the comparative histology and physiology of the spleen, with reference chiefly to its cellular constituents. *J Anat* **63**: 314–344.

Yu M-L, Sarot DA, Filazzola RJ and Perlmutter A (1970).

Effects of splenectomy on the immune response of the blue gourami *Trichogaster trichopterus* to infectious pancreatic necrosis (IPN) virus. *Life Sci* G Pt II: 749–755.

Yu M-L, Kiley CW, Sarot DA and Perlmutter A (1971). Regulation of haemosiderin to erythropoiesis in the blue gourami *Trichogaster trichopterus*. *J Fish Res Board Can* **28**: 47–48.

Zapata A (1980). Ultrastructure of elasmobranch lymphoid tissue. I. Thymus and spleen. *Dev Comp Immunol* **4**: 459–472.

Zapata A (1982). Lymphoid organs of teleost fish. III. Splenic lymphoid tissue of *Rutilus rutilus* and *Gobio gobio*. *Dev Comp Immunol* **6**: 87–94.

Zapata A, Villena A and San Miguel R (1979). Estudio ultra-structural de los microambientes hematopoieticos de *Pleurodeles waltlii*. *Morf Norm Patol* **3**: 445–456.

Zapata A, Leceta J and Barrutia MG (1981a). Ultrastructure of splenic white pulp of the turtle *Mauremys caspica*. *Cell Tissue Res* **220**: 845–855.

Zapata A, Leceta J and Solas MT (1981b). The spleen of *Mauremys caspica*. A histophysiological model for comparative immunology. *Dev Comp Immunol* **5** (Suppl. 1): 137–142.

Zapata A, Gomariz RP, Garrido E and Cooper EL (1982). Lymphoid organs and blood cells of the caecilian *Icthyophis kohtaoensis*. *Acta Zool (Stockh)* **63**: 11–16.

Zwillenberg HHL (1964). *Bau and funktion der Forellenmilz*. Hans Huber: Bern.

7

Lymph Nodes

INTRODUCTION

During the evolution of the circulatory system, as blood pressure increased more liquids and plasma proteins escaped from the capillaries into the interstitial fluid than was returned to it by the veins. To accommodate this condition, a separate lymphatic system evolved. The lymphatic system plays a role in returning fluid and plasma proteins from tissues to the main part of the circulatory system. Since foreign, antigenic material which is potentially pathogenic may enter, both the circulatory and lymphatic systems simultaneously evolved organs of the immune system—the spleen and lymph nodes—which can therefore filter blood and lymph.

The lymphatic system has reached its greatest development in eutherian or placental mammals, where lymphatic capillaries occur in most tissues of the body. Lymphatic capillaries are more permeable and pressures within them are lower than blood capillaries which lie between arteries and veins. Since lymphatic capillaries are highly permeable, they are the most likely route for the spread of microorganisms or cancer cells within the body. Lymph nodes lie at many points where small lymphatic vessels converge. As small, well-defined bodies, lymph nodes possess the two anatomical and functional divisions of the immune system, T and B areas, where lymphocytes are found. In addition, there are numerous macrophages which trap and phagocytose antigen in both non-specific as well as specific immune responses. The evolution of lymph nodes from fish to monotreme mammals will be the subject of this chapter.

FISH

Teleost fish are endowed with a thymus, spleen and an interesting organ—the pronephros or head kidney. It should be mentioned in this chapter that controversy exists concerning where to categorize the head kidney. Whereas some comparative immunologists have considered the pronephros a homolog of lymph nodes, you have read earlier that we have chosen to classify it as an equivalent of bone marrow. This classification is mostly due to the fact that every line of hemopoietic differentiation has been observed in the pronephros, including the capacity for that which is more closely related to the immune system, i.e. lymph- and plasma-cytopoiesis.

AMPHIBIANS

General Considerations

Amphibians occupy a critical point in the evolution of terrestrial vertebrates and are convenient models for explaining the ontogeny and phylogeny of functional components of vertebrate immune systems. For this reason, numerous studies have focused on the potentialities of their immune systems (Borysenko, 1976; Cooper, 1976a; Cohen, 1977). The anuran lymphoid system consists principally of the thymus and spleen. Moreover, bone marrow and aggregations of lymphoid cells in structures which resemble mammalian lymph nodes have evolved for the first time in anurans. The most important lymphomyeloid organs of anuran larvae are the lymph glands and ventral cavity bodies. In adult anurans they are the jugular, procoracoid and prepericardial bodies. The anatomy and histology of these organs were first reanalyzed in *Rana catesbeiana* (Cooper, 1965, 1966a, b, 1976b; Baculi and Cooper, 1968), in *Bufo marinus* (Kent *et al.*, 1964; Evans *et al.*, 1966; Diener and Nossal, 1966) and in other diverse, anuran species (Baculi *et al.*, 1970). Their ontogeny has been studied in *Rana pipiens* (Horton, 1971b). These organs are situated in the branchial region of larvae and in throat and axillary regions of adults. They are composed of small to large lymphocytes, plasma cells, granulocytes and monocytes. These more solid parenchymal components are broken by intervening sinusoids which are lined by phagocytic cells (Baculi and Cooper, 1968; Horton, 1971b). With respect to their functional significance, comparative immunologists consider them precursors of mammalian hemolymph nodes (Baculi and Cooper, 1968) and the lymph nodes which are first observed in primitive mammals (Diener and Nossal, 1966).

Anuran Larvae

The tadpoles of many higher anurans possess a lymphomyeloid node different from that found in adults. This is the larval lymph gland, a bilateral structure located in the branchial chamber near the developing anterior limb (Cooper, 1967a, b). The lymph glands are attached to the membranes which separate the gill cavity from the lymphatic sinuses and grow deeply into the temporal lymphatic sinuses (Szarski, 1938). The lymph glands of *Rana catesbeiana* and *Rana pipiens* disappear after metamorphosis (Riviere and Cooper, 1973; Cooper, 1976a, b) but these organs persist in *Rana esculenta* and are localized within the accumulations of fat immediately under the skin (Szarski, 1938). Unexpectedly, the lymph gland is absent in another representative of the genus *Rana*, i.e. *R. temporaria* (Plytycz and Bigaj, 1982). The lymph gland does not exist in other anuran genera, e.g. in *Alytes* (Du Pasquier, 1968), *Xenopus* (Manning and Horton, 1969), *Bufo* or *Bombina* (Plytycz and Bigaj, 1982). Clearly experimental results have revealed that the lymph gland may house stem cells that can differentiate into T- and B-lymphocytes (Cooper *et al.*, 1975). Its functional equivalent in animals which do not possess the lymph gland is unknown (Cooper, 1976a, b).

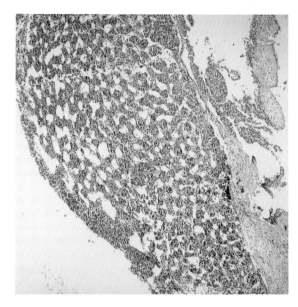

Figure 7.1 Larval lymph gland showing lymphocytes, sinusoids and reticuloendothelial cells ($\times$ 150).

The larval lymph gland, like its adult equivalents, is composed of lobules of mostly lymphoid cells which surround blood sinusoids lined by reticuloendothelial cells (Figure 7.1). The lymph gland's parenchyma is supported by stromal cells as well as macrophages, granulocytes and plasma cells (Baculi and Cooper, 1968). Some of the macrophages and reticuloendothelial cells can phagocytose injected carbon particles of India ink that circulate through the lymph gland from its blood sinusoids (Baculi and Cooper, 1968). However, it should be noted that the larval lymph gland lies in the anterior lymphatic sinus (Horton, 1971a, b; and unpublished morphological observations), which suggests that cells on the outer surface of the gland, next to this lymphatic sinus, are capable of taking up ink directly from the body fluids. The lymph gland may thus be both a blood- and lymph-filtering organ (Cooper, 1976b).

The larval lymph gland plays a role in humoral immunity. Blast cell transformation and plaque-forming cells have been observed in lymph glands of larvae injected with foreign erythrocytes (Moticka *et al.*, 1973; Cooper *et al.*, 1975). Tadpoles with lymph glands removed fail to synthesize antibody but are able to reject allografts (Cooper, 1968; Cooper *et al.*,

1971). However, the gland can not only restore antibody synthesis to foreign erythrocytes, but it can also partially restore transplantation immunity in larvae rendered immunologically incompetent by total body irradiation (Cooper *et al.*, 1975). These results lead to the postulation that the lymph gland is a source of both T- and B-stem cells.

Other organs, larval branchial bodies, are ideally situated to deal with pathogens which are present in the water and can pass through the gills or gain entry via the operculum opening (Horton, 1971a, b). Four pairs of ventral cavity bodies and two pairs of dorsal cavity bodies occur constantly in the branchial region of *Xenopus laevis* (Tochinai, 1975), while *Rana pipiens* larvae possess the extreme number (maximum 30) of ventral cavity bodies (Horton, 1971a, b). During early metamorphic stages, the number of branchial bodies diminishes rapidly and at the end of metamorphosis they have disappeared (Horton, 1971a, b).

Adult Anurans—The Lymphomyeloid Organs, Notably the Jugular Bodies

General Morphology

The jugular body of adult *Rana pipiens* is a bilateral organ that lies lateral to the sternohyoideus muscle and ventromedial to the parathyroids, external jugular veins, hypoglossal nerve and external carotid artery. The organ is encapsulated by a thin mesothelium and an underlying connective tissue layer formed by fibroblasts and collagenous fibres. Numerous fat cells surround the capsule and sometimes appear inside the jugular body. The parenchyma is composed of cell cords arranged between sinusoidal blood vessels (Figure 7.2). The cords consist of supporting reticular cells and fibers and free lymphoid elements (Figure 7.3).

Reticular Cells

Reticular cells are large, branched, electron-dense elements that exhibit a round nucleus and cytoplasm with numerous vesicles, small, electron-dense granules and Golgi bodies (Figure 7.4). Some small mitochondria and many free or membrane-associated ribosomes are also present. Bundles of cytoplasmic filaments and zonulae adherens-type cell junctions join the reticular cells, a most remarkable feature. Reticular fibers appear in the intercellular spaces, sometimes in close association with the reticular cells.

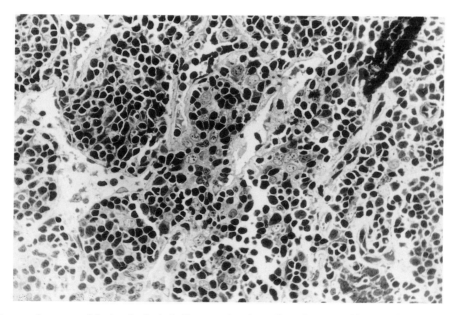

Figure 7.2 Panoramic survey of the jugular body in *Rana* sp. showing cell cords arranged between blood sinuses. The cords are composed mainly of lymphoid cells. The sinuses are lined by flat endothelial cells ($\times$ 320).

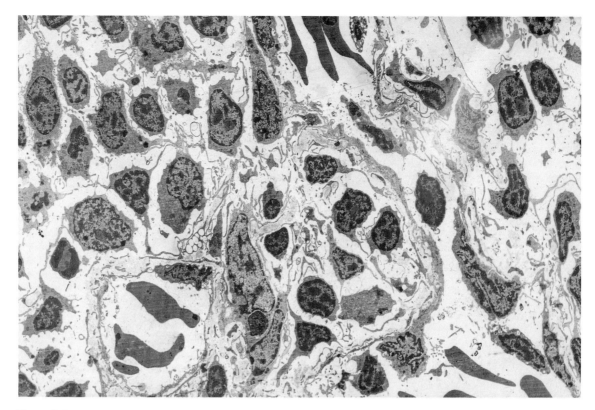

Figure 7.3 Ultrastructural organization of the parenchyma in the jugular body. Cell cords containing small and medium lymphocytes, macrophages and supporting reticular cells occur between blood sinuses formed by irregular endothelial cells (× 2250).

Lymphoid Cells

Small and medium lymphocytes, lymphoblasts and developing and mature plasma cells are the most frequently observed free cells (Figure 7.5). Small lymphocytes are electron dense, with a high nucleo-cytoplasmic ratio, and abundant condensed chromatin. The cytoplasm contains numerous free ribonucleoproteins and scant membranous organelles. In contrast, medium lymphocytes have a smaller nucleo-cytoplasmic ratio, the amount of condensed chromatin is decreased and there is a prominent nucleolus. The cytoplasm exhibits characteristics similar to those found in smaller lymphocytes. Lymphoblasts are numerous and may represent precursors of plasma cells. They show a low electron density, scant, condensed chromatin and a large nucleolus. In their cytoplasm there are free polysomes, light electron-dense mitochondria, and few, small granules. Developing plasma cells contain numerous elements of rough endoplasmic reticulum arranged in parallel fashion, large mitochondria and a few cytoplasmic granules. Frequently, these cells appear to be in mitosis. Mature plasma cells exhibit an electron-dense nucleus with abundant, condensed chromatin and an inactive nucleolus. Their cytoplasm is filled with a well-dilated, rough endoplasmic reticulum that contains an electron-dense material (Figure 7.6).

Other Free Cells

There are smaller numbers of other free cells, which are mainly macrophages, neutrophils and eosinophils. Macrophages are large, with an irregular nucleus and cytoplasm filled with slightly electron-dense vesicles, Golgi bodies, elements of smooth endoplasmic reticulum and residual dense bodies. Neutrophils have a

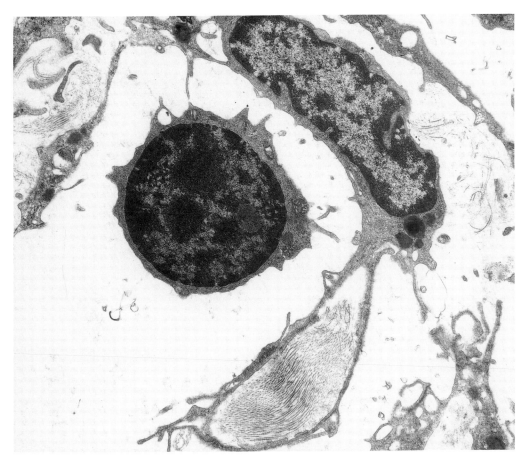

Figure 7.4 Reticular cells constitute the supporting apparatus of the parenchyma in the jugular body of *Rana* sp. These cells show numerous, irregular processes embracing collagenous fibers. Electron-dense granules appear in the cytoplasm. Note the small lymphocyte near the reticular cell ($\times$ 12500).

lobulated nucleus and long, or rounded, granules of variable electron density that seem to correspond to a single granular type. Eosinophils are electron dense, and contain two granular types, both devoid of crystalline inclusions; one is small, round and electron dense, and the other is larger, round or polygonal, and exhibits less electron density (Figure 7.7).

Vascularization

Jugular bodies are well vascularized by blood sinusoids which are found between cell cords. Sinusoids are lined by electron-dense, sometimes irregular endothelial cells which contain numerous cytoplasmic filaments. They are joined by cell interdigitations and junctional complexes, and show a discontinuous basement membrane. Occasionally, lymphatic vessels are found in the jugular bodies of *Rana pipiens* and are characterized by extremely thin irregular walls without a basement membrane (Figure 7.8). Innervation, although mainly vasomotor, does involve nerve endings within cell cords near reticular cells and lymphoid cells.

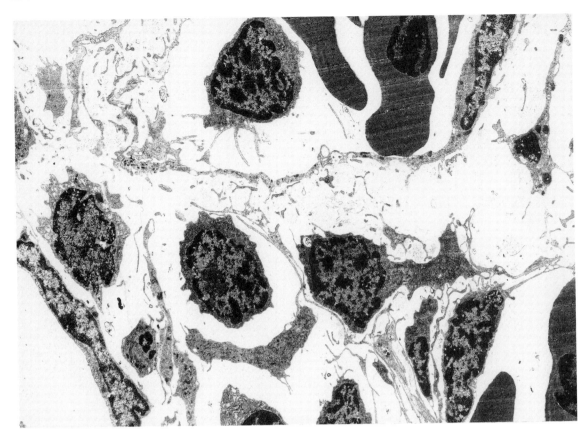

Figure 7.5 Note small and medium lymphocytes and plasma cells which occur between the processes of reticular cells. The lymphocytes are characterized by their high electron density, abundant condensed chromatin, patent nucleolus and scarce nucleo-cytoplasmic ratio. Note the nerve endings scattered among the cellular elements ($\times$ 6880).

Relationship to Immunity

The ultrastructure of jugular bodies in adult leopard frogs (Villena and Zapata, 1981; Zapata *et al.*, 1981a) confirms the structure revealed by light microscopy in other diverse anuran species (Cooper, 1965, 1966a, b, 1967a, b; Evans *et al.*, 1966; Diener and Nossal, 1966; Baculi and Cooper, 1967, 1968; Baculi *et al.*, 1970; Horton, 1971a, b). However, there are important differences in the parenchymal organization, vascularization and functional significance. These include differences in relation to phagocytic function of sinusoidal lining cells and reticular cells (Baculi *et al.*, 1970; Horton, 1971a, b). According to ultrastructural analyses, the phagocytic capacity is localized exclusively in macrophages which occur free in the parenchyma. Sinusoidal endothelia and fixed reticular cells do not exhibit numerous phagosome-like bodies. By contrast, sinusoidal lining cells are characterized by abundant pinocytotic vesicles on both sides; reticular cells have cytoplasmic filaments and cell junctions.

Reticular cells. Reticular cells appear to function exclusively to support free cells, whereas free macrophages are responsible for binding antigens. Earlier, however, in the jugular body of *Bufo marinus*, Diener and Marchalonis (1970) found that the surfaces of reticular cells bind flagellar antigens. In higher vertebrates, two types of antigen localization occur in lymph nodes (Nossal, 1967). One type is found in macrophages typical of medullary areas, while a second type, termed follicular localization, involves

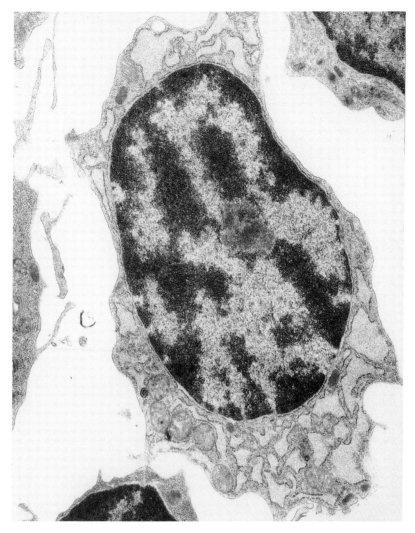

Figure 7.6 Mature plasma cells are the most frequent elements in the jugular body of *Rana* sp. Note the peripheral arrangement of the condensed chromatin in the nucleus, and active nucleolus. In the cytoplasm, clearly there are dilated cisternae of rough endoplasmic reticulum which contains electron dense material (× 17000).

the attachment of antigen to reticular cell surfaces in lymphoid follicles. These discrepancies may be due to the absence of any follicular organization in anuran jugular bodies and perhaps species variability. Thus it is possible to consider that binding may occur by free macrophages.

Lymphocytes and plasma cell precursors. Ultra-structural results confirm the abundance of lympho-cytes, and few plasma cells, granulocytes and

monocytes in anuran jugular bodies (Baculi and Cooper, 1968; Baculi *et al.*, 1970; Horton, 1971a, b). However, the existence of dividing precursors of plasma cells and proplasmatocytes underscores the important plasmacytopoietic capacity of the jugular body. Moreover, in another species, the fine structure of *Bufo* plasma cells resembles that of typical mam-malian-type plasma cells, with extensive intracisternal enlargement of the rough endoplasmic reticulum, apparently where large amounts of Ig are stored

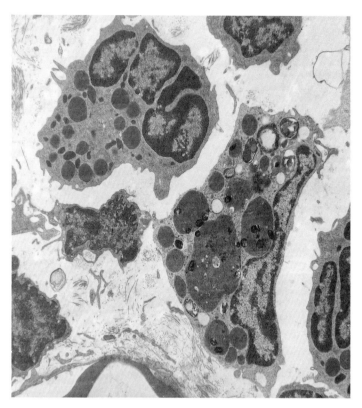

Figure 7.7 Eosinophilic granulocytes and macrophages in the jugular body of *Rana* sp. The eosinophil shows a lobulated nucleus with abundant, condensed chromatin and round or polygonal electron-dense cytoplasmic granules of various sizes. Macrophages are characterized by numerous, electron-dense bodies which fill the cytoplasm (× 7125).

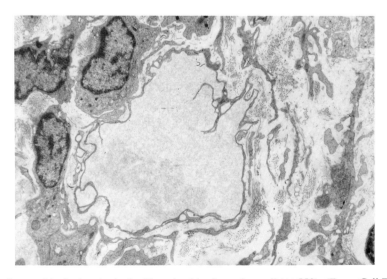

Figure 7.8 Lymphatic vessel in the jugular body. Note the thin, irregular wall (× 550). (From *Cell Tissue Res* **221**: 193, 1981, reproduced by permission.)

(Cowden and Dyer, 1971). Although the significance of increased Ig synthesis is not clear, the role of temperature must be considered (Wright *et al.*, 1978). Several authors (Kent *et al.*, 1964; Diener and Nossal, 1966; Ambrosius and Hanstein, 1971) have demonstrated antibody-forming cells in anuran jugular bodies which develop after challenge by different antigens. However, the functional significance of these organs is still not well understood.

Changes following immunization. Jugular bodies change following immunization (Diener and Nossal, 1966). There is a marked increase in pyroninophilia accompanied by the appearance of antibody-producing plasma cells to soluble antigens (Kent *et al.*, 1964; Evans *et al.*, 1966) and plaque-forming cells to sheep erythrocytes (SRBC) (Minagawa *et al.*, 1975; Wright and Cooper, 1980). Second, antigen is retained extracellularly on the processes of dendritic cells, as in the spleen (Diener and Marchalonis, 1970), antigen trapping occurs randomly throughout the lymphocytic nodules of the organ and pyroninophilia is similarly widespread. Despite these changes, there seems to be no germinal center formation similar to that which occurs in the mammalian lymph node (Diener and Nossal, 1966).

These findings support yet another view, that at the anuran amphibian stage of evolution jugular bodies may not be true nodes but are organs with sinusoidal blood flow which provide another site where lymphoid cells can accumulate and respond to stimulation by antigens. In *Rana pipiens*, however, the jugular bodies, rather than the spleen, are sites where long-term antigen retention occurs (M. J. Manning, unpublished observations). Thus, HGG appeared in jugular bodies during the first week after injection (via either intramuscular, intraperitoneal or dorsal lymph sac route), and only began to disappear after about week 9.

In another species, *Rana bermeja*, changes in the jugular body have been studied in relation to immunization with a T-dependent antigen, SRBC (Zapata *at al.*, 1981a, b). On day 7 after antigen stimulation, there are four apparent morphological changes. First, there is an active cellular diapedesis and extravasation, followed by frequent appearances of lymphoblasts with a small amount of condensed chromatin and an electron-light cytoplasm. Second, actively dividing proplasma cells as well as many mature plasma cells

have been observed. Third, there is a remarkable increase in eosinophils under the capsule concomitant with an apparent increase in immature myelocytes. Moreover, there is a high number of eosinophils and some remains of degranulated eosinophils near the capsule. On day 14, plasma cells were less numerous in the stroma and areas of eosinophil accumulation and degranulation occurred in cellular cords. On day 21, the jugular body again showed lymphoblasts and developing plasma cells.

Some evolutionary considerations. Diener and Nossal (1966) found that the nodes of *Bufo marinus* filter lymph and are apparently homologous to primitive lymph nodes in the monotreme mammal, the echidna. In contrast, Baculi *et al.* (1970) concluded after extensive studies in *R. catesbeiana* and other anurans that all lymphomyeloid organs are interposed between blood vessels and not between lymphatic vessels. Thus, they are not comparable to the lymphatic system of mammals. Our fine-structural analyses reveal the importance of sinusoidal blood vascularization, but there are also lymphatic vessels in the jugular bodies. These organs may therefore filter blood- and lymph-borne antigens, responding by producing numerous plasma cells. Still, the organ is not homologous to mammalian lymph nodes or hemolymph nodes. To resolve this controversy further investigations combining structural and immunological analysis are necessary for understanding the phylogenetic significance of these primitive organs.

REPTILES

With respect to lymph nodes, the situation in reptiles appears to be more advanced. The gecko, *Gehyra variegata*, is interesting because of the discovery by Johnston (1973) of lymphoid tissue in the axillae closely associated with the lymphatic and blood systems. Within the perivascular space—a part of the lymphatic system—perivascular lymphoid tissue occurs in both axillary sinuses. This lymphoid tissue invests the veins draining the body wall as they cross the axillary sinus to join the lateral vein. As in all lymphoid tissues, gecko lymphocytes are provided with an internal support composed of reticular cells and fibers.

The axillary sinus, because of its location, may be

continuous with the lateral lymphatics; it is lined with endothelium. All lymphatics and blood vessels are lined by simple squamous, flattened epithelial cells, through which mobile leukocytes can squeeze by diapedesis. Lymph is carried in the lateral lymphatics, flows into the sinus, and bathes the vein and perivascular lymphoid tissue before continuing to the lymphaticovenous junction. Such an arrangement represents a fundamental difference in structure and function between the gecko's organs and analogous amphibian organs which, despite controversy, appear to be blood filtering, since all blood cells, erythrocytes and leukocytes must pass through them. Of even more importance to immunity is how mature lymphocytes can enter either the lymphatic or circulatory systems. One difference lies in the fact that the lymph on the lymphatic end should consist only of lymphocytes, with no myeloid leukocytes or granulocytes, or erythrocytes. Thus, in regard to lymph filtration, the gecko lymph nodule is apparently functionally close to that of mammals.

The axillary position of the gecko's node-like structure, interesting as it is, recalls such locations of primary nodes in mammals; primary nodes lack germinal centers. The basic architecture of the gecko node, i.e. lymphoid tissue supported by a reticular framework surrounding a blood vessel and all enclosed within a lymphatic, confirms its striking similarity to that of the monotreme mammal, the echidna (see Monotreme mammals). In the snake, *Elaphe*, lymphoid tissue occurs in the wall of the cardinal lymphatic vessel, giving it superficial resemblance to nodes in the domestic fowl (Kotani, 1959; Biggs, 1957). Modern analyses of reptilian lymphoid organs raise the issue of the possible evolution of avian and mammalian lymph nodes from a common, extant reptilian ancestor.

BIRDS

General Considerations

The presence of lymph nodes in birds has to some extent been a matter of controversy, at least during recent times. This may be due to the fact that relevant observations were made fairly early during the history of modern immunology (Manabe, 1930a, b, c; Kihara and Naito, 1933; Kondo, 1937a, b, c; Biggs, 1957).

Second, a great deal of focus in avian immunology has been on the thymus and bursal system peculiar to birds which results in less experimental information dealing with other components such as the bone marrow, spleen, lymph nodes and organs described in Chapter 8 on GALT, BALT, UALT, etc. In birds, lymphoid aggregations have become more complex and there seems to have evolved, for the first time, a separation into organs that filter lymph and not blood, known as lymphoid aggregates (LA) (Olah and Glick, 1983).

These authors have described three types of LA based on histology, which may reflect different developmental stages and correlate with their functional activity. Although Biggs (1957) distinguished three types of nodes on the basis of size, Olah and Glick (1983) conclude that size of LA does not reflect its structural framework since size may be a function of sinuses. The presence or absence of sinuses may determine whether they will respond to the injection of antigen into the foot-pad (McCorkle *et al.*, 1979). The smallest LA appear as lymphoid infiltrations embedded in fat tissue. According to Biggs (1957), these accumulations seem to be non-encapsulated. A second type of LA differs from the small LA in that it possesses germinal centers, which seem to develop in response to antigen stimulation. These two types do not contain lymphatic sinuses and germinal centers are located far from the lymphatic trunk. Thus, these LA may receive an antigenic stimulus from the blood via blood vessels located in the fat which surrounds the LA instead of the lymphatics.

Structure of Lymphoid Aggregations

Circulation

The most complex LA will be referred to as a lymph node (LN), which possesses well-developed sinuses which are absent in the other LA. LN are comparable to the cervicothoracic lymph node of water fowls (Kampmeier, 1969). The surface of sinuses is smooth, but in several places along the endothelium hairy macrophages occur which render these sinuses competent for lymph filtration and antigen trapping. With respect to circulation, anatomical analyses have been performed. When perfusion fixation was carried out 30 minutes after ligature of the femoral artery and vein, the sinuses and intersinusoidal substance of the LN were filled with erythrocytes. Thus, after blocking venous circulation, blood may enter the lymphatic system. This observation by Olah and Glick may confirm Kampmeier's (1969), who proposed the existence of a lymphaticovenous anastomosis in the periphery.

Location of B and T Areas

The existence of functional lymphocyte subtypes has been considered. These well-developed LN possess a compartmentalization which contains T- and B-lymphocytes. For example, after foot-pad injection of PHA, certain nodes developed large areas containing mainly lymphoblasts, while other regions possessed only small lymphocytes. According to one interpretation, the lymphoblast-containing area was originally a 'T-dependent' one which responds to stimulation by PHA, while the area containing small lymphocytes may be a 'B-dependent' area. That lymphocytes may migrate through sinus walls suggests the presence of T- and B-cell compartmentalization, as in mammalian lymph nodes, a finding previously confirmed by Berens von Rautenfeld and Budras (1983).

The condition of the capsule is controversial. According to Biggs (1957), nodes lack a capsule, but Olah and Glick (1983) found one. Assuming that the lymphoid tissue is well developed, it may reach the capsule. However, if lymphoid tissue is scarce the space beneath the capsule is filled by fat cells and the node appears to lack a capsule. Thus the delicate connective tissue capsule may determine the presence of a distinct compartment, which is filled by fat cells and lymphocytes. In the presence of antigen or mitogen, lymphoid areas increase and fat decreases. The relationship between lymphoid and adipose tissues may be similar to that of the bone marrow. Instead of lymphoid tissue, myeloid tissue is present.

MAMMALS (MONOTREME)

Basic Structure Differs from Eutherian Mammals

The interesting organ of the echidna's immune system has been referred to as the lymph nodule. By means of a lymphogram, injections of an X-ray-detectable, radio-opaque dye, the patterns of the thoracic duct

and clusters of lymph nodules of the echidna become obvious. A comparison of the echidna's lymph nodules with those of a placental mammal, the rat, shows that they are fundamentally different. Whereas a single rat node is composed of many nodules and lies in the path of a lymphatic vessel with afferent and efferent channels, several echidna nodules lie within the lumen of a lymphatic vessel suspended by a vascular bundle. A large circular sinus represents the interspace between the lymphatic vascular wall and the lymph nodule.

There are other obvious differences. Echidna nodules are composed primarily of small lymphocytes, located in the periphery, that are vascularized by post-capillary venules; there are no primary lymphoid follicles in the periphery of the nodule. In eutherian or placental mammals, primary nodules such as these are composed of densely packed lymphocytes arranged in the outer portion of the node and referred to as the cortex. The medulla, the inner area of a eutherian mammalian node, is absent in the echidna.

FINAL COMMENT

Formation of Germinal Centers

Labelling echidna nodes with tritiated thymidine after antigen stimulation reveals the presence of highly active germinal centers, usually one per nodule. Antigen is localized first around the entire nodule, but later it appears in the germinal center. Occasionally germinal centers are located eccentrically. Thus, the eutherian mammals may be more efficient after encountering the same antigen a second time, producing therefore both primary and secondary responses. In other words, in eutherian nodes, germinal centers, characteristic of secondary follicles, seem to stand ready for encounter with antigens. Such complexity of follicular arrangement into a single node is absent in monotremes; this difference may account for the atypical secondary or memory response of monotremes. It is assumed that the monotreme lymph node represents a primitive stage in the phylogeny of placental mammalian lymph nodes. It recalls the fish, amphibian, reptile and even avian lymph node condition.

REFERENCES

Ambrosius H and Haustein R (1971). Beitrage zur Immunobiologie poikilothermer Wilbeltiere. VI Die Dynamik antikorperproduzierender Zellen in den lymphoiden organen des Wasserfrosches *Rana esculenta* L. *Acta Biol Med Ger* **27**: 771–782.

Baculi BS and Cooper EL (1967). Lymphomyeloid organs of amphibia. II. Vasculature in larval and adult *Rana catesbeiana*. *J Morph* **123**: 463–479.

Baculi BS and Cooper EL (1968). Lymphomyeloid organs of amphibia. IV. Normal histology in larval and adult *Rana catesbeiana*. *J Morph* **126**: 463–476.

Baculi BS, Cooper EL and Brown BA (1970). Lymphomyeloid organs of amphibia. V. Comparative histology in diverse anuran species. *J Morph* **131**: 315–328.

Berens von Rautenfeld D and Budras K-D (1983). Topography, ultrastructure and phagocytic capacity of avian lymph nodes. *Cell Tissue Res* **228**: 389–403.

Berens von Rautenfeld D, Budras K-D, Manthey H and Stenzel H (1981). Zur feinstruktor und funktion der aviarem lymphknoten. *Verh Anat Ges* **75**: 741–743.

Biggs PM (1957). The association of lymphoid tissue with the lymph vessels in the domestic chicken *Gallus domesticus*. *Acta Anat* **29**: 36–47.

Borysenko M (1976). Phylogeny of immunity: an overview. *Immunogenetics* **3**: 305–326.

Cohen N (1977). Phylogenetic emergence of lymphoid tissues and cells. In Marchalonis JJ (Ed), *The Lymphocyte, Structure and Function*. Part I. Marcel Dekker: New York. pp 115–205.

Cooper EL (1965). Some aspects of the reticuloendothelial system in *Rana catesbeiana* (Abstract). *Anat Rec* **151**: 448

Cooper EL (1966a). Algunos aspectos de inmunidad en invertebrados, peces y anfibios (Abstract). *Acta Med* **2**: 1–5.

Cooper EL (1966b). The lympho-myeloid organs of *Rana catesbeiana* (Abstract). *Anat Rec* **154**: 456.

Cooper EL (1967a). Lymphomyeloid organs of amphibia. I. Appearance during larval and adult stages of *Rana catesbeiana*. *J Morph* **122**: 381–398.

Cooper EL (1967b). Some aspects of the histogenesis of the amphibian lymphomyeloid system and its role in immunity. In Smith RT, Good RA and Miescher PA (Eds), *Ontogeny of Immunity*. University of Florida Press: Gainesville. pp 87–102.

Cooper EL (1968). Lymphomyeloid organs of amphibia. III. Antibody synthesis and lymph glands in larval bullfrogs. *Anat Rec* **162**: 453–458.

Cooper EL (1976a). *Comparative Immunology*. Prentice Hall: Englewood Cliffs, New Jersey. p 336.

Cooper EL (1976b). Immunity mechanisms. In Lofts B (Ed), *Physiology of the Amphibia*. Vol III. Academic Press: New York. pp 164–272

Cooper EL, Brown BA and Baculi BS (1971). New observations on lymph gland (LM1) and thymus activity in larval bullfrogs *Rana catesbeiana*. In Lindahl-Kiessling, K,

Alm G and Hanna Jr MG (Eds), *Morphological and Fundamental Aspects of Immunity*. Advances in Experimental Medicine and Biology, Vol 12. Plenum Press: New York. pp 1–10.

Cooper EL, Brown BA and Wright RK (1975). New ideas on amphibian immunity: the lymph gland: a generator of both T and B cells. *Am Zool* **15**: 85–92.

Cowden RR and Dyer RF (1971). Lymphopoietic tissue and plasma cells in amphibians. *Am Zool* **11**: 183–192.

Diener E and Marchalonis J (1970). Cellular and humoral aspects of the primary immune response of the toad *Bufo marinus*. *Immunology* **18**: 279–293.

Diener E and Nossal GJV (1966). Phylogenetic studies on the immune response. Localization of antigens and immune response in the toad *Bufo marinus*. *Immunology* **10**: 535–542.

Du Pasquier L (1968). Les proteines seriques et le complexe lymphomyeloide chez le tetard d' *Alytes obstetricans* normal et thymectomise. *Ann Inst Pasteur Paris* **114**: 490–502.

Evans EE, Kent SP, Bryant RE and Moyer M (1966). Antibody formation and immunological memory in the marine toad. In Smith RT, Good RA and Miescher PA (Eds), *Phylogeny of Immunity*. University of Florida Press: Gainesville. pp 218–226

Horton JD (1971a). Histogenesis of the lymphomyeloid complex in the larval leopard frog *Rana pipiens*. *J Morphol* **134**: 1–19.

Horton JD (1971b). Ontogeny of the immune system in amphibians. *Am Zool* **11**: 219–228.

Johnston MRL (1973). Perivascular lymphoid tissue associated with the axillary lymph sinus and lateral vein of *Gehyra variegata* (Reptilia: Gekkonidae). *J Morph* **139**: 431–438.

Kampmeier OF (1969). *Evolution and Comparative Morphology of the Lymphatic System*. Charles C Thomas: Springfield, Illinois.

Kent SP, Evans EE and Attleberger MH (1964). Comparative immunology: lymph nodes in the amphibian *Bufo marinus*. *Proc Soc Exp Biol Med* **116**: 456–459.

Kihara T and Naito E (1933). Uber den einlagerungsund verbreitungsmodus des lymphatischen gewebes im lymphgefasssystem der ente. *Okijamas Fol Anat Jap* **11**: 405–413.

Kondo M (1937a). Die lymphatischen gebilde im lymphgefasssystem des huhnes. *Okijamas Fol Anat Jap* **15**: 309–325.

Kondo M (1937b). Die lymphatische gebilde im lymphgefasssystem der verschiedensen vogelarten. *Okijamas Fol Anat Jap* **15**: 329–348.

Kondo M (1937c). Die entwicklung der lymphknotchen um lymphgefasssystem des huhnes. *Okijamas Fol Anat Jap* **15**: 349–355.

Kotani M (1959). Lymphgefasse, lymphatische apparate und extravasculare saftbahnen der Schlange (*Elaphe quadrivirgata* Boie). *Acta Sch Med Univ Kioto Japan* **36**: 121–171.

Manabe S (1930a). Untersuchung uber das vogel lymph-gefasssystem. 1. Uber das lymphgefasssystem der ente. *Kaibogaku Zasshi* **3**: 119−131.

Manabe S (1930b). Untersuchung uber das vogel lymphge-fasssystem. 2. Uber den ban und entwicklung der enter-lymphknoten. *Kaibogaku Zasshi* **3**: 282−297.

Manabe S (1930c). Untersuchung uber das vogel lymphge-fasssystem. 3. Uber das vorkommen der lymphknoten an verschiedenen vogelarten. *Kaibogaku Zasshi* **3**: 349−360.

Manning MJ and Horton JD (1969). Histogenesis of lymphoid organs in larvae of the South African clawed toad, *Xenopus laevis* (Daudin). *J Embryol Exp Morphol* **22**: 265−277.

McCorkle FM, Stinson RS, Olah I and Glick B (1979). The chicken's femoral lymph nodules: T and B cells and the immune response. *J Immunol* **123**: 667−669.

Minagawa Y, Ohnishi K and Murakawa S (1975). Structure and immunological function of lymphomyeloid organs in the bullfrog *Rana catesbeiana*. In Hildemann WH and Benedict AA (Eds), *Immunologic Phylogeny*. Plenum Press: New York. pp 257−266.

Moticka EJ, Brown BA and Cooper EL (1973). Immuno-globulin synthesis in bullfrog larvae. *J Immunol* **110**: 855−861.

Nossal GJV (1967). Mechanisms of antibody production. *Ann Rev Med* **18**: 81−96.

Olah I and Glick B (1983). Avian lymph node: light and electron microscopic study. *Anat Rec* **205**: 287−299

Plytycz B and Bigaj J (1982). Tadpoles of *Rana temporaria* do not possess the lymph gland. *Dev Comp Immunol* **6**: 781−784.

Riviere HB and Cooper EL (1973). Thyroxine induced regression of tadpole lymph glands. *Proc Soc Exp Biol Med* **143**: 320−322.

Szarski H (1938). The blood vessel of the thymus gland in some of the urodela. *Bull Acad Polon Sci* **BII**: 305−315.

Tochinai S (1975). Distribution of lympho-epithelial tissues in the larval South African clawed toad *Xenopus laevis* Daudin. *J Fac Sci Hokkaido Univ Ser VI Zool* **19**: 803−811.

Villena A and Zapata A (1981). Ultrastructure of the jugular body of *Rana pipiens*. In Solomon JB (Ed), *Aspects of Developmental and Comparative Immunology. I.* Pergamon Press: Oxford. pp 491−492.

Wright RK and Cooper EL (1980). Temperature and immunological memory in anuran amphibians. In Manning MJ (Ed), *Phylogeny of Immunological Memory*. Elsevier/North-Holland: Amsterdam. pp 155−160.

Wright RK, Eipert EF and Cooper EL (1978). Regulatory role of temperature on the development of ectothermic vertebrate lymphocyte populations. In Gershwin ME and Cooper EL (Eds), *Animal Models of Comparative and Developmental Aspects of Immunity and Disease*. Pergamon Press: New York. pp 80−92.

Zapata A, Villena A and Cooper EL (1981a). Ultrastructure of the jugular body of *Rana pipiens*. *Cell Tissue Res* **221**: 193−202.

Zapata A, Villena A, Rasquin B and Cooper EL (1981b). The jugular body in anuran amphibians: role in immunity. *Dev Comp Immunol* **5** Suppl 1: 129−135.

8

Lymphoid Aggregations Associated with the Gut, Lungs and Urogenital System

INTRODUCTION

In mammals, gut-associated lymphoid tissue (GALT), bronchial lymphoid aggregates (BALT) and lymphoid tissue contained in other mucosal organs, such as urinary and genital tracts, mammary glands and salivary glands, constitute an integrated, mucosal-associated lymphoid system (Bienenstock *et al.*, 1978; McDermott and Bienenstock, 1979). Whether indeed a similar system occurs in ectothermic vertebrates is unclear, but some evidence suggests that, at least from a morphological viewpoint, non-mammalian vertebrates contain lymphoid tissues equivalent to those of the mammalian mucosae.

In this present chapter we review the phylogeny of gut-associated lymphoid tissue (GALT), with special attention given to that of reptiles as well as to the structure of avian cecal tonsils. No references on the organization of bronchus-associated lymphoid tissue (BALT) are available but Borysenko and Cooper (1972) have described a dense lymphoid aggregate in the connective tissue layer between the epithelium and the tracheal cartilage of the snapping turtle, *Chelydra serpentina*. Moreover, some few accumulations of small lymphocytes are commonly found in the reptilian (Borysenko and Cooper, 1972) and anuran lung (Manning and Horton, 1969; Zapata, unpublished observations). Finally, we will describe other diffuse lymphoid aggregations, mainly lymphoid tissue, in the avian pineal system and Harderian gland.

THE GUT-ASSOCIATED LYMPHOID TISSUE (GALT)

Fish

Development of GALT in Primitive Fish

All vertebrates possess isolated lymphoid cells scattered in the lamina propria and epithelium of the gut, but more or less organized cell aggregates only occur in certain intestinal regions. Cyclostomes (myxinoids and lampreys) show intestinal lymphocytes but true lymphoid aggregates occur for the first time in the Chondrichthyes. In hagfish, *Eptatretus burgeri* and *Myxine glutinosa*, migrations of lymphoid cells through the epithelium have been reported (Tomonaga *et al.*, 1973; Ostberg *et al.*, 1976) and small groups of lymphocytes occur in the esophageal lamina propria and epithelium of the ammocoetes of *Petromyzon marinus* (Ardavin *et al.*, 1984). Small lymphoid aggregates (Figure 8.1) have been found in the spiral valve of various elasmobranchs (Drzewina, 1905; Jacobshagen, 1915; Kanesada, 1956; Fichtelius *et al.*, 1968; Zapata, 1977). Moreover, Hart *et al.* (1986) have recently studied the ontogenetic development of GALT in the spiral valve of the dogfish, *Scyliorhinus canicula*.

At stage 1 of development (external gills) spiral valves occur as an outpouching of the gut, but without lymphoid tissue. A lymphoid kidney and the thymic

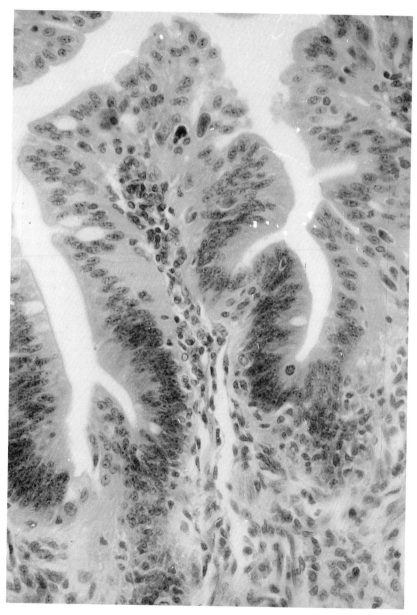

Figure 8.1 Mucosal fold found in the spiral valve of the skate *Raja clavata*. A few lymphoid cells occur in the lamina propria and inside the intestinal epithelium (× 2000).

primordium occur at that stage but not the spleen, Leydig or epigonal organs. At stage 2, when fish are ventilated by sea water and hence potentially vulnerable to antigens, the spiral valve begins to differentiate, when it contains areas of connective tissue, packed with lymphoid cells and occasional macrophages. By stage 3, the spiral valve has reached a stage of development compatible with the adult form. Then GALT is recognizable in the spiral valve lamina of individual cells as accumulations of lymphocytes and macrophages. Cells cross blood vessel walls of the lamina propria but there is no cell traffic across the epithelial basement membrane. As fish are dependent upon the yolk sac for nourishment at this stage, some authors suggest that the presence of these cells is not induced by exogenous antigen.

Stages 4 and 5 differ from stage 3 in that intraepithelial populations of leukocytes are identifiable. Likewise, lymphoid accumulations in the lamina propria, recorded at stage 3 and subsequently found in the upper spiral valve, increase in size and relevance with age. These authors suggest that while the organism is contained within the so-called mermaid's purse, although it is ventilated by sea water it gains nutrients solely from the yolk sac; it is unlikely that antigenic challenge of the spiral valve will occur. Conversely, the free-living stage, once partaking of any exogenous food, would be challenged by antigen and leukocytic development would therefore be affected by antigen. Fish observed after stage 5, at 4½ weeks, 6 months and 2 years, have increasing intraepithelial and intralaminal leukocyte populations in the spiral valve.

In Dipnoi, lymphoid accumulations occur along the gut tract (Jordan and Spiedel, 1931), whereas the paddlefish, *Polydon spathula*, possesses lymphocytic nodules in the region of the ileocecal valve and in the gut (Fichtelius *et al.*, 1968; Weisel, 1973). Sparse lymphocytes have been found in the intestine of another chondrostean, *Scapirhynchus plathorhynchus* (Good *et al.*, 1966; Weisel, 1979) and abundant lymphoid tissue occurs in the gut of gars (Figure 8.2). Teleosts show lymphoid cells in the epithelium as well as in the lamina propria of the gut (Fichtelius *et al.*, 1968; Pontius and Ambrosius, 1972; Kimura and Kudo, 1975; Zapata, 1979). The GALT of *Rutilus* appears as a small non-encapsulated infiltrate in the lamina propria and in the basal portion of the intestinal epithelium (Figure 8.3). It consists of small and

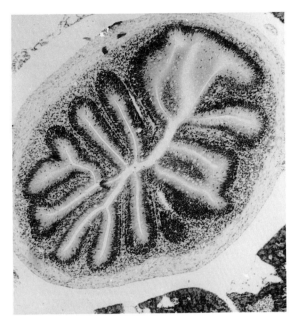

Figure 8.2 Cross-section of the small intestine in the teleost *Rutilus rutilus*. Note the single, large lymphoid aggregate in the lamina propria (× 50).

medium lymphocytes (Figure 8.4), lymphoblasts (Figure 8.5), immature and mature plasma cells, some basophils, heterophils and numerous large macrophages (Figure 8.4). In *Barbus conchonius* and *Cyprinus carpio*, GALT contains mainly lymphocytes and heterophilic granulocytes, occasional macrophages and PAS-positive granulocytes (Davina *et al.*, 1980).

The Teleosts

Pontius and Ambrosius (1972) demonstrated antibody-secreting cells in the lamina propria of the pyloric region in perch after immunization with sheep erythrocytes (SRBC). Feeding of plaice with heat-killed *Vibrio anguillarum* resulted in observable antibody titers in the intestinal mucus (Fletcher and White, 1973). Likewise, oral administration of *Vibrio* bacteria resulted in a considerable increase in intraepithelial leukocytes within 30 minutes in the entire intestine of *Barbus conchonius* and *Cyprinus carpio*, where they were most pronounced in the bulbus and second segment (Davina *et al.*, 1980, 1982). This short

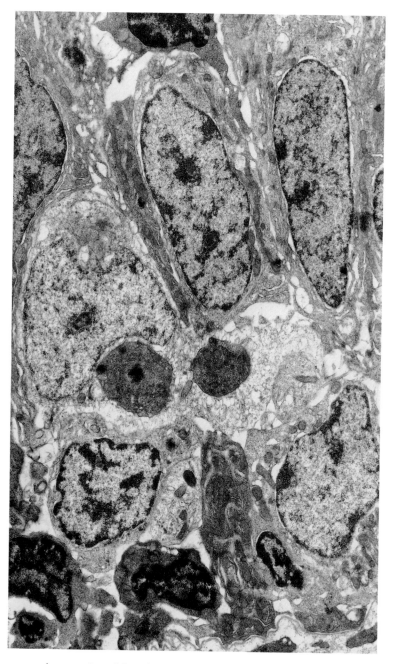

Figure 8.3 Migrating macrophages and small lymphocytes in the intestinal epithelium of *Rutilus rutilus* (× 9950). (From *Morf Normal y Patolgica* Sec A **3**: 23, 1979, reproduced by permission.)

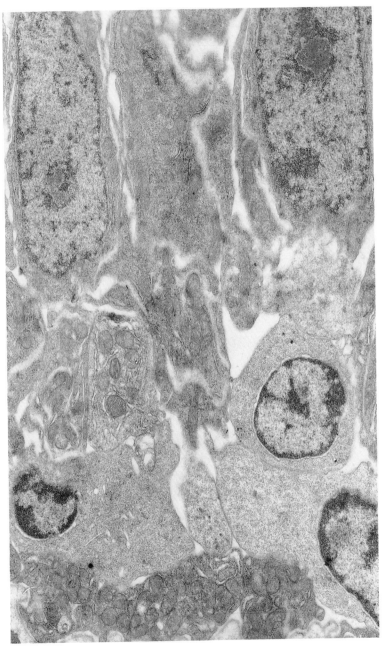

Figure 8.4 Intraepithelial lymphocytes and lymphoblasts in the bases of the intestinal epithelium in the teleost *Rutilus rutilus* (× 12 100).

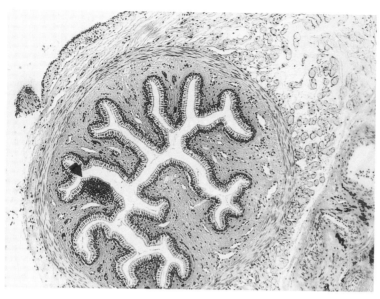

Figure 8.5 Note the small lymphoid aggregate in the lamina propria of the esophagus of *Pleurodeles waltlii* (× 90). (From *J Morphol* **173**: 35, 1982, reproduced by permission.)

time interval suggests, however, that it is a non-immune reaction and leukocytes, possibly representing heterophils, frequently occur in the GALT of these teleosts. Although the functional significance of GALT in lower vertebrates will be discussed later, according to its ultrastructural organization (Zapata, 1979), ontogenetic development (Davina *et al.*, 1980; Hart *et al.*, 1986) and immunological capacity (Pontius and Ambrosius, 1972; Fletcher and White, 1973; Davina *et al.*, 1980), fish GALT seems to be related to the immunological, intestinal barrier found in mammals.

Specific antibody responses have been induced in both elasmobranchs and teleosts by per-oral and per-anal antigenic exposure (Harris, 1972; Fletcher and White, 1973; Rombout *et al.*, 1986; Hart *et al.*, 1987). Uptake of both bacterial antigens and whole bacteria and viruses occurs in the gut of various teleosts (Davina *et al.*, 1982; Buras *et al.*, 1985; Nelson *et al.*, 1985; Rombout *et al.*, 1986). In other, non-teleostean fish, uptake of macromolecules has been demonstrated (Langille and Youson, 1985 in cyclostomes; Hart, 1987 in larval elasmobranchs). Contrary to the anal route, often the oral administration of antigens produced undetectable immune responses, probably as a consequence of the antigenic breakdown by gastric hydrolysis and enzyme digestion. In this regard, the importance of GALT in trapping antigenic materials and in developing vaccines has recently been emphasized (Hart *et al.*, 1988). Conversely, hypersensitive reactions, probably mediated by gut PAS-positive granules and eosinophilic granular cells have been reported in teleost fish although IgE is absent from fish and their mast cells lack histamine (Ellis, 1982, 1986).

Amphibians

Introduction

Amphibian GALT consists of small, non-encapsulated aggregations of densely packed lymphocytes in the lamina propria just beneath the mucosal epithelium. Such GALT has been found in *Rana*, *Bufo*, *Xenopus* and *Bombina* (Goldstine *et al.*, 1975; Plytycz and Slezek, 1981; Hussein *et al.*, 1984) as well as in the urodeles *Triturus* (Plytycz and Slezek, 1981) and *Pleurodeles* (Ardavin *et al.*, 1982a) but not in other urodeles such as *Salamandra* (Goldstine *et al.*, 1975). In addition, Wong (1972) described encapsulated lymphoid tissue in the esophagus of *Bufo melanostictus*.

Urodeles

In *Pleurodeles waltlii* lymphoid aggregates appear throughout the gut as true infiltrates (Figures 8.6, 8.7) located between the muscle and connective tissue elements (Figure 8.8). They are found predominantly in the small intestine, where accumulations are located opposite the region of the mesenteric attachment (Figure 8.7) (Bloom and Fawcett, 1975). There is no notable development of lymphoid tissue in the large intestine and cloaca of urodeles and it is lacking in the stomach (Ardavin *et al.*, 1982a). In these intestinal lymphoid accumulations, small and medium-sized lymphocytes are the most frequently observed cellular elements (Figure 8.8). Immature and mature plasma cells, granulocytes and macrophages occur in these lymphoid accumulations.

Infiltration of lymphoid cells from underlying accumulations into the intestinal epithelium produces a decrease in epithelial mucus cells and disappearance of the basement membrane (Figure 8.9). This modification of the intestinal epithelium as a consequence of a massive intraepithelial invasion by lymphoid elements shows an homology with mammalian Peyer's

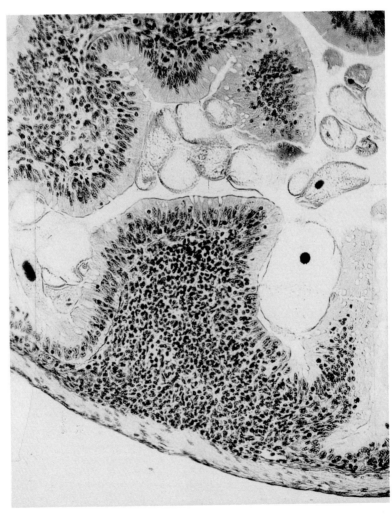

Figure 8.6 Large lymphoid aggregate in the lamina propria of the small intestine of *Pleurodeles waltlii*. The lymphoid accumulation enlarges the intestinal villus ($\times$ 230).

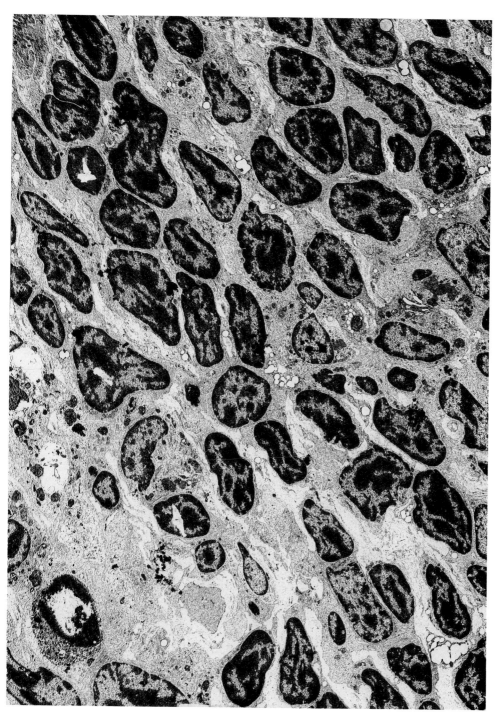

Figure 8.7 Small and medium lymphocytes, together with macrophages, are the main cell components of a lymphoid aggregate which occurs in the gut lamina propria of *Pleurodeles waltlii* (× 2304).

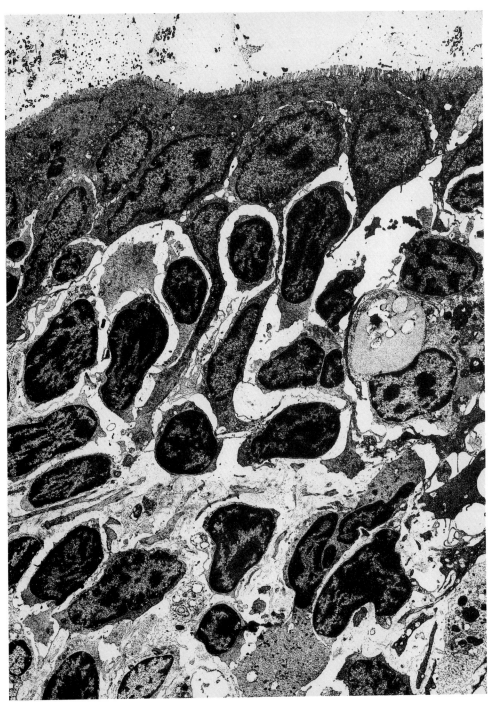

Figure 8.8 Numerous lymphocytes infiltrate the intestinal epithelium of *Pleurodeles waltlii* (× 3080). (From *Cell Tissue Res* **224**: 663, 1982, reproduced by permission.)

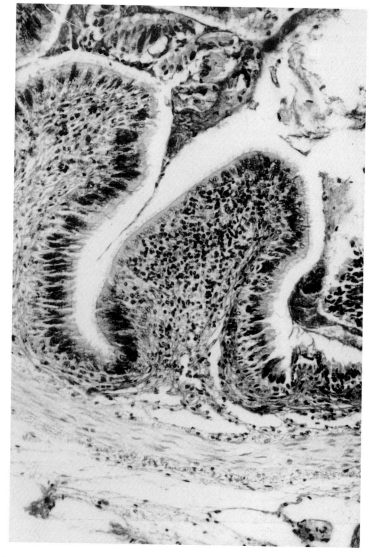

Figure 8.9 Small lymphoid aggregate in the lamina propria of the esophagus of the natterjack, *Bufo calamita*. Note the asymmetry induced in the villus by the occurrence of lymphoid aggregates and in the modified surface epithelium (× 500).

patches (Olah *et al.*, 1975). The intraepithelial cells are similar to cell types found in lymphoid accumulations of the lamina propria: small and medium-sized lymphocytes and macrophages (Figure 8.9) which are distributed between but are not found inside the epithelial cells. Ardavin *et al.* (1982a) made two observations and one conclusion on the basis of ultrastructural images, by showing migrating lymphocytes through the blood vessel's endothelia from lymphoid accumulations in the intestinal lamina propria of *Pleurodeles*

waltlii; lymphoblasts, in mitosis, were also present. They concluded that, although the gut-associated lymphoid populations arise extrinsically in *Pleurodeles*, amplification of this intestinal lymphoid tissue took place *in situ*.

Anurans

General considerations. In anurans, development of GALT is greater than in urodeles but it shows similar histological organization, with an asymmetric arrangement in the gut villi and profound modifications in the epithelium, including loss of mucus cells and epithelial disorganization (Figure 8.10). *Xenopus laevis* has apparently the least GALT of all the anuran species that have been examined (Goldstine *et al.*, 1975). These authors described a diffuse pattern of nodules in the duodenum and a single row of nodules opposite the mesenteric attachment of the ileum. No nodules were found in the esophagus but Jurd (1977) reported them in the colon and rectum. In *Bufo regularis*, lymphoid aggregates, either moderate or minute in size, are readily detected in small and large intestine but not in the esophageal or stomach regions (Hussein *et al.*, 1984).

Embryonic development. Embryonic development of GALT has been studied in some anurans. In stage V and all succeeding larval stages of development in *Rana pipiens* (Horton, 1971), lymphoid accumulations are closely associated with the epithelium of the whole gastrointestinal tract from the oral cavity through the intestine to the cloaca. In these locations, lymphocytes are found alongside the intestinal epithelium and also in the underlying connective tissue in association with blood capillaries and few granulocytes. In larval *Alytes obstetricans*, Du Pasquier (1968) described many nodular lymphoid formations, with accompanying capillaries, along the small intestine and large esophageal lymphoid organ. In contrast, Manning and Horton (1969) found a negligible amount of lymphoid tissue associated with the post-pharyngeal region of the larval *Xenopus gut*, although Horton (1969) has described such accumulations in the post-metamorphic clawed toad.

Role in immunity. The GALT nodules of *Bufo melanostictus* contain phagocytic cells which trap carbon (Chin and Wong, 1977) and respond to antigenic stimulation followed by the appearance of pyroninophilic and plasma cells (Goldstine *et al.*, 1975 in *Xenopus laevis*; Minagawa *et al.*, 1975 in *Rana catesbeiana*). Responses to antigenic stimulation have also been examined histologically in GALT of *Pleurodeles waltlii* (Ardavin, 1981). Primary, intra-oral immunization with SRBC did not produce modifications in number or size of lymphoid accumulations in any regions of the gastrointestinal tract, due probably to enzymatic degradation of erythrocytes in the stomach. Primary stimulation within the cloaca gave rise to increasing numbers of lymphoid aggregates in small and large intestine but not in the upper intestinal areas. Moreover, lymphoid aggregates showed a greater development in both regions of the gut. Finally, intraperitoneal immunization induced a significant increase in number and size of lymphoid accumulations in intestinal segments, even in the cloaca. A second intraperitoneal challenge of SRBC, but not the primary dose, produced increased numbers of gut−lymphoid aggregates in comparison to control animals injected with saline.

Adult *Xenopus laevis* bile and alimentary canal secretions contain IgM and IgRAA (the 7-S, non-mu chain containing Ig of non-mammalian tetrapods;

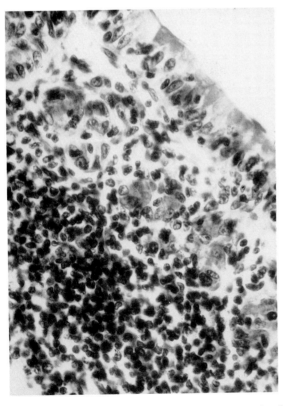

Figure 8.10 Lymphoid infiltration in the lamina propria of the ileocecal junction in the turtle *Mauremys caspica* (× 665).

Jurd, 1977). According to Jurd, lymphoid cells from the intestinal nodules which express surface IgM (51−68%) were approximately the same as those in the peripheral blood, while a small proportion (less than 4%) of the cells expressed IgRAA. Besides in *Xenopus* GALT lymphocytes are cytoplasmic Ig-positive cells (Michea-Hamzehpour, 1977). On the other hand, Tochinai (1976) has pointed out that GALT is not affected by early thymectomy.

Reptiles

General Considerations and Distribution

The GALT of reptiles has been studied extensively in the last few years and much information on its structure and function is now available. First reports (Jolly, 1915; Paltzel, 1936; Kotani, 1959; Sidky and Auerbach, 1968) considered gut-associated lymphoid aggregates, mainly those in the turtle anal sacs, present in various reptilian species, as phylogenetic precursors of the avian bursa of Fabricius. More recent studies which have combined ultrastructural, immunological analyses after antigenic stimulation have, in contrast, confirmed their relationships to the mammalian mucosal immune system, despite the fact that Vaerman *et al.* (1975) were unable to find IgA in bile and intestinal secretions of the tortoise *Testudo hermanni*, or within immunocytes present in the intestinal lamina propria. Numerous lymphoid aggregates containing densely packed lymphocytes occur throughout the gut, although they predominate mainly in some regions. In alligators, the esophagus, ileocolic region and cloaca contain the largest lymphoid accumulations (McCauley, 1956). In the lizards *Iguana iguana*, *Gekko gekko*, *Basiliscus basiliscus* (Fichtelius *et al.*, 1968), *Chalcides ocelatus*, *Scincus scincus*, *Eumeces schneideri*, *Mabuya quinquetaeniata*, *Tarentola annularis*, *Uromastyx aegyptia* (El Ridi *et al.*, 1981) and *Psammodromus algirus* (Zapata and Solas, 1979) numerous aggregates occur along the entire gut but especially abundant lymphoid tissue is located in the ileocecal junction (Figure 8.11) of *Chalcides ocellata* (El Ridi *et al.*, 1981) and *Psammodromus algirus* (Zapata and Solas, 1979).

In contrast, no GALT has been found in the lizards *Agama stellio* and *Chamaeleon chamaeleon* (El Ridi *et al.*, 1981). In snakes, lymphoid aggregates appear in all regions of the gut except the stomach (El Ridi *et al.*, 1981, in *Spalerosophis diadema*, *Psammophis schokari* and *Psammophis sibilans*; Zapata and Solas, 1979, in *Natrix maura*). Of special interest is the snake gut, where there are peculiar, elongate patches in the small intestine which consist of two lymphoid accumulations (Figure 8.12). In boid snakes (*Python molurus bivittatus*, *P. reticulatus*, *P. sebae*, *P. regius*, *P. curtus*, *Constrictor constrictor*), Jacobson and Collins (1980) described esophageal lymphoid structures which seem to be related to mammalian tonsils.

Common Structural Pattern

In turtles and tortoises, GALT is highly developed in the ileum and cloaca (Sidky and Auerbach, 1968; Borysenko and Cooper, 1972; Goldstine *et al.*, 1975; Zapata and Solas, 1979; Hameed, 1980). In the cloacal lamina propria of *Mauremys caspica*, lymphoid tissue is arranged according to two models: one as large lymphoid accumulations protruding into the cloacal lumen, and another as lymphoid infiltrates of lesser size (Figure 8.13). In both cases, the intestinal epithelium appears to be modified at the level of lymphoid tissue. By electron microscopy, these modifications consist of cell infiltrations between the epithelial cells, mainly of lymphocytes, lymphoblasts and, in lesser amounts, plasma cells, phagocytes and granulocytes. The intestinal epithelial cells also show less mucous material and shorter apical microvilli than those showing no lymphoid infiltrates. Mucosal lymphoid accumulations contain lymphocytes, lymphoblasts and immature and mature plasma cells in a connective tissue network of collagenous fibers and fibroblasts (Figure 8.14).

Ontogeny

The ontogenetic development of GALT has also been studied in some reptiles. Lymphoid aggregates in the cloacal complex of snapping turtles, *Chelydra serpentina*, are first evident at the time of hatching (Sidky and Auerbach, 1968). In the lizard *Calotes versicolor*, the cloacal lymphoid aggregates do not appear until two months post-hatching (Pitchappan and Muthukkaruppan, 1977), whereas in *Chalcides ocellatus* small lymphoid accumulations are sharply delimited in the esophagus and large intestine in four of

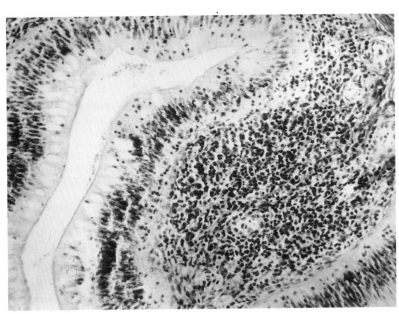

Figure 8.11 Note a large lymphoid infiltration occurs in two intestinal villi in the jejunum of the snake *Natrix maura* (× 280).

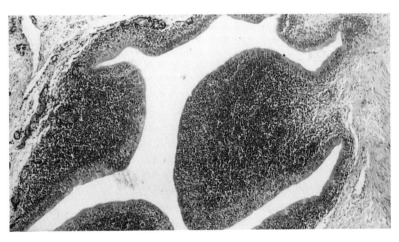

Figure 8.12 Large lymphoid infiltration in the cloaca of the turtle *Mauremys caspica* (× 100).

five lizards investigated on the day of birth. Esophageal and colic aggregates increase slightly in number with age from day 0 to 30. Accumulations appear in the stomach at day 15, while more are detected in the small intestine of all age groups. No GALT lymphopoiesis has been found in the embryos of *Chalcides ocellatus* (El Deeb, 1983).

Function in Relation to Lymphocyte Populations

There is evidence for the function of GALT, although its role in reptilian immune responses is controversial. The lymphocytes of GALT in *Chalcides ocellatus* are highly vulnerable to whole-body gamma irradiation. Moreover, an intraperitoneal injection of 1 mg hydro-

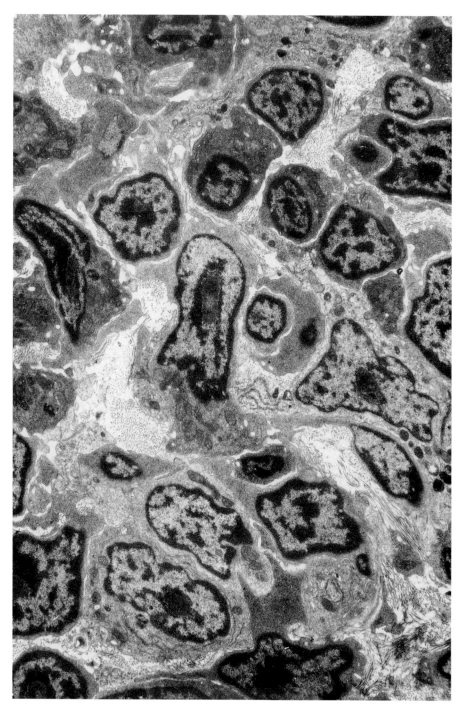

Figure 8.13 Lymphoblasts, lymphocytes and macrophages scattered between the connective tissue of the lamina propria are the principal cell components occurring in the small intestine of the lizard *Lacerta lepida* (× 7360).

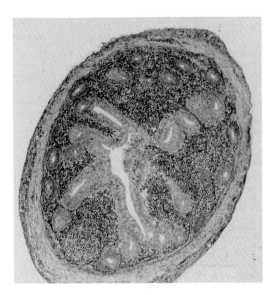

Figure 8.14 Cross-section of the cecal tonsil of the spotless starling *Sturnus unicolor*. Note abundant lymphoid follicles in the lamina propria, some of which show germinal centers (× 40).

cortisone acetate per gram body weight induces a severe depletion of lymphocytes in esophageal aggregates but does not affect lymphoid accumulations in small and large intestines (Akef, 1978). Likewise, adult thymectomy induces a significant decrease in number and size of esophageal accumulations, while the rest of GALT is totally unaffected. Both results suggest that the esophageal aggregates of *Chalcides ocellatus* contain thymus-derived cells sensitive to hydrocortisone treatment, while lymphocytes of small and large intestine are probably not thymus-derived and resistant to corticosteroids.

The Condition of the Immune Response in GALT Versus GALT-less Species

Since splenectomy in some GALT-rich lizards (e.g. *Chalcides ocellatus*) has no apparent effects on humoral responses, it has been suggested that GALT plays an important role in those immune reactions. Moreover, a direct correlation has been observed consistently in different lizard species between number of gut-associated lymphoid aggregates and antibody production against rat erythrocytes injected intraperitoneally (El Deeb, 1978). *Agama stellio*, a lizard

without GALT, rejects skin allografts in a manner and tempo similar to those reported in the GALT-rich lizards. However, *Agama stellio* and *Chameleon chameleon*, both GALT-less lizards, are able to produce but a negligible amount of immune antibodies when confronted with various mammalian erythrocytes or human serum albumin (HSA) over a wide dose range, via intraperitoneal, intramuscular or subcutaneous routes, and whether or not the antigen is incorporated into Freund's adjuvant. Nevertheless, *Agama stellio* possesses small amounts of 2-mercaptoethanol (2-ME)-sensitive hemagglutinin and forms 2-ME-sensitive antibodies when stimulated with *Salmonella typhimurium*. These results suggest that GALT in lizards plays a crucial role in humoral immunity (El Ridi *et al.*, 1981).

Appearance of Immune Cells After Immunization

Plaque-forming cells (PFC) are scarce in the reptilian cloacal complex (Rothe and Ambrosius, 1968; Kanakambika and Muthukkaruppan, 1972) and in the intestine (Sidky and Auerbach, 1968), although numerous plasma cells have been observed at the ultrastructural level in both locations (Solas and Zapata, 1980; Zapata and Solas, 1979).

In this sense, intracloacal, primary immunization of the turtle *Mauremys caspica* with SRBC induces, after 10 days, a significant increase in lymphoid accumulations in all cloacal areas, appearing even in submucosal aggregates. At 20 days post-immunization, lymphoid accumulations decrease to original levels. A second challenge three months after the first one elicits greater increases in cloacal lymphoid tissue. Even after 20 days post-secondary immunization, the development of cloacal lymphoid accumulations is greater than in control, saline-injected turtles (Solas *et al.*, 1981).

Some Evolutionary Considerations

The development of reptilian GALT is greater than in any other ectothermic vertebrates, which suggests a trend toward increasing GALT throughout phylogeny, culminating in more definite organs of mammals such as tonsils, Peyer's patches and appendix. Ingram and Molyneux (1983), in a study on the immune response of *Lacerta viridis*, against the parasitic antigens of *Leishmania agumae* reported that oral immunization induced higher antibody titers than intraperitoneal or cutaneous injections. Antigen residues detected by the PAP method occurred in lymphoid aggregates in the stomach and ileum especially in lizards producing high antibody levels after oral administration of promastigotes. This suggests a role for GALT of *Lacerta viridis* in the trapping and processing of antigens and in antibody formation.

Birds

Introduction

Due to its key immunological function, the bursa of Fabricius has monopolized the thoughts and work of many immunologists, thus obviating to some extent the importance and therefore the need to study other lymphoid organs associated with the avian gastrointestinal tract. However, in birds, GALT is extensive, including, in addition to the bursa of Fabricius, the cecal tonsil, Peyer's patches and other lymphoid aggregates in the urodeum and proctodeum (Bryant *et al.*, 1973) and elsewhere in the gut (Payne, 1971; Toner, 1965; Back, 1970a, b, 1972a, b; Bjerregaard, 1975). Because of their quantitative importance and phylogenetic significance, Peyer's patches and cecal tonsils deserve special attention.

Peyer's Patches

Microscopic structure. McGarry and Bourns (1980), who described annular bands of lymphoid tissue in the intestine of the duck, and Befus *et al.* (1980) in chickens, have analyzed the histology and function of Peyer's patches in birds. Peyer's patches in chickens can be detected as intestinal areas with a rich supply of blood vessels, where the shape of the villi is broader and leaf-like. By light microscopy, the villi show a marked thickening due to heavy lymphoid cell infiltration, follicles and a distinct lymphoepithelium. The morphological organization of Peyer's patches resembles that of the cecal tonsil (see above) in that there is an underlying subepithelial zone, heavily infiltrated by lymphocytes, and a more central area of lymphoid tissue where primary follicles and/or germinal centers predominate. Blood vessels with endothelial cells containing large round nuclei, perhaps analogous to mammalian high endothelial postcapillary venules,

occur also in the diffuse, non-follicular tissue of the central region. Certain regions of the epithelium which cover the chicken's Peyer's patches have apparently a mature lymphoepithelium with an abundance of lymphocytes, few if any goblet cells and certain cells without microvilli that give an appearance similar to M-cells (Befus *et al.*, 1980). Other workers, however, have not found a lymphoepithelium in the intestinal lymphoid aggregates of geese (Perey, 1971) or ducks (McGarry and Bourns, 1980).

Ontogeny and senescence. The ontogeny of chicken Peyer's patches has also been studied (Befus *et al.*, 1980). At 10 days of age but not after hatching, Peyer's patches as well as cecal tonsils can be identified. They increase in size until approximately 12 weeks, after which they involute with age. The epithelium is often disrupted, the lymphoid follicles become less distinct and fewer in number, appearing relatively depopulated of lymphoid elements in the subepithelial zones. Nevertheless, in some chickens, even after one year some aggregates remain, showing an unmodified morphology. Moreover, abundance and distribution of chicken Peyer's patches change with age. By day 10 and thereafter, one Peyer's patch is present consistently in approximately 10% of the total length of the gut anterior to the cloaca. In contrast, birds between 52 and 58 weeks old possess only a single Peyer's patch anterior to the ileocecal junction.

Immunological responses. Information is scarcely available on immunological aspects of chicken Peyer's patches. Peyer's patches, although present in bursectomized birds sacrificed at 4 weeks of age, show depopulated subepithelial zones and smaller numbers of lymphoid follicles. In contrast, the numbers of pyronin positive cells (perhaps plasma cells) do not appear to be different from those in sham and normal birds. Orally administered carbon can be found later in the germinal centers of Peyer's patches, but if it is administered anally there are two patterns of uptake. Peyer's patches do not appear to contain significant quantities, whereas the follicular-associated epithelium and medulla of the bursa of Fabricius are heavily infiltrated (Befus *et al.*, 1980). These same workers found no Ig-containing cells in chicken Peyer's patches using immunofluorescent techniques.

Cecal Tonsils

Introduction. Although the existence of cecal tonsils in birds has been known for more than 100 years (Basslinger, 1858), only some aspects of their structure and function have been studied in chickens and recently in the spotless starling, *Sturnus unicolor.* The cecal tonsil is lymphoid tissue that usually appears in the chicken as an enlargement at the proximal region of each cecum (Muthmann, 1913; Looper and Looper, 1929; Calhoun, 1932; Payne, 1971), but it can show many variants (Thompson, 1925). Thus, long cecae, typical of herbivorous or omnivorous animals, are hollow and similar histologically to those of the intestine, while the short cecae of carnivorous birds are 'closed' and glandular in nature (Magnan, 1911). In any case, germinal centers occur in both the cecal tonsil (Looper and Looper, 1929; Jankovic *et al.*, 1966; Jankovic and Mitrovic, 1967) and in the distal portion of the cecum, the cecal pouch (Looper and Looper, 1929; Calhoun, 1932), with a greater concentration in the distal portion (Glick *et al.*, 1978).

General considerations of structure. The cecal tonsil in chickens and spotless starlings consists of a diffuse mass of lymphoid tissue which occupies almost the whole intestinal lumen (Figure 8.15). The diffuse lymphoid tissue contains large, encapsulated and partially encapsulated, small germinal centers (Figures 8.15, 8.16) located deep, near the muscle layer of the tunica propria (Figure 8.16). All authors (Hegde and George, 1973; Jankovic and Mitrovic, 1967; Olah and Glick, 1979; Hoshi and Mori, 1973), after examining light and electron microscopic evidence, agree on several different histological regions in the cecal tonsils: lymphoepithelium which covers the lymphoid aggregates; lymphoid tissue just beneath the epithelium, the subepithelial zone, primary follicles and germinal centers, and diffuse interfollicular lymphoid tissue.

Distribution of lymphoid cells. By scanning electron microscopy, Glick *et al.* (1978) found no marked differences between surface morphology of cecal tonsils and the remaining proximal region of the cecum. In the lumen, numerous villi showed bacteria adherent to their surfaces (Calhoun, 1932; Whitlock *et al.*, 1975; Glick *et al.*, 1978). The epithelium which covers the lymphoid aggregates, infiltrated by numerous lym-

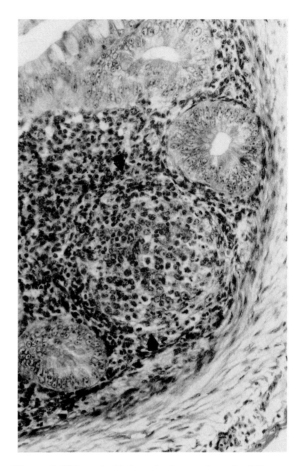

Figure 8.15 Lymphoid tissue in the cecal tonsil of *Sturnus unicolor* showing a germinal center in the basal region near the muscularis mucosae. Note the absence of a peripheral mantle of dense-stained, small lymphocytes in the germinal center (× 150).

phoid elements, contains smaller numbers of goblet cells than the neighboring epithelium (Hoshi and Mori, 1973). Electron-lucent cells which show characteristics of the mammalian M-cells occur in the epithelium of the cecal tonsil of *Sturnus unicolor* (Figure 8.17). They show few villi, abundant mitochondria and smooth vesicles in the apical cytoplasm (Figure 8.18). Finger-like processes anchor these cells to their neighboring, normal epithelium (Figure 8.19). They are mainly small and medium lymphocytes and lymphoblasts, plasma cells (Hoshi and Mori, 1973) and granular lymphocytes. Granular lymphocytes occur frequently in the epithelium which covers the cecal

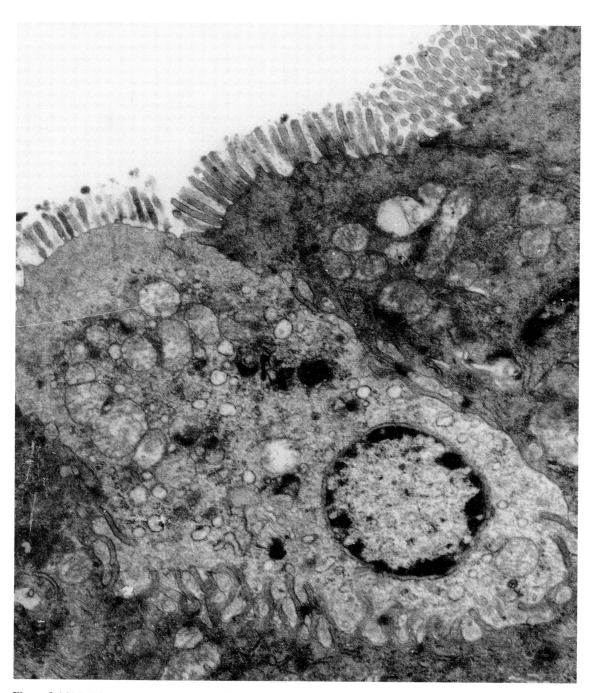

Figure 8.16 Modified cell (M cell) in the epithelium covering the lymphoid follicle in the cecal tonsil of *Sturnus unicolor*. Note the numerous infoldings which, coming from the neighboring cells, appear in the cytoplasm (× 13 750).

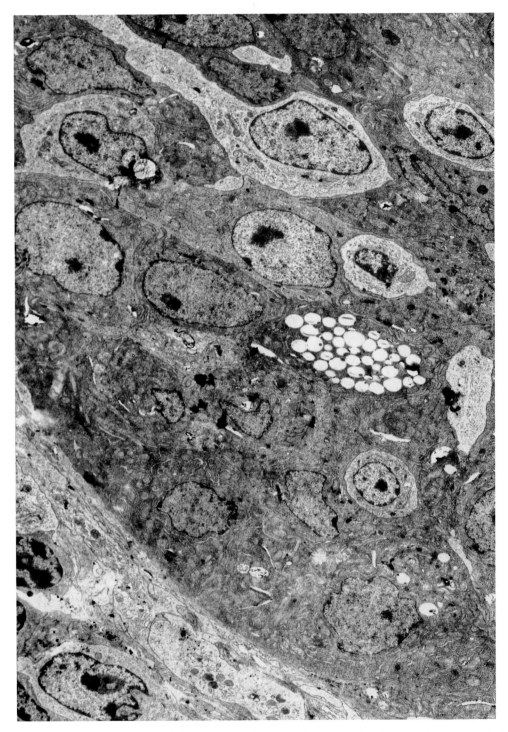

Figure 8.17 Lymphocytes invading the epithelium of the cecal tonsil of *Sturnus unicolor*. They are electron-lucent with scant cytoplasmic organelles (× 5700).

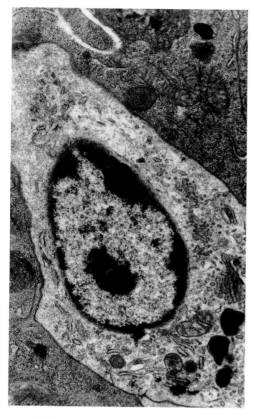

Figure 8.18 Intraepithelial granular lymphocyte in the cecal tonsil of *Sturnus unicolor*. Three or four round polygonal, electron-dense granules appear in the cytoplasm together with smooth tubules, small Golgi apparatus and profiles of rough endoplasmic reticulum (× 11200).

tonsil of *Sturnus unicolor*. These cell types are quite similar to medium or large lymphocytes in size and electron density but always contain three to five electron-dense granules near the Golgi apparatus, few mitochondria, abundant smooth endoplasmic reticulum and short profiles of rough endoplasmic reticulum (Figure 8.20).

The origin, nature and functional significance of these granular lymphocytes are, however, obscure. Intraepithelial granular cells have been described in the small intestine of chickens (Back, 1970a; Bjerregaard, 1975) which relates them to granular leukocytes that, at least in mammals, seem to be intraepithelial mast cells (Ernst *et al.*, 1985).

Mammalian intraepithelial lymphocytes contain a uniquely large proportion (60%) of granular lymphocyte-like cells whose morphology is quite similar to that of certain intraepithelial cells of the cecal tonsil of *Sturnus unicolor*. However, despite morphological and histochemical similarities between the granules of this intraepithelial cell population and those of cytotoxic T-cells and NK cell clones or lines, only a small percentage of intraepithelial lymphocytes are cytotoxic T-cells or have NK activity in several mammals (Ernst *et al.*, 1985). Moreover, remarkable associations between interdigitating cells and small lymphocytes have been found in the intestinal epithelium of the cecal tonsil in the spotless starling.

Interdigitating cells, a non-lymphoid element present in the thymus and T-dependent areas of the peripheral lymphoid organs in mammals, have been recently described in the thymus and spleen of *Sturnus unicolor* (Fonfria *et al.*, 1982). These cells are numerous in the diffuse interfollicular lymphoid tissue of the tonsil. This intraepithelial association between interdigitating cells and small lymphocytes (Figure 8.21) has also been observed in the mammalian GALT (Sminia *et al.*, 1983) and might be important for immune responses which occur in the cecal tonsil.

Non-follicular diffuse lymphoid tissue. The non-follicular diffuse lymphoid tissue of cecal tonsils in *Sturnus unicolor* consists of large masses of lymphoid elements arranged between reticular cells, fibroblasts, collagenous fibers and smooth muscle elements located in the intestinal lamina propria; it contains mainly large lymphocytes (Figure 8.22). Large lymphoblasts show electron-lucent nuclei and cytoplasm with few clumps of condensed chromatin, numerous large mitochondria and significant amounts of cytoplasmic-free ribosomes (Figure 8.22). Small and medium lymphocytes are heavily electron-dense cells with abundant condensed chromatin and scarce cytoplasm (Figure 8.22). Moreover, numerous immature and mature plasma cells occur in this interfollicular diffuse lymphoid tissue mainly in the subepithelial zone (Figure 8.23). They are typically characterized by extensive development of profiles of rough endoplasmic reticulum in the cytoplasm. In the most mature cells, the cisternae of rough endoplasmic reticulum appear enlarged and contain a medium electron-dense material (Figure 8.23). Macrophages are also evident

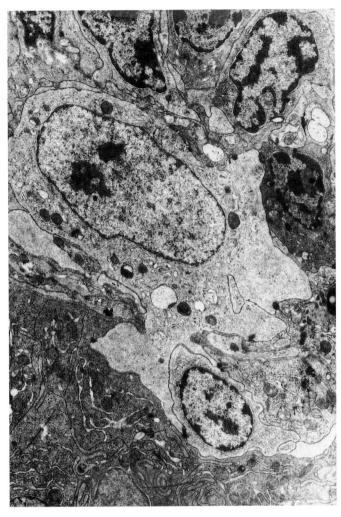

Figure 8.19 Interdigitating cells and small lymphocytes migrating together into the epithelium which covers lymphoid tissue of the cecal tonsil in *Sturnus unicolor* (× 10 000).

in the interfollicular lymphoid tissue and are associated with plasma cells in the subepithelial zone (Figure 8.24). They are irregular pale cells with scant, condensed chromatin and a patent nucleolus which contains, in the cytoplasm, remains of engulfed, defenestrated cells, electron-dense granules and smooth vesicles and tubules associated with the Golgi region (Figure 8.24).

Interdigitating cells are a common feature of interfollicular lymphoid tissue in the cecal tonsil of *Sturnus unicolor* and might be considered as a morphological

marker of T-lymphoid areas in peripheral lymphoid organs (Figure 8.25). They are large irregular cells with an electron-lucent nucleus and cytoplasm which contains small amounts of condensed chromatin and abundant, membranous organelles arranged near the nucleus. The electron-lucent peripheral cytoplasm, with no organelles, shows labyrinthine contacts with narrow cell processes from the neighboring lymphoid and non-lymphoid cells (Figure 8.25). Finally, high endothelial venules, suggested in previous studies by light microscopy in chickens (Hoshi and Mori, 1973),

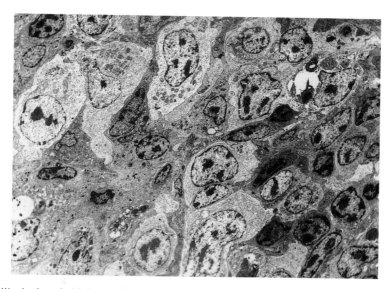

Figure 8.20 Interfollicular lymphoid tissue, which consists mainly of small lymphocytes, lymphoblasts and macrophages in the cecal tonsil of *Sturnus unicolor* (× 3800).

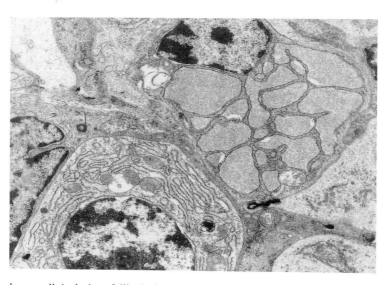

Figure 8.21 Mature plasma cells in the interfollicular lymphoid tissue of the cecal tonsil in *Sturnus unicolor*. Note the variable development of the rough endoplasmic reticulum (× 9900).

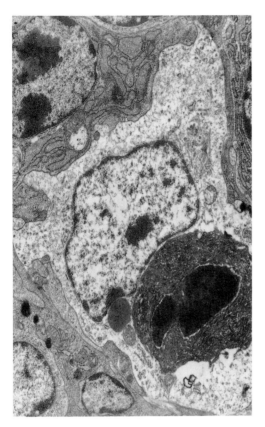

Figure 8.22 Macrophages in the interfollicular lymphoid tissue of the cecal tonsil in the spotless starling, which shows phagocytosed plasma cells in the cytoplasm (× 15 000).

have been confirmed ultrastructurally in the interfollicular, diffuse lymphoid tissue of the cecal tonsil in *Sturnus unicolor* (Figure 8.26). They occur as pale, sometimes closed areas formed by electron-lucent endothelial cells. They have an irregular nucleus which shows scarce, condensed chromatin and a prominent nucleolus. Sometimes small lymphocytes have been observed to pass through their walls (Figure 8.26).

Germinal centers. Encapsulated and partially encapsulated germinal centers occur deep in lymphoid tissues of the chicken and starling cecal tonsils. Partially encapsulated germinal centers may represent a specific site for proliferation and differentiation of uncommitted stem cells (Olah and Glick, 1979). The

germinal centers represent pale areas (Figure 8.16) where the numbers of reticular fibers, as revealed after silver impregnation, are higher in the periphery as well as in the surrounding interfollicular lymphoid tissue than in the middle of the germinal center (Figure 8.27). Their capsule consists of several layers of flat reticular cells (Figure 8.28) which are lacking in some places where lymphoid elements are close to the muscle cells of the muscularis mucosa (Figure 8.29). In chickens (Jankovic and Mitrovic, 1967; Hedge and George, 1973; Hoshi and Mori, 1973; Olah and Glick, 1979) as well as in the spotless starling, germinal centers of cecal tonsils contain mainly lymphoblasts, lymphocytes and macrophages (Figures 8.27, 8.28). Plasma cells are few, if any, in the germinal centers (Jankovic and Mitrovic, 1967; Olah and Glick, 1979).

Lymphoblasts are the most frequent cells in the germinal centers. They consist of two types: one smaller, containing polyribosomes and some mitochondria, and the other more mature, with a prominent nucleolus, polyribosomes and profiles of rough endoplasmic reticulum. Sometimes lymphoblasts occur in mitosis, being located predominantly in the cortical zone (Figure 8.28). Macrophages, which are always present, represent tingible bodies containing cells which show numerous, engulfed, degenerated cells in their cytoplasm (Figure 8.29). Small lymphocytes, some of them with pycnotic signs, are also frequent (Figures 8.28, 8.29), although a mantle of peripheral small lymphocytes, typical of mammalian germinal centers, is lacking. In chickens, Olah and Glick (1979) have found in the central part of germinal centers secretory-like cells of unknown significance which contain large granules with electron-dense material.

Ontogenetic development. The ontogenetic development of cecal tonsils has also been analyzed in chickens (Looper and Looper, 1929; Jankovic and Mirovic, 1967; Hoshi and Mori, 1973). In chick embryos of 18−19 days, the cecal tonsils contain reticular cells, few lymphocytes but no plasma cells (Looper and Looper, 1929; Jankovic and Mitrovic, 1967). Foci of four to nine pyroninophilic blasts, however, occur (Jankovic and Mitrovic, 1967). On hatching, only small infiltrates of lymphocytes are found in the lamina propria in the proximal region of the cecum where the cecal tonsil will be formed (Looper and Looper, 1929; Jankovic and Mitrovic, 1967;

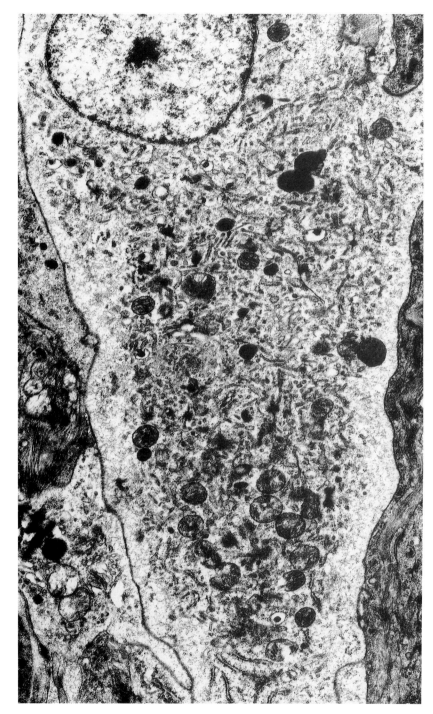

Figure 8.23 Mature interdigitating cell in the interfollicular lymphoid tissue of the cécal tonsil in *Sturnus unicolor*. Note the central arrangement of cytoplasmic organelles, mainly fragments of smooth and rough endoplasmic reticulum, small electron-dense granules and mitochondria and the emptied cytoplasm (× 12800).

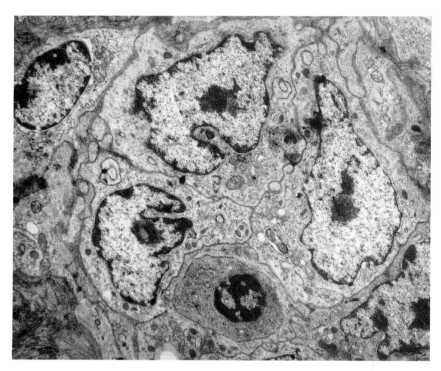

Figure 8.24 High endothelial, postcapillary venule in the interfollicular lymphoid tissue of the cecal tonsil of *Sturnus unicolor*. The lumen of the vessel is closed by high endothelial cells. Note a small lymphocyte migrating through the vessel walls (× 10 000).

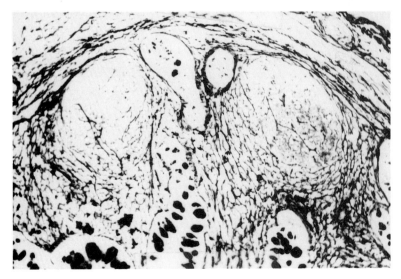

Figure 8.25 Reticular fiber arrangement in the lamina propria of *Sturnus unicolor*. Areas devoid of fibers represent germinal centers (× 150).

Hoshi and Mori, 1973). About 24 hours after hatching, increased numbers of lymphocytes appear in the mid and deep layers of the lamina propria, some of which aggregate immediately under the epithelium of the basal portion of villi. In this location, the mucous membrane is apparently hypertrophic and is covered by irregular villi.

On the tenth day, the cecal tonsil is almost fully developed, germinal centers are still scarce, but the whole thickness of the lamina propria is occupied by a large accumulation of lymphocytes. Moreover, the intestinal epithelium, especially that overlying the subepithelial zone, appears to be penetrated by lymphoid elements (Hoshi and Mori, 1973). Plasma cells first appear on the sixth day. Around the eighth day after hatching, germinal center formation occurs. The earliest stage in plasma cell development is characterized by the appearance of intensely basophilic, large lymphocytes, which become grouped, forming cell clusters. This event is accompanied by the concurrent, local proliferation of reticular cells. Finally, there is an increase in size and extent of these masses and their encapsulation by flat reticular cells, thus completing the process (Hoshi and Mori, 1973).

Thymus-dependent and bursa-dependent lymphocytes. Cecal tonsils in chickens apparently contain both thymus-dependent and bursa-dependent lymphocytes (Back, 1970a, b, 1972a, b; Hoshi and Mori, 1973), and Albini and Wick (1974) demonstrated the presence of T- and B-cells. Bienenstock *et al.* (1973) also found cells which contain cytoplasmic Ig, and *in vitro* studies on the synthesis of Ig by chicken cecal tonsils showed that IgA was the product (Bienenstock *et al.*, 1973). Hyperimmunization induces abundant proliferation of plasma cells in tonsils (Jankovic and Mitrovic, 1967), and antibodies against BSA have also been reported (Jankovic and Mitrovic, 1967; Jankovic, 1968; Orlans and Rose, 1970).

Apparently there is a relationship between the bursa of Fabricius and the thymus and these lymphoid accumulations. Bursectomy causes depletion of lymphocytes in subepithelial zones, which leads to decreased numbers of lymphoid follicles (Befus *et al.*, 1980; Hoshi and Mori, 1973; Jankovic and Mitrovic, 1967). Likewise after bursectomy, Jankovic and Mitrovic (1967) reported moderate diminution of blasts and plasma cells but not small lymphocytes. In contrast,

Befus *et al.* (1980) found no variations in the numbers of pyronin-positive cells after bursectomy. Neonatal thymectomy affects the numbers of lymphocytes but not those of blasts and plasma cells (Jankovic and Mitrovic, 1967). The number of germinal centers is also fewer in thymectomized chickens (Jankovic and Mitrovic, 1967; Hoshi and Mori, 1973). According to these results, lymphoid tissue in germinal centers of cecal tonsils may be at least partially bursal dependent and the interfollicular, diffuse lymphoid tissue is thymus dependent.

Evolutionary considerations. The question of antigen entrance is somewhat problematic but highly relevant in antibody-producing organs. Olah and Glick (1979) have described two routes for the arrival of antigen to chicken tonsils: the surface epithelium and the vascular system. As in the chicken Peyer's patches, after intra-oral but not intra-anal carbon administration the germinal centers of cecal tonsils contain deposits (Befus *et al.*, 1980). In this regard Sorvari *et al.* (1977) suggested that the bursa of Fabricius might play an important role in the initial response against environmental antigens reaching the gastrointestinal tract 'per anum'. The cecal tonsils might be important after bursal involution. Truly the phylogenetic significance of the chicken cecal tonsils is unclear. Thus, whereas Glick *et al.* (1981) have reported that the histological organization is different from that of mammalian Peyer's patches but quite similar to tonsils, Jankovic and Mitrovic (1967) considered them as a large aggregate of Peyer's patches.

THE PINEAL SYSTEM

Henle suggested as early as 1871 that the pineal system was a lymphatic ganglion. Although presence of lymphocytes has occasionally been reported in numerous studies devoted to the cytology and histology of the pineal gland, mainly in chickens and rats, only recently has attention been focused on its functional significance. We will review the available evidence, with special reference to avian pineal glands.

The lymphoid tissue is absent from the parenchyma of chick pineal system for the first few days post-hatching (Spiroff, 1958; Campbell and Gibson, 1970; Boya and Calvo, 1978; Cogburn and Glick, 1981, 1983).

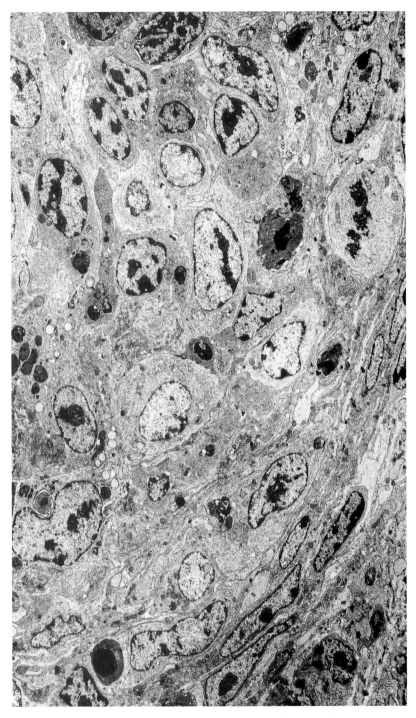

Figure 8.26 Basal zone of a germinal center in the cecal tonsil of *Sturnus unicolor*. Note the connective tissue capsule formed by several layers of flat reticular cells which surround lymphoid cells; some of them are in mitosis (× 4920).

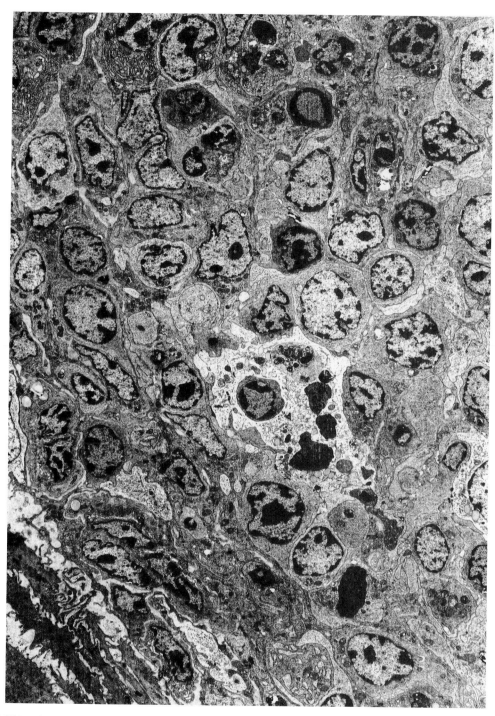

Figure 8.27 Medium lymphocyte and tingible body macrophages in a germinal center of the cecal tonsil of *Sturnus unicolor*. Note the absence of a connective tissue capsule in this area; lymphoid cells appear near the muscle elements (× 5440).

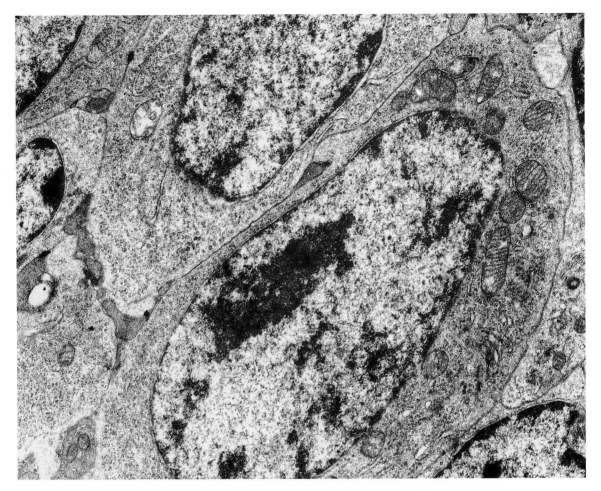

Figure 8.28 Lymphoblasts in a germinal center of the cecal tonsil of *Sturnus unicolor*. Different electron density in both cells, numbers of cytoplasmic ribosomes and presence/ absence of nucleolus suggest that they represent two distinct stages of differentiation (× 32 250).

Maximal accumulation occurs during the first month of life (Campbell and Gibson, 1970; Boya and Calvo, 1978; Cogburn and Glick, 1981, 1983), although Spiroff (1958) reported the peak in 3-month-old chickens. Workers agree on the disappearance of lymphoid tissue from chick pineal system at 4−6 months of life (Spiroff, 1958; Campbell and Gibson, 1970; Boya and Calvo, 1978; Cogburn and Glick, 1981, 1983), although Boya and Calvo (1978) have reported lymphoid tissue in pineal stroma of chickens even at 3 years of age.

In chickens (Romieu and Jullien, 1942; Quay, 1965; Cogburn and Glick, 1981; Olah and Glick, 1984), as in house sparrows and sandpipers (Quay, 1965), pineal lymphoid tissue appears to be associated mainly with connective tissue of the capsule (Figure 8.29), trabeculae and vascular channels, but scattered lymphocytes have been identified utrastructurally among the pinealocytes (Figure 8.30; Olah and Glick, 1984). The lymphoid accumulations of chicken pineal gland contain germinal centers (Quay, 1965; Campbell and Gibson, 1970; Cogburn and Glick, 1981) the expression of which seems to be synchronized with their formation in other peripheral lymphoid tissues (Cogburn and Glick, 1981).

In contrast, the origin and functional significance of

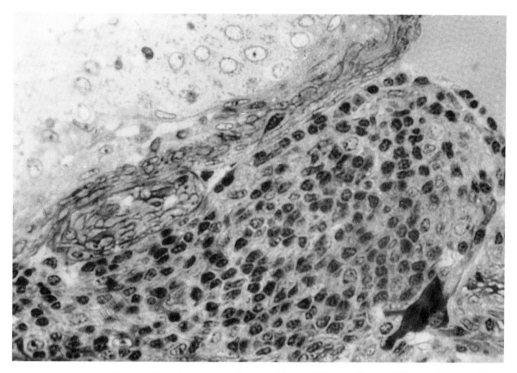

Figure 8.29 Presence of lymphoid accumulations under the connective tissue capsule of 2-month-old chicken pineal gland (× 450).

pineal lymphoid elements is a matter of controversy. Romieu and Jullien (1942) suggested that they differentiate *in situ,* but cell migration in both directions, from the blood vessels to pineal parenchyma and vice versa, has been reported (Cogburn and Glick, 1981; Olah and Glick, 1984). Cogburn and Glick (1979) have indicated that the pineal lymphoid tissue is composed of nearly equal proportions of bursal (42%) and thymic lymphocytes (51%). Thus, surgical bursectomy, thymectomy or their combination at hatching followed by whole-body irradiation inhibited the initial influx of lymphoid elements to the chicken's pineal gland (Cogburn and Glick, 1981). Furthermore, cyclophosphamide treatment prevented normal expression of pineal lymphoid tissue (Cogburn and Glick, 1981). Agammaglobulinemic birds lacked lymphoid tissue in both pineal parenchyma and choroid plexus (Cogburn and Glick, 1981). Consequently, these workers speculated that a functional bursa is essential to development of pineal lymphoid tissue (Coburn and Glick, 1981). Pineal lymphocytes also seem to be able to respond to antigens (Cogburn and Glick, 1981, 1983).

Romieu and Jullien (1942) suggested that pineal lymphoid tissue was the source of lymphocytes seen in cerebrospinal fluid and meninges, and Cogburn and Glick (1981) reported that pineal lymphocytes invaded ependymal cells and were found exterior to the choroid plexus in cerebrospinal fluid. In addition, Olah and Glick (1984) claimed, from ultrastructural evidence, that the pineal gland is a suitable microenvironment for proliferation and differentiation of lymphoid cells, and Mede *et al.* (1981) reported accumulations of T-lymphocytes in the pineal gland of aged rats. In any case, the immunological significance of pineal lymphoid accumulations must be conclusively clarified.

HARDERIAN GLAND

Numerous vertebrates possess a Harderian gland. It is a compound tubulo-acinar paired gland located in the eye's orbit, where it produces a lubricating secretion for the cornea. In some vertebrates, especially birds, the Harderian gland participates in immune responses.

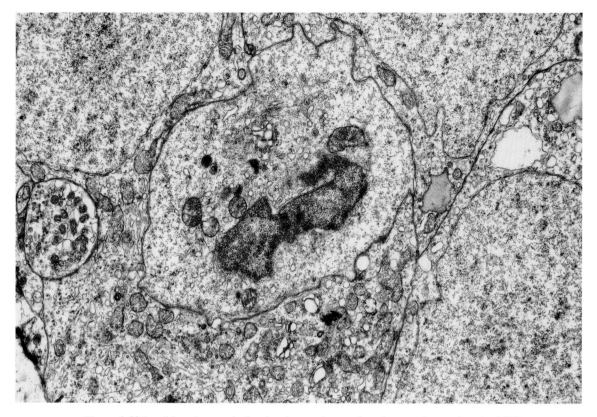

Figure 8.30 Small lymphocytes in the pineal parenchyma of an ultrasound-treated rat ($\times$ 7600).

The avian Harderian glands represent the largest discrete accumulation of lymphoid tissue in the paraocular area, although other glands in the ocular region, such as lateral nasal glands and lacrimal glands, contain also lymphoid cells (Bang and Bang, 1968; Mueller et al., 1971; Wight et al., 1971; Sundiek et al., 1973; Albini et al., 1974; Burns, 1975; Darelaar and Kouwenhoven, 1976; Aitken and Survashe, 1977; Survashe and Aitken, 1977; Glick et al., 1977; Glick, 1979; Pejkovski et al., 1979; Powell et al., 1979; Survashe et al., 1979). Variations between distinct avian species are, however, important. The lymphoid infiltration of the nasal area is prominent in chickens, moderate in pheasants and turkeys and only slight in 57 other species examined (Aitken and Survashe, 1977).

The avian Harderian glands are formed by lobules separated from each other by a small amount of connective tissue which contains a few blood vessels and nerves. Furthermore, connective tissue trabeculae project into the lobules, interspersed between the glandular parenchyma, formed by a single layer of secretory epithelium. Within the intralobular trabeculae there are numerous plasma cells, macrophages and lymphocytes, especially in the central parts of the lobules (Bang and Bang, 1968; Mueller et al., 1971; Wight et al., 1971; Rothwell et al., 1972; Burns, 1975; Kittner et al., 1978; Niedorf and Wolters, 1978; Schramm, 1980). Heterophils (Bang and Bang, 1968; Wight et al., 1971; Burns, 1975) and eosinophils (Schramm, 1980) are also occasionally present. Apparently, there is an age-dependent increase of the plasma cell infiltration of the Harderian gland (Bang and Bang, 1968; Burns, 1975; Glick et al., 1977; Niedorf and Wolters, 1978; Wight et al., 1971).

A paucity of plasma cells has been reported in the Harderian gland of newly hatched chicks (Wight et al., 1971; Albini et al., 1974). Maximum concentrations occur after 4 weeks of age (Burns, 1975; Neidorf and Wolters, 1978; Wight et al., 1971). Gallego and Glick (1988) claimed recently that the Harderian gland contains the highest concentration of plasma cells when compared to all the avian lymphoid organs. During the first weeks after hatching, sIgM[+] cells are numerous in the gland (Albini *et al.*, 1974). IgG and IgA appear between 5 and 9 weeks, with the IgA isotype becoming dominant by 11 weeks (Albini *et al.*, 1974). Additionally, u[+], Ia[+] and T-cells have been recently identified in the chicken Harderian gland (Gallego and Glick, 1988), confirming previous immunofluorescence findings (Albini and Wick, 1973; Albini *et al.*, 1974; Glick *et al.*, 1977). Finally, a significant proportion of degenerating plasma cells occurs also in the chicken Harderian gland (Burns, 1975; Zicca *et al.*, 1982). The lymphoid tissue of these Harderian glands plays an important immunological role in providing local protection for this area. Ig secreted from the Harderian gland's lymphoid components reach the conjunctival sac and subsequently the nasal cavities (Mueller *et al.*, 1971; Burns, 1977; Burns and Maxwell, 1979). Thus, the Harderian gland produces antibodies to particulate antigens applied locally (Mueller *et al.*, 1971; Powell *et al.*, 1979) and antibodies to infectious bronchitis virus. Newcastle disease virus and *Mycoplasma gallisepticum* have been detected in Harderian gland extracts and secretions (Powell *et al.*, 1979). Moreover, surgical removal of the Harderian gland leads to lower levels of IgM production (Neumann and Kaleta, 1977).

It is unknown whether Harderian gland plasma cells represent an *in situ* differentiated cell population from B-cells in response to antigenic stimulation or the Harderian gland is a site of concentration for maturing B-cells. This second possibility is supported by the observation that plasma cells are largely predominant over B-cells (Sundick *et al.*, 1973; Albini *et al.*, 1974) in the gland, and the percentage of plasma cells producing different Ig isotypes is fairly stable in adult chickens (Lydyard *et al.*, 1981). Alternatively, Gallego and Glick (1988) proposed that B-cell migration to the Harderian gland may occur prior to 2 weeks of age and the continued presence of plasma cells after this period could be attributed, at least in part, to the persistence of a small population of long-lived B-cells and the proliferative capacity of plasmacytic cells. The role played by other avian lymphoid organs in the colonization of Harderian gland lymphoid tissue is also controversial. Although bursectomy interferes with the normal development of Harderian gland lymphoid

tissue (Mueller *et al.*, 1971; Dohms *et al.*, 1981) and suppresses the size of the plasma cell compartment, the suppression is, however, not complete, suggesting a partial bursal-independent origin for the plasma cells in Harderian glands (Wolters *et al.*, 1977).

Plasma cells are also present in avian lacrimal glands, although are fewer in number and their appearance does not seem to be age dependent (Burns, 1976). Remarkably, the elimination of the Harderian gland evokes an increased immunological activity of the lacrimal gland. Functional detection of the Harderian gland increases the number of plasma cells in the lacrimal glands (Survashe and Aitken, 1977; Burns, 1979). Furthermore, BSA immunization of intact birds restricts anti-BSA activity to the Harderian gland, but in fowls without Harderian glands anti-BSA activity was found in the lacrimal glands (Burns, 1979).

FINAL COMMENT

There are primary lymphoid organs where lymphocytes originate and mature up to a certain stage. It is in the secondary lymphoid organs where further maturation occurs and where immunological responses are initiated once immunocompetent cells are selected by antigen. The secondary centers are not restricted to the spleen and lymph nodes that are intimately associated with the circulatory and lymphatic systems. In addition, there are other accumulations (perhaps tertiary) of lymphoid cells, chiefly in association with highly vulnerable epithelial surfaces that provide the other subepithelial component of the body's defense armamentarium enbarium. This renders an animal totally covered by a network of protection from invading potentially pathogenic microorganisms.

REFERENCES

Aitken ID and Survashe BD (1977). Plasma cells in vertebrate paraocular glands. *Int Arch Allergy Appl Immunol* **53**: 62–67.

Akef M (1978). Immunological studies in some Egyptian reptiles. MSc thesis, Faculty of Sciences, Cairo University.

Albini B and Wick G (1973). Immunoglobulin determinants on the surface of chicken lymphoid cells. *Int Arch Allergy* **44**: 804–822.

Albini B and Wick G (1974). Delineation of B and T lymphoid cells in the chicken. *J Immunol* **112**: 444–450.

Albini B, Wick G, Rose E and Orlans E (1974). Immunoglobulin production in chicken Harderian gland. *Int Arch Allergy* **47**: 23–24.

Ardavin CF (1981). Tejido linfoide asociado al tubo digestivo en el anfibio urodelo *Pleurodeles waltlii*. Efecto de la immunization primaria y secondaria. Master's thesis, Complutense University (Madrid).

Ardavin CF, Zapata A, Villena A and Solas MT (1982a). Gut-associated lymphoid tissue (GALT) in the amphibian urodele *Pleurodeles waltlii*. *J Morph* **173**: 35–41.

Ardavin CF, Zapata A, Garrido E and Villena A (1982b). Ultrastructure of gut-associated lymphoid tissue (GALT) in the amphibian urodele *Pleurodeles waltlii*. *Cell Tissue Res* **224**: 663–671.

Ardavin CF, Gomariz RP, Barrutia MG, Fonfria J and Zapata A (1984). The lympho-hemopoietic organs of the anadromous sea lamprey *Petromyzon marinus*. A comparative study throughout its life span. *Acta Zool Stockh* **65**: 1–15.

Back O (1970a). Studies on the lymphocytes in the intestinal epithelium of the chicken. III. Effect of thymectomy. *Int Arch Allergy Appl Immunol* **39**: 192–200.

Back O (1970b). Studies on the lymphocytes in the intestinal epithelium of the chicken. IV. Effect of bursectomy. *Int Arch Allergy Appl Immunol* **39**: 342–351.

Back O (1972a). Studies of the lymphocytes in the intestinal epithelium of the chicken. I. Ontogeny. *Acta Pathol Microbiol Scand Sect A* **80**: 84–90.

Back O (1972b). Studies on the lymphocytes in the intestinal epithelium of the chicken. II. Kinetics. *Acta Pathol Microbiol Scand Sect A* **80**: 91–96.

Bang BB and Bang FB (1968). Localized lymphoid tissues and plasma cells in paraocular and paranasal organ systems on chickens. *Am J Pathol* **53**: 735–751.

Basslinger J (1858). Die peyerischen inseln (plaques) der vogel. *Z Wiss Zool* **9**: 299–300.

Befus AD, Johnston N, Leslie GA and Bienenstock J (1980). Gut associated lymphoid tissue in the chicken. I. Morphology, ontogeny and some functional characteristics of Peyer's patches. *J Immunol* **125**: 2626–2632.

Bienenstock J, Gauldie J and Perey DY (1973). Synthesis of IgG, IgA, IgM by chicken tissues: immunofluorescent and ^{14}C amino acid incorporation studies. *J Immunol* **111**: 1112–1118.

Bienenstock J, McDermott M, Befus D and O'Neill M (1978). A common mucosal immunologic system involving the bronchus, breast and bowel. *Adv Exp Med Biol* **107**: 53–59.

Bjerregaard P (1975). Lymphoid cells in chicken intestinal epithelium. *Cell Tissue Res* **161**: 485–495.

Bloom W and Fawcett D (1975). *A Textbook of Histology*. WB Saunders: Philadelphia.

Borysenko M and Cooper EL (1972). Lymphoid tissue in the snapping turtle *Chelydra serpentina*. *J Morph* **138**: 487–498.

Boya J and Calvo J (1978). Post-hatching evolution of the pineal gland of the chicken. *Acta Anat* **101**: 1–9.

Bryant BJ, Adler JE, Cordy DR, Shifrine M and DaMassa AJ (1973). The avian bursa-independent humoral immune system: serologic and morphologic studies. *Eur J Immunol* **3**: 9–15.

Buras N, Duek L and Niv S (1985). Reactions of fish to micro-organisms in wastewater. *Appl Environ Microbiol* **50**: 989–995.

Burns RB (1975). Plasma cells in the avian Harderian gland and the morphology of the gland in the rook. *Can J Zool* **53**: 1258–1269.

Burns RB (1976). The structure of the lacrimal glands of the domestic fowl and of the ducks. *Res Vet Sci* **21**: 291–299.

Burns RB (1977). Possible route of antigen uptake by the Harderian gland of the domestic fowl. *Br Poultry Sci* **18**: 407–409.

Burns RB (1979). Histological and immunological studies on the fowl lacrimal gland following surgical excision of Harder's gland. *Res Vet Sci* **27**: 69–75.

Burns RB and Maxwell MH (1979). The structure of the Harderian gland and lacrimal gland ducts of the turkey, fowl and duck. A light microscope study. *J Anat* **128**: 285–292.

Calhoun ML (1932). The microscopic anatomy of the digestive tract of *Gallus domesticus*. *Iowa State College J Sci* **7**: 261–281.

Campbell E and Gibson MA (1970). A histological and histochemical study of the development of the pineal gland in the chick *Gallus domesticus*. *Can J Zool* **48**: 1321–1328.

Chin KN and Wong WC (1977). Some ultrastructural observations on the intestinal mucosa of the toad *Bufo melanostictus*. *J Anat* **123**: 331–339.

Cogburn LA and Glick B (1979). The pineal gland: a prominent lymphoid tissue in young chickens (Abstract). *Physiologist* **22**: 20.

Cogburn LA and Glick B (1981). Lymphopoiesis in the chicken pineal gland. *Am J Anat* **162**: 131–142.

Cogburn LA and Glick B (1983). Functional lymphocytes in the chicken pineal gland. *J Immunol* **130**: 2109–2112.

Darelaar FG and Kouwenhoven B (1976). Changes in the Harderian gland of the chicken following conjunctival and intranasal infection with infectious bronchitis virus in one and 20-day old chickens. *Avian Pathol* **5**: 39–50.

Davina JHM, Rijkers GT, Rombout JH, Timmermans LPM and van Muiswinkel WB (1980). Lymphoid and nonlymphoid cells in the intestine of cyprinid fish. In Horton JD (Ed), *Development and Differentiation of Vertebrate Lymphocytes*. Elsevier/North-Holland: Amsterdam. pp 126–140.

Davina JHM, Parmentier HK and Timmermans LPM (1982). Effect of oral administration of *Vibrio* bacteria on the intestine of cyprinid fish. *Dev Comp Immunol* Suppl **2**: 157–166.

Dohms JE, Lee KP and Rosenberger JK (1981). Plasma cell changes in the gland of Harder following infectious bursal disease virus infection of the chicken. *Avian Dis* **25**: 683–695.

Drzewina A (1905). Contribution a l'etude du tissue lymphoide des Ichthyopsides. *Archs Zool Exp Gen* **4**: 145−338.

Du Pasquier L (1968). Les proteines seriques et le complexe lymphomyeloide chez le tetard d' *Alytes obstetricans* normal et thymectomise. *Ann Inst Pasteur Paris* **114**: 490−502.

El Deeb SO (1978). Study of the immune system of some Egyptian lizards. MSc thesis, Faculty of Science, Cairo University.

El Deeb SO (1983). Ontogeny of the immune system of the lizard *Chalcides ocellatus*. PhD thesis, Faculty of Science, Cairo University.

El Ridi R, El Deeb S and Zada S (1981). The gut-associated lymphoepithelioid tissue (GALT) of lizards and snakes. In Solomon JB (Ed), *Aspects of Developmental and Comparative Immunology I.* Pergamon Press: Oxford. pp 233−239.

Ellis AE (1982). Histamine, mast cells and hypersensitivity responses in fish. *Dev Comp Immunol* Suppl **2**: 147−155.

Ellis AE (1986). The function of teleost fish lymphocytes in relation to inflammation. *Int J Tissue React* **4**: 263−270.

Ernst PB, Befus AD and Bienenstock J (1985). Leukocytes in the intestinal epithelium: An unusual immunological compartment. *Immunol Today* **6**: 50−55.

Fichtelius KE, Finstad J and Good RA (1968). Bursa equivalents of bursaless vertebrates. *Lab Invest* **19**: 339−351.

Fletcher TC and White A (1973). Antibody production in the plaice *Pleuronectes platessa* L. after oral and parenteral immunization with *Vibrio anguillarum* antigens. *Aquaculture* **1**: 417−428.

Fonfria J, Barrutia MG, Villena A and Zapata A (1982). Ultrastructural study of interdigitating cells in the thymus of the spotless starling *Sturnus unicolor*. *Cell Tissue Res* **225**: 687−691.

Gallego M and Glick B (1988). The proliferative capacity of the cells of the avian Harderian gland. *Dev Comp Immunol* **12**: 157−166.

Glick B (1979). The immune response of the chicken: Lymphoid development of the bursa of Fabricius and thymus and an immune response role of the gland of Harder. *Poultry Sci* **57**: 1441−1444.

Glick B, Subba-Rao DSV, Stinson R and McDuffie FC (1977). Immunoglobulin positive cells from the gland of Harder and bone marrow of the chicken. *Cell Immunol* **31**: 177−181.

Glick B, Holbrook, KA, Olah I, Perkins WD and Stinson R (1978). A scanning electron microscope study of the caecal tonsil: The identification of a bacterial attachment to the villi of the caecal tonsil and the possible presence of lymphatics in the caecal tonsil. *Poultry Sci* **57**: 1408−1416.

Glick B, Holbrook KA, Olah I, Perkins WD and Stinson R (1981). An electron and light microscope study of the caecal tonsil: The basic unit of the caecal tonsil. *Dev Comp Immunol* **5**: 95−104.

Goldstein SN, Manickavel V and Cohen N (1975). Phylogeny of gut-associated lymphoid tissue. *Am Zool* **15**: 107−118.

Good RA, Finstad J, Pollara B and Gabrielsen AE (1966). Morphologic studies on the evolution of the lymphoid tissues among the lower vertebrates. In Smith RT, Miescher PA and Good RS (Eds), *Phylogeny of Immunity*. University of Florida Press: Gainesville. pp 149−170.

Hameed NSS (1980). Studies on the distribution of the gut-associated lymphoid tissues (GALT) in vertebrates. MPh thesis, Madurai University, Tamilnadu (India).

Harris JE (1972). The immune response of a cyprinid fish to infections of the acanthocephalan, *Pomphorhynchus laevis*. *Int J Parasitol* **2**: 459−469.

Hart S (1987). Immunity in the alimentary tract and other mucosae of the dogfish *Scyliorhinus canicula* L. PhD thesis, Plymouth Polytechnic (UK).

Hart S, Wrathmell AB and Harris JE (1986). Ontogeny of gut-associated lymphoid tissue (GALT) in the dogfish *Scyliorhinus canicula* L. *Vet Immunol Immunopathol* **12**: 107−116.

Hart S, Wrathmell AB, Doggett TA and Harris JE (1987). An investigation of the biliary and intestinal immunoglobulin and the plasma cell distribution in the gall bladder and liver of the common dogfish *Scyliorhinus canicula* L. *Aquaculture* **67**: 147−155.

Hart S, Wrathmell AB, Harris JE and Grayson TH (1988). Gut immunology in fish: A review. *Dev Comp Immunol* **12**: 453−480.

Hedge SN and George CJ (1973). The nature of the lymphoid tissue in the caecum of the domestic fowl. *Curr Sci* **42**: 645−647.

Henle (1871). *Handbuch der Systematische Anatomie des Menschen*. Nervenlehre 3 (cited by Romieu and Jullien, 1942).

Horton JD (1969). Ontogeny of the immune response to skin allografts in relation to lymphoid organ development in the amphibian *Xenopus laevis* Daudin. *J Exp Zool* **170**: 449−466.

Horton JD (1971). Histogenesis of the lymphomyeloid complex on the larval leopard frog *Rana pipiens*. *J Morph* **134**: 1−19.

Hoshi H and Mori T (1973). Identification of bursa-dependent and thymus-dependent areas in the tonsilla caecalis of chickens. *Tohoku J Exp Med* **111**: 309−322.

Hussein MF, Badir N, Zada S, El Ridi R and Zahran W (1984). Effect of seasonal changes on immune system of the toad *Bufo regularis*. *Bull Fac Sci Cairo Univ* **52**: 181−192.

Ingram GA and Molyneux DH (1983). The immune response of *Lacerta viridis* to *Leishmania agamae*. *Dev Comp Immunol* **7**: 717−718.

Jacobshagen E (1915). Zur morphologie des spiraldarms. *Anat Anz* **48**: 188−254.

Jacobson ER and Collins BR (1980). Tonsil-like esophageal lymphoid structures of boid snakes. *Dev Comp Immunol* **4**: 703−712.

Jankovic BD (1968). The development and function of immunologically reactive tissue in the chicken. *Wiss Z Friedrich Schiller Univ Jena Math Naturwiss Reihe* **17**: 137 ff.

Jankovic BD and Mitrovic K (1967). Germinal centers in the tonsilla caecalis— relationship to the thymus and the bursa of Fabricius. In Cottier H, Odartchenko N, Schnidler R and Congdon CC (Eds), *Germinal Centers in the Immune Responses*. Springer-Verlag: Berlin. pp 34 – 37.

Jankovic BD, Mitrovic K, Popeskovic L and Milosevic D (1966). Tonsilla caecalis: An immunologically active tissue in the chicken. *Yugoslav Physiol Pharmacol Acta* **2**: 71 – 75.

Jolly J (1915). La bourse de Fabricius et les organes lympho-epitheliaux. *Arch d'anat Micr Par* **16**: 363 – 547.

Jordan HE and Speidel CC (1931). Blood formation in the African lungfish under normal conditions and under conditions of prolonged estivation and recovery. *J Morphol Physiol* **51**: 319 – 371.

Jurd RD (1977). Secretory immunoglobulins and gut-associated lymphoid tissue in *Xenopus laevis*. In Solomon JB and Horton JD (Eds), *Developmental Immunobiology*. Elsevier/North-Holland: Amsterdam. pp 307 – 314.

Kanakambika P and Muthukkaruppan VR (1972). The immune response to sheep erythrocytes in the lizard, *Calotes versicolor*. *J Immunol* **109**: 415 – 419.

Kanesada A (1956). A phylogenetic survey of hemocytopoietic tissues in submammalian vertebrates. *Bull Yamaguchi Med School* **4**: 1 – 35.

Kimura N and Kudo S (1975). Fine structure of the stratum granulosum in the pyloric caeca of the rainbow trout. *Jap J Ichthyol* **22**: 16 – 22.

Kittner Z, Olah I and Toro I (1978). Histology and ultra-structure of the Harderian glands— accessory lacrimal gland— of the chicken. *Acta Biol Acad Sci Hung* **29**: 29 – 41.

Kotani M (1959). Lymphgefasse, lymphatische apparate und extravasculare softbahnen der Schlange *Elaphe quadrivirgata* Boie. *Acta Sch Med Univ Kioto Japan* **36**: 121 – 171.

Langille RM and Youson JH (1985). Protein and lipid absorption in the intestinal mucosa of adult lampreys (*Petromyzon marinus*) following induced feeding. *Can J Zool* **63**: 691 – 702.

Looper JB and Looper MH (1929). A histological study of the colic caeca in the bantam fowl. *J Morph* **48**: 585 – 609.

Lydyard PM, Millo R, De Barbieri A, Cardoni A and Grossi CE (1981). Some aspects of B cell maturation in the chicken. In Solomon JB (Ed), *Aspects of Developmental and Comparative Immunology I*. Pergamon Press: Oxford. pp 241 – 252.

Magnan A (1911). Morphologie des caecoms chez des orseaux en fonction du regime alimentaire. Annales des Sciences Naturelles. *Zoologie T* 14, g-serie.

Manning MJ and Horton JD (1969). Histogenesis of lymphoid organs in larvae of the South African clawed toad *Xenopus laevis* (Dandin). *J Embryol Exp Morphol* **22**: 265 – 277.

McCauley WMJ (1956). The gross anatomy of the lymphatic system of *Alligator mississippiensis*. *Am J Anat* **99**: 189 – 209.

McDermott MR and Bienenstock J (1979). Evidence for a common mucosal immunologic system. I. Migration of B immunoblasts into intestinal, respiratory and genital tissues. *J Immunol* **122**: 1892 – 1898.

McGarry RC and Bourns TKR (1980). Annular bands of lymphoid tissue in the intestine of the mallard duck *Anas platyrhynchos*. *J Morph* **163**: 1 – 8.

Michea-Hamzehpour M (1977). Indirect immunofluorescent identification of 19S immunoglobulin-containing cells in the intestinal mucosa of *Xenopus laevis*. *J Exp Zool* **201**: 109 – 114.

Minagawa Y, Ohuishi K and Murakawa S (1975). Structure and immunological function of lymphomyeloid organs in the bullfrog *Rana catesbeiana*. In Hildermann WH and Benedicts AA (Eds), *Immunologic Phylogeny*. Plenum Press: New York. pp 257 – 266.

Mueller AP, Sato K and Glick B (1971). The chicken lacrimal gland, gland of Harder, caecal tonsil and accessory spleens as sources of antibody producing cells. *Cell Immunol* **2**: 140 – 152.

Muthmann E (1913). Beitrage fur vergluchende anatomie der blind darmes der lymphoiden organe des darmkanales ber saugetieren und vogeln. *Anat Hefte* **48**: 67 – 114.

Nelson JS, Rohovec JS and Fryer JL (1985). Tissue location of *Vibrio anguillarum* bacterin delivered by intraperitoneal injection, immersion and oral routes to *Salmo gairdneri*. *Fish Pathol* **19**: 263 – 270.

Neumasen V and Kaleta ET (1977). Untersuchungen zur immunologischen funktion der Harderschen druse des Huhnes. *Zentrabl Veterinaer Med Reihe B* **24**: 331 ff.

Niedorf HR and Wolters B (1978). Development of the Harderian gland in the chicken; light and electron microscopic investigations. *Invest Cell Pathol* **1**: 205 – 215.

Olah I and Glick B (1979). Structure of the germinal centers in the chicken caecal tonsil: Light and electron microscopic and autoradiographic studies. *Poultry Sci* **58**: 195 – 210.

Olah I and Glick B (1984) Lymphopineal tissue in the chicken. *Dev Comp Immunol* **8**: 855 – 862.

Olah I, Rohlich P and Toro I (1975). *Ultrastructure of Lymphoid Organs*. Masson: Paris.

Orlans E and Rose ME (1970). Antibody formation by transferred cells in inbred fowls. *Immunology* **18**: 473 – 482.

Ostberg Y, Fange R, Mattisson A and Thomas NW (1976). Light and electron microscopical characterization of heterophilic granulocytes in the intestinal wall and islet parenchyma of the hagfish *Myxine glutinosa* (Cyclostomata). *Acta Zool Stockh* **57**: 89 – 102.

Paltzel V (1936). Der darm. In Mollendorff MW (Ed), *Handbuch der Mikroskopischen Anatomie des Menschen*. Vol 5, No. 3. Julius Springer: Berlin. pp 1 – 448.

Payne LN (1971). The lymphoid system. In Bell DJ and Freeman BM (Eds), *Physiology and Biochemistry of the Domestic Fowl*. Academic Press: New York. pp 988 – 1037.

Pejkovski C, da Velaar FG and Kouwenhoven B (1979). Immunosuppressive effect of infectious bursal disease virus of vaccination against infectious bronchitis. *Avian Pathol* **8**: 95 – 106.

Perey DYE (1971). Mammalian analogues of the bursal – thymic systems. In *Cellular Interactions in the Immune Response*. Karger: Basel.

Pitchappan RM and Muthukkaruppan VR (1977). Analysis of the development of the lizard *Calotes versicolor*. II. Histogenesis of the thymus. *Dev Comp Immunol* **1**: 217 – 230.

Plytycz B and Slezek J (1981). Gut-associated lymphoid tissue in several amphibian species. *Folia Biol (Krakow)* **29**: 93 – 101.

Pontius H and Ambrosius H (1972). Contribution to the immune biology of poikilothermic vertebrates. IX. Studies on the cellular mechanism of humoral immune reactions in perch *Perca fluviatilis* L. *Acta Biol Med Ger* **29**: 319 – 339.

Powell JR, Aitken ID and Survashe BD (1979). The response of Harderian gland of the fowl to antigen given by the ocular route. *Avian Pathol* **8**: 363 – 373.

Quay WB (1965). Histological structure and cytology of the pineal organ in birds and mammals. *Prog Brain Res* **10**: 49 – 86.

Rombout JW, Block LJ, Lamers CH and Egberts E (1986). Immunization of carp (*Cyprinus carpio*) with *Vibrio anguillarum* bacteria: indications for a common mucosal immune system. *Dev Comp Immunol* **10**: 341 – 351.

Romieu M and Jullien G (1942). Sur l'existence d'une formation lymphoide dans l'epiphyse des Gallinaces. *CR Soc Biol* **136**: 626 – 628.

Rothe F and Ambrosius H (1968). Beitrage zur immuno-biolilige poikilothermer Wirbeltiere: V. Die Proliferation Antikorper bildender Zellen bei Schildkoten. *Acta Biol Med Ger* **21**: 525 – 536.

Rothwell B, Wight PAL, Burns RB and MacKenzie GM (1972). The Harderian glands of the domestic fowl. III. Ultrastructure. *J Anat* **112**: 233 – 250.

Schramm M (1980). Lymphoid cells in the Harderian gland of birds. An electron microscopical study. *Cell Tissue Res* **205**: 85 – 94.

Sidky YA and Auerbach R (1968). Tissue culture analysis of immunological capacity of snapping turtles. *J Exp Zool* **167**: 187 – 196.

Sminia T, Wilders MM, Janre EM and Hoefsmit ECM (1983). Characterization of non-lymphoid cells in Peyer's patches of the rat. *Immunobiology* **164**: 136 – 143.

Solas MT and Zapata A (1980). Gut-associated lymphoid tissue (GALT) in reptiles: intraepithelial cells. *Dev Comp Immunol* **4**: 87 – 99.

Solas MT, Laceta J and Zapata A (1981). Structure of the cloacal lymphoid complex of *Mauremys caspica*. *Dev Comp Immunol* Suppl **1**: 151 – 156.

Sorvari R, Naukkarinen A and Sorvari T (1977). Anal suck-ing-like movements in the chicken and chick embryo followed by the transportation of environmental material to the bursa of Fabricius, caeca and caecal tonsils. *Poultry Sci* **56**: 1426 – 1429.

Spiroff BEN (1958). Embryonic and post-hatching develop-ment of the pineal body of the domestic fowl. *Am J Anat* **103**: 375 – 401.

Sundick RS, Albini B and Wick G (1973). Chicken Harder's gland: Evidence for a relatively pure bursa-dependent lymphoid cell population. *Cell Immunol* **7**: 332 – 335.

Survashe BD and Aitken ID (1977). Further observations on functional selection of paraocular glands in the fowl *Gallus domesticus*. *Res Vet Sci* **23**: 217 – 223.

Survashe BD, Aitken ID and Powell JR (1979). The response of the Harderian gland of the fowl to antigen given by the ocular route. I. Histological changes. *Avian Pathol* **8**: 77 – 93.

Thompson JA (1925). *Biology of Birds*. Cited by J.B. Looper and M.H. Looper, 1929. pp 108 – 110.

Tochinai S (1976). Lymphoid changes in *Xenopus laevis* following thymectomy at the initial stage of its histo-genesis. *J Fac Sci Hokkaido Univ Ser* **6**: 20 – 175.

Tomonaga S, Hirokane T and Awaya K (1973). The primi-tive spleen of the hagfish. *Zool Mag* **82**: 215 – 217.

Toner PG (1965). The fine structure of the globule leucocyte in the fowl intestine. *Acta Anat* **61**: 321 – 330.

Uede T, Ishi Y, Matsome A, Shimagawara J and Kikuchi K (1981). Immunohistochemical study of lymphocytes in rat pineal gland. Selective accumulation of T lymphocytes. *Anat Rec* **199**: 239 – 247.

Vaerman JP, Picard J and Heremans JF (1975). Structural data on chicken IgA and failure to identify the IgA of the tortoise. In Hildemann WH and Benedict AA (Eds), *Immunologic Phylogeny*. *Adv Exp Med Biol* **64**: 185 – 195.

Weisel GF (1973). Anatomy and histology of the digestive system of the paddlefish *Polydon spathula*. *J Morph* **140**: 243 – 256.

Weisel GF (1979). Histology of the feeding and digestive organs of the shovelnose sturgeon *Scaperhynchus platorhynchus*. *Copeia* **1979**: 518 – 525.

Whitlock DR, Lushbaugh WB, Danforth HD and Ruff MD (1975). Scanning electron microscopy of the caecal mucosa in *Eimeria tenella* infected and uninfected chickens. *Avian Dis* **19**: 293 – 304.

Wight PAL, Burns RB, Rothwell B and Mackenzie GM (1971). The Harderian gland of the domestic fowl. I. Histology with reference to the genesis of plasma cells and Russell bodies. *J Anat* **110**: 30 – 33.

Wolters G, Hultshe R and Niedorf HR (1977). Bursa-independent plasma cells in the Harderian gland of the chicken *Gallus domesticus*. Histomorphometrical investi-gations. *Beitr Pathol* **160**: 50 – 57.

Wong WC (1972). Lymphoid aggregations in the oeso-phagus of the toad *Bufo melanostictus*. *Acta Anat* **83**: 461 – 478.

Zapata A (1977). Estructura de los organos linfoides y linfo-mieloides de peces. PhD thesis, Universidad Complutense, Madrid.

Zapata A (1979). Ultraestructura del tejido linfoide asociado al tubo digestivo (GALT) de *Rutilus rutilus*. *Morf Norm*

Patol Sec A **3**: 23 – 29.

Zapata A and Solas MT (1979). Gut-associated lymphoid tissue (GALT) in reptilia: Structure of mucosal accumulations. *Dev Comp Immunol* **3**: 477 – 487.

Zicca A, Cadoni A, Leprini A, Millo R, Lydyard PM and Grossi CE (1982). Immunofluorescent and ultrastructural analysis of plasma cell degeneration in the chicken Harder's gland. *Dev Comp Immunol* **6**: 131 – 139.

9

Seasonal Variations in the Immune System

INTRODUCTION

In previous chapters we presented those most relevant aspects concerning the histophysiology of lymphoid organs. That coverage is clearly an oversimplification since these organs undergo seasonal variations which affect their structure and function. We have known for many years that there are influences such as low temperature, stress or pollution which affect fish immunoreactivity, but the underlying mechanisms are essentially unknown. More recently, endogenous neuroendocrine rhythms which regulate the immune system have been assumed to be present (based on limited data) especially in reptiles but also in fish and amphibians. Furthermore, mutual influences between the immune and endocrine systems as well as seasonal activities of lymphoid organs, including the thymus and spleen, have been observed in embryonic and adult birds.

Information on seasonal variations which affect the immune system of ectothermic vertebrates can be summarized in three basic categories: (1) different vertebrate classes or species undergo similar immune changes during distinct annual seasons; (2) individual genetic features might be important in explaining variable results (although there is minimal if any exhaustive evidence); (3) different causative agents, such as temperature, photoperiod, and/or internal, homeostatic mediators—hormones, neuromodulators, neuropeptides, etc.—may be involved (Zapata et al., 1983).

In this chapter we will review current evidence supporting the effects of these environmental variables. In the broadest sense, we will first analyze seasonal changes in numbers of circulating leukocytes, as well as those that occur in the structure of central and peripheral lymphoid organs, and then how these changes affect cell-mediated and humoral immune responses. The possible causative agents of these seasonally dependent variations will be presented first from a double viewpoint of direct effects produced by environmental agents such as temperature, photoperiod, nutrition, etc., and second, the indirect effects which environmental parameters exert on the immune system via interactive variations in homeostatic mechanisms. In this regard, special attention will be focused on the role of steroids in season-dependent immune mechanisms.

SEASON-DEPENDENT CHANGES IN THE NUMBER OF CIRCULATING LYMPHOCYTES

There have been numerous reports concerning seasonal and annual variations in absolute and relative numbers of circulating blood cells: mainly leukocytes in vertebrates (Murachi, 1959; McKnight, 1966; Gardner and Yevich, 1969; Ezzat et al., 1974; Denton and Yousef, 1975; McLeay, 1975; Bridges et al., 1976; Fourie and Hattingh, 1976; van Vuren and Hattingh, 1978; Mahajan and Dheer, 1979; Srivastava and Agrawal, 1981; Pickering, 1986; Alvarez *et al.*, 1988 in teleosts; Duguy, 1970; Harris, 1972 in amphibians; Duguy, 1970; Cuchens *et al.*, 1976; Hussein *et al.*, 1978a, 1979a; El Ridi *et al.*, 1981 in reptiles; Dieterich and Feist, 1980; Jakubow *et al.*, 1984 in wild mammals).

Although there are important variations in data, even in the same species (cited by van Vuren and Hattingh, 1978), a notable reduction in numbers of peripheral blood lymphocytes during the winter season is claimed to occur for most species which have been examined; however, maximum levels seem to occur during the warm months (McLeay, 1975; Cuchens *et al.*, 1976; El Ridi *et al.*, 1980; Alvarez *et al.*, 1988). Yet low numbers of small and large lymphocytes have been reported in the middle of summer, but granulocytes increased in winter and summer, in brown trout, *Salmo trutta fario* (Alvarez *et al.*, 1988). Decreased numbers of circulating lymphocytes have also been observed and they occur when the breeding season begins (Mahajan and Dheer, 1979 in *Channa punctatus*; Alvarez *et al.*, 1988 in *Salmo trutta fario*). Other comparative immunologists have, however, found a negative correlation between lymphocyte numbers and pituitary—interrenal axis activity (McLeay, 1975 in *Oncorhynchus kisutch*).

In contrast, there is little available information on seasonal variations which distinctly functional lymphocyte populations may undergo. In the lizard *Chalcides ocellatus*, for example, proportions of peripheral blood lymphocytes recognized by an antithymocyte antiserum declined progressively, so that in winter no reactive cells were detected, but by the end of spring they reach 90% of the total peripheral blood lymphocytes (El Ridi *et al.*, 1980). However, lymphocytes bearing surface Ig remain in the peripheral blood (El Ridi *et al.*, 1980). Perhaps distinct lymphoid subpopulations are affected differentially by circumannual rhythms, a point which will be presented in more detail later.

SEASONAL CHANGES IN LYMPHOID ORGANS OF ECTOTHERMIC VERTEBRATES

Fish

A substantial regression followed by a further disappearance of the thymus after sexual development has been reported in annual fish, Koayu (*Plecoglossus altivelis*), the ice goby (*Leucopsarion petersi*) and Pacific salmon (*Oncorhynchus keta*) (Robertson and Wexler, 1960; Tamura and Honma, 1970; Honma and Tamura, 1972). In contrast, fish that can survive after spawning show no thymic regression even during sexual maturation (Tamura and Honma, 1973), but seasonal thymic changes reach peak activity in June—July (Tamura and Honma, 1977). This peak is independent of the breeding season in most species (Tamura and Honma, 1973, 1974, 1975, 1977, 1979; Tamura, 1978; Tamura *et al.*, 1981). In the rock-fish, *Sebasticus marmoratus*, Nakanishi (1986) described, however, the lowest thymic weight for both sexes in September but peak activity in February and April for male and female thymus, respectively. Moreover, the female thymus in this species is extremely atrophied shortly before and after spawning, whereas the male thymus is well developed (Nakanishi, 1986).

On the other hand, a slight increase in the thymic volume has been observed in surf-perch, *Ditrema temmincki* (Tamura *et al.*, 1981) and other species of fish observed in October (Tamura and Honma, 1974, 1975, 1977; Tamura, 1978). Alvarez *et al.* (1987) reported histological changes in the thymus of wild brown trout, *Salmo trutta fario*, caught throughout the year. Increased numbers of thymocytes occur in spring and summer (Figure 9.1), whereas pale, degenerated lymphoid cells were found at the beginning of autumn and in winter (Figure 9.2). Changes in thymic stromal components, including reticuloepithelial cells and macrophages, affected the subcapsular inner and outer thymic zones. Furthermore, erythropoietic foci occupied the thymic inner zone from June to September. A season-dependent erythropoietic activity of the thymus has been reported in other vertebrates, mainly birds (Kendall, 1980), and will be analyzed later.

These diverse variations in thymus which occur during seasonal changes described in the teleosts take place one to two months earlier than those observed in the spleen, especially in the periphery of the splenic artery and lymphoid tissue of the head kidney (Tamura and Honma, 1977). In wild brown trout, *Salmo trutta fario*, Alvarez *et al.* (1987) reported remarkable histological and ultrastructural changes, so that in some seasons degenerated lymphoid cells filled the splenic and renal lymphoid tissue. During winter and

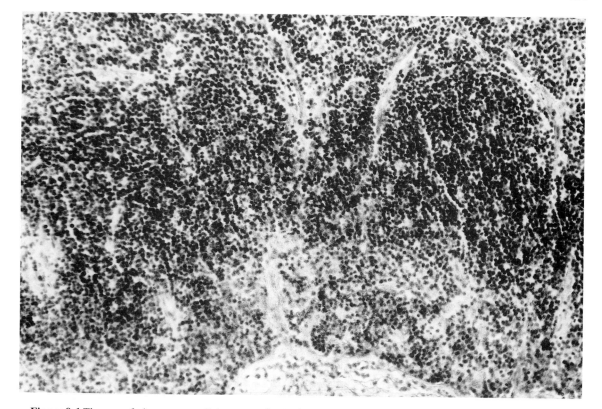

Figure 9.1 Thymus of a brown trout, *Salmo trutta farrio*, in May. Note the abundance of lymphoid elements (× 270).

early spring (December – March, depending on river water temperature) lymphoid tissue decreases considerably (Figure 9.3) and presumptive, degenerated, pale lymphoid cells abound, especially during late winter and early spring (February – March) in spleen, pro- and mesonephros (Figure 9.4).

In agreement with these results, under experimental conditions, goldfish acclimated at 4 °C have a 46% reduction in mononucleated spleen cell numbers when compared to fish acclimated at 22 °C (Azzolina, 1978). During spring (from April to the middle of May) the number of degenerated lymphoid cells diminished but this was followed by a gradual recovery of lymphoid tissue which occurs until May – June, when lymphoid components peak in peripheral lymphoid organs (Figure 9.5). Only then do true lymphoid follicles, containing numerous developing and mature plasma cells, appear in the splenic parenchyma. During summer, lymphoid tissue decreases again in both spleen and kidney, a change which resembles the condition in February – March (Figure 9.6). In

September, numerous pyknotic lymphocytes appear to have been engulfed in the cytoplasm of macrophages. Actually autumn (September – November) represents an intermediate stage when pycnotic cells and some lymphoid recovery are coincident in trout lymphoid organs. Finally in November, the amount of lymphoid tissue reaches a new peak although it is lower than that which has been observed in May – June (Figure 9.7).

Amphibians

Sporadic analyses of seasonal variations affecting the amphibian immune system which span some 60 years have been focused mostly on the thymus (von Braumulh, 1926; Holzapfel, 1937; Kapa *et al.*, 1968; Toro *et al.*, 1969; Balduzzi, 1976; Bazan-Kubik and Skrzypiec, 1980; Wright and Cooper, 1980; Bigaj and Plytycz, 1981, 1984; Plytycz and Bigaj, 1983; Hussein *et al.*, 1984b). In *Rana temporaria* (Plytycz and Bigaj, 1983) and *Rana ridibunda* (Bazan-Kubik and Skrzypiec, 1980) a maximum thymic weight as well as

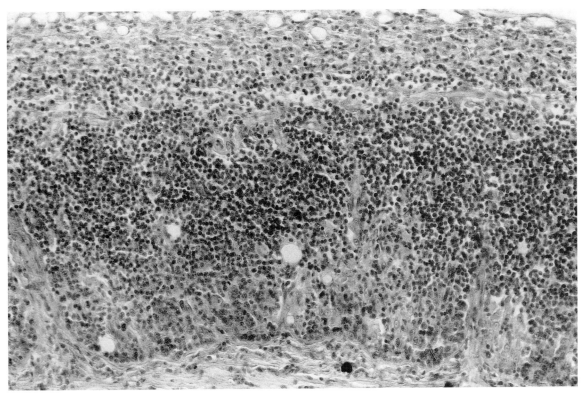

Figure 9.2 Thymus of a brown trout in February. Scant thymocytes occur ($\times$ 270).

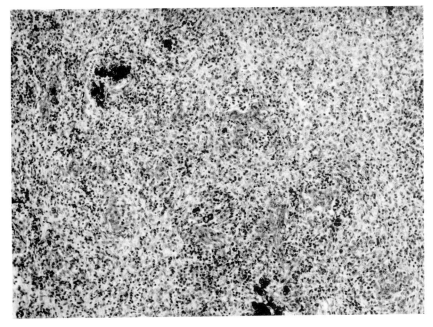

Figure 9.3 Survey of the spleen of a brown trout, caught in winter. Note the scarce development of lymphoid tissue ($\times$ 185).

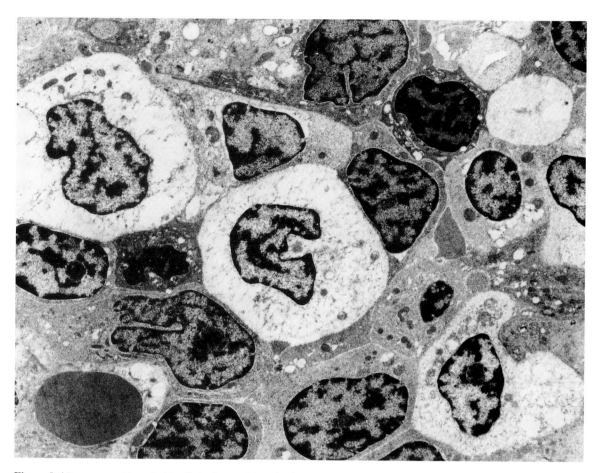

Figure 9.4 Degenerated lymphoid cells in the renal lympho-hemopoietic tissue of a brown trout in February – March. Note the absence of membranous organelles in the cytoplasm although the ultrastructure of the nucleus remains apparently normal (× 6840).

lymphocyte content have been recorded during the summer months, while a marked winter involution is followed by gradual recovery which ends in May. These workers presume that the autumnal decrease in thymic weight is related to lymphocyte emigration and/or death, while vernal increase could be due to lymphocyte influx and/or mitotic activity. Furthermore, ultrastructural analysis demonstrated scant secretory granule-containing cells and abundant inter-digitating-like cells during frog active life, but the reverse condition occurs during the hibernation period (Plytycz and Bigaj, 1983).

Remarkably, experimental manipulations of external temperature did not affect significantly the season-specific morphology of the frog thymus gland (Bigaj and Plytycz, 1984). Thymuses of experimental animals forced to lead an active life during winter months show the 'winter-like' appearance. They possess an abundant population of secretory cells and numerous thymic cysts. Nevertheless, the number of thymocytes is considerably greater than that in thymus glands of hibernating frogs. Likewise, thymus glands of frogs obtained immediately after capturing them in the field in May and June are clearly divided into a lymphocyte-rich cortex and an epithelial medulla. Such 'summer' thymic morphology is still evident in frogs kept in a refrigerator, which produces an artificial hibernation, from the end of May until the end of June.

Figure 9.5 Maximal development of lymphoid tissue in peripheral lymphoid organs of brown trout in May—June. Note the abundance of lymphoid follicles in the spleen (× 185).

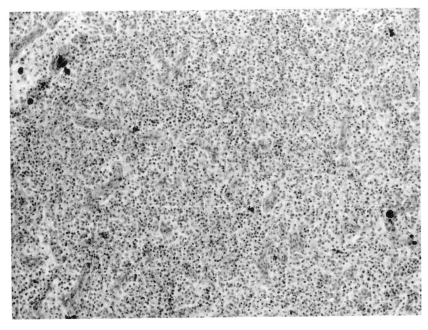

Figure 9.6 Low numbers of lymphocytes in the spleen of a brown trout during summer (× 185).

Figure 9.7 Abundant lymphoid tissue in the spleen of a brown trout in November. After the decrease in lymphoid tissue found in summer, splenic lymphocytes reach a new peak in the middle of autumn ($\times$ 185).

These results suggest that endogenous biological rhythms, which probably govern the seasonal histophysiology of the thymus gland (see below) are independent of environmental temperature.

In other species, the pattern of seasonal variations found in lymphoid organs is slightly different. In *Bufo regularis*, lymphoid depletion has been described in the thymus, spleen and gut-associated lymphoid tissue (GALT) during winter, a condition followed by degeneration in the spring (Hussein *et al.*, 1984b). From summer through autumn a gradual and slow involution has been observed but this disagrees with the above-mentioned condition in *Rana temporaria* and *Rana ridibunda* (Hussein *et al.*, 1984b). On the other hand, a lower activity in the thymus in frogs (*Rana perezi*) observed in February than in those of November has been reported recently (Garrido *et al.*, 1988). Remarkably, thymuses of February show degeneration of the stromal reticuloepithelial cells (Figure 9.8), a condition which could be related to the high levels of circulating sex steroids, as well as variations in numbers of pycnotic and mitotic thymocytes (Garrido *et al.*, 1988). In addition, frogs sacrificed in February exhibit decreased splenic lymphoid tissue

without apparent signs of pycnosis, and high numbers of lymphocytes in the peripheral blood and bone marrow. These observations suggest a redistribution of lymphocytes between the different peripheral lymphoid compartments of *Rana perezi* (Garrido *et al.*, 1988).

Reptiles

Season-dependent histological changes have been found in lymphoid organs of most reptiles, including lizards (Hussein *et al.*, 1978a in *Chalcides ocellatus*; Hussein *et al.*, 1978b in *Mabuya quinquetaeniata* and *Uromastyx aegyptia*; Hussein *et al.*, 1979b in *Scincus scincus*), snakes (Hussein *et al.*, 1979a in *Spalerosophis diadema*; El Ridi *et al.*, 1981 in *Psammophis diadema*) and turtles (Leceta and Zapata, 1985 in *Mauremys caspica*). Nevertheless, Hussein *et al.* (1984a) reported that lymphoid tissues in the gecko *Tarentola annularis* are not affected by seasonal rhythms, although humoral responses are influenced by seasons. Thus, the lymphoid components of thymus, spleen and GALT are not drastically depleted in winter and only undergo a slight increase during summer (Hussein *et al.*, 1984a).

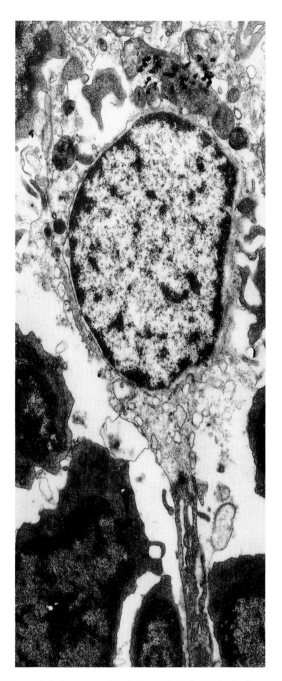

Figure 9.8 Degenerated reticuloepithelial cells in the thymus of *Rana perezi* in February. Most cytoplasmic components show a pale, electron-lucent aspect but desmosomes maintain adherence of these reticulo-epithelial cells with others, without signs of degeneration ($\times$ 11 800).

In general, reptilian thymus observed during the winter is small, difficult to locate and profoundly involuted. It displays a poor cell architecture, so that cortical lymphocytes are few, but the medulla is partially depleted (Hussein *et al.*, 1978a in *Chalcides ocellatus*; Hussein *et al.*, 1978b in *Mabuya quinquetaeniata* and *Uromastyx aegyptia*; Hussein *et al.*, 1979a in *Spalerosophis diadema*; Hussein *et al.*, 1979b in *Scincus scincus*; El Ridi *et al.*, 1981 in *P. schokari*). Slight involution has also been described in the turtle *Mauremys caspica* (Leceta and Zapata, 1985; Leceta *et al.*, 1988). During other seasons, mainly in the summer, important species-specific differences have been observed in thymic morphology. Increased thymic lobes, containing tightly packed lymphocytes in the cortex and medulla, have been observed in several reptilian species examined during spring (Hussein *et al.*, 1978a, b, 1979a, b; El Ridi *et al.*, 1981).

At the beginning of spring, the thymic cortex of the turtle *Mauremys caspica* was reduced and pale, but no variations were found in the medulla (Leceta and Zapata, 1985). Morphometric analyses at this season showed a slight decrease in thymic size and the lowest lymphocytic density in the cortex (Leceta and Zapata, 1985), variations recently confirmed by electron microscopy (Leceta *et al.*, 1988). Ultrastructural analyses reveal that numerous reticuloepithelial cells which form the cortical thymic stroma show degenerative modifications, which exhibit an electron-lucent cytoplasm, tonofilaments and desmosomes (Figure 9.9). Reticuloepithelial cells in the medulla, however, showed an electron-dense cytoplasmic matrix without degenerative signs and with abundant electron-dense granules and vacuoles. Mature interdigitating cells were absent and only macrophages, monocytes and presumptive pro-interdigitating cells could be found during this season (Leceta *et al.*, 1984, 1988).

In this species, at the end of spring, the thymic cortex increased considerably, reaching then the highest proportions of thymic – somatic cell index, lymphocyte density and mitotic index in the cortical area, while the medulla remained pale, leaving the characteristic thymic demarcation between the two regions clear (Leceta and Zapata, 1985, 1986). A high phagocytic activity was associated with monocytes and macrophages; mature interdigitating cells were found in the cortex. The thymic parenchyma contained then

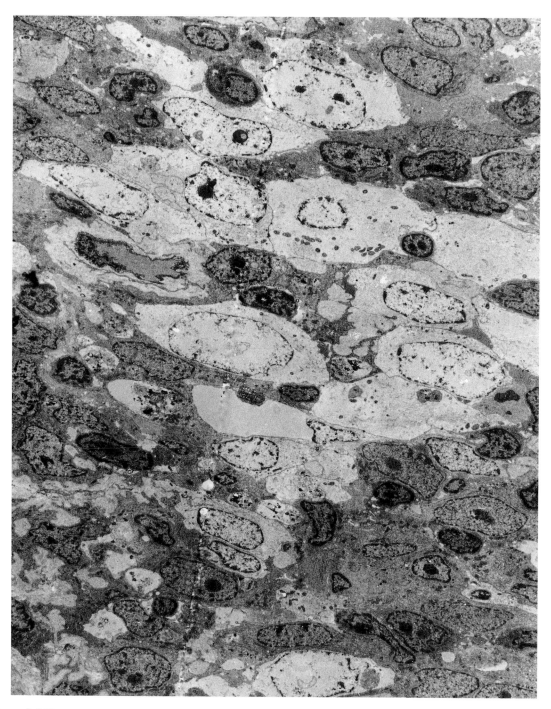

Figure 9.9 Numerous degenerated reticuloepithelial cells in the thymic cortex of a turtle, *Mauremys caspica*, during the mating period (April–May) (× 25 000).

substantial cell debris engulfed in the cytoplasm of these cells (Leceta *et al.*, 1984, 1988). A well-developed thymus with abundant thymocytes and clearly delimited cortex and medulla appear in lizards during summer (Hussein *et al.*, 1978a in *Chalcides ocellatus*; Hussein *et al.*, 1978b in *Mabuya quinquetaeniata* and *Uromastix aegyptia*; Hussein *et al.*, 1979b in *Scincus scincus*). In contrast, in the snake *Psammophis schokani* (El Ridi *et al.*, 1981) and the turtle *Mauremys caspica* (Leceta and Zapata, 1985) entirely involuted thymi have been found in summer (Figure 9.10).

Ultrastructural studies of non-lymphoid thymic components of *Mauremys caspica* in the summer revealed spindle-shaped or polygonal reticuloepithelial cells with an electron-dense cytoplasm containing few membranous organelles and electron-dense granules (Leceta *et al.*, 1988). Non-presumptive, pro-interdigitating cells, not mature interdigitating cells, were found and only occasionally were macrophages detected (Leceta *et al.*, 1988). An intermediate condition within thymic lobes decreased in size but numerous thymocytes exist in the snake *Spalerosophis diadema* (Hussein *et al.*, 1979a). With few quantitative variations, the thymi of all reptiles studied up to now contain a well-delimited cortex and medulla and moderate to rich lymphocyte numbers during autumn, gradually involuting thereafter (Hussein *et al.*, 1978a, b, 1979a, b; El Ridi *et al.*, 1981; Leceta and Zapata, 1985) (Figure 9.11).

Seasonal variations which affect splenic structure reflect those just described in the thymus. In the lizards *Chalcides ocellatus* (Hussein *et al.*, 1978a), *Mabuya quinquetaeniata*, *Uromastyx aegyptia* (Hussein *et al.*, 1978b) and *Scincus scincus* (Hussein *et al.*, 1979b) splenic lymphoid tissue is depleted in winter but extensively developed during warm months (spring and summer). In winter, the lizard white pulp is composed of few, small distinct lymphoid follicles which surround a central arteriole. They are formed by loosely aggregated lymphocytes, reticular cells and macrophages. In spring and summer, splenic lymphoid tissue becomes large, containing abundant lymphocytes that, in some cases, constitute a continuous phase throughout the splenic parenchyma. In these lizards, during autumn, although the amount of lymphoid tissue is generally less than in spring and summer, there still are lymphocytes distributed throughout the parenchyma. In snakes, conditions are somewhat different and

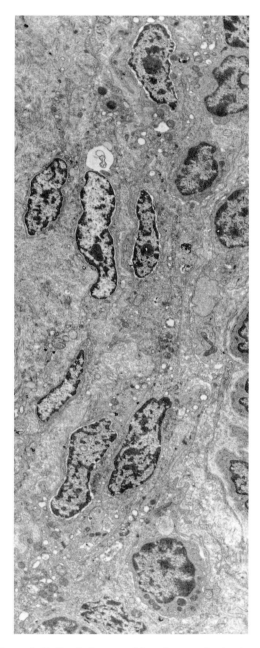

Figure 9.10 Total absence of lymphocytes in the thymic cortex of a turtle, *Mauremys caspica*, sacrificed during summer (× 4100).

splenic lymphoid tissue is scant (Hussein *et al.*, 1979a in *Spalerosophis diadema*) or not developed (El Ridi *et al.*, 1981 in *Psammophis schokari*) in both winter and summer. In contrast, during spring and autumn the

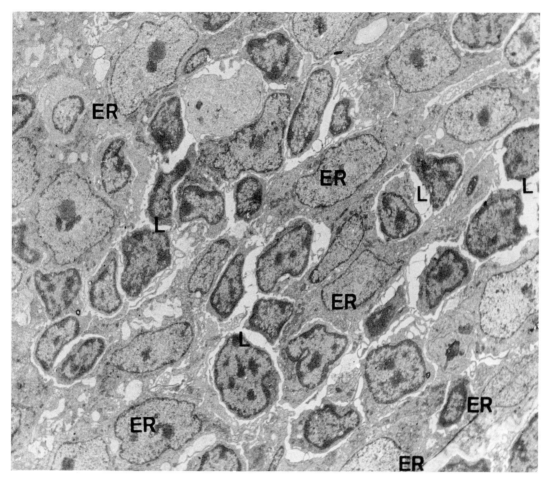

Figure 9.11 Condition of the thymic cortex in turtles during autumn, in contrast to the condition in spring and summer. Note the epithelial reticular cells (ER) and lymphocytes (L) (× 3500).

spleen is well developed and is rich in lymphoid components (Hussein *et al.*, 1979a; El Ridi *et al.*, 1981).

A more detailed description of seasonal histological changes in splenic lymphoid tissue has been achieved in the turtle *Mauremys caspica* (Leceta and Zapata, 1985). In summer, splenic white pulp only consists of small groups of loosely packed lymphocytes. The periellipsoidal lymphoid sheaths (PELS) show a narrow external zone and the periarterial lymphoid sheaths (PALS) possess many areas devoid of lymphocytes (Figure 9.12). Remarkably, involution of PALS during this period begins before that of PELS. During autumn, there is a gradual increase in splenic lymphoid

tissue and both PALS and PELS contain densely packed lymphocytes (Figure 9.13). Nevertheless, increases in the outer region of PELS are not clearly distinguishable until the end of the season. No further variations found during winter in the splenic white pulp were evident, but when spring begins, although there are no changes in size of either of the lymphoid sheaths (PALS and PELS), lymphocyte numbers decrease, mostly in the inner region of PELS, which then appear pale (Figure 9.14). At the end of spring there is a considerable increase in white pulp, especially in the outer region of PELS, where there are abundant lymphoid cells (Figure 9.15).

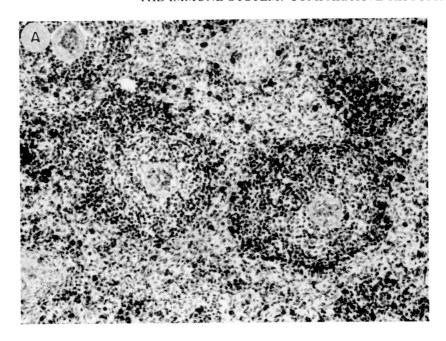

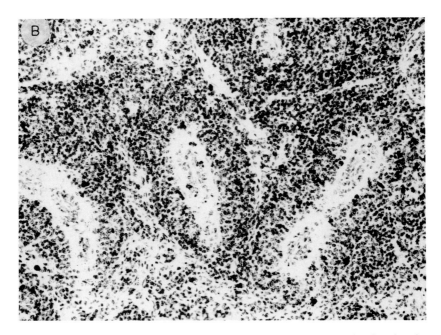

Figure 9.12 Small groups of loosely packed lymphocytes constitute the splenic white pulp of turtles observed in summer. The PALS (a) as well as the outer zone of the PELS (b) show many areas devoid of lymphocytes ($\times$ 100 (a), $\times$ 100 (b)).

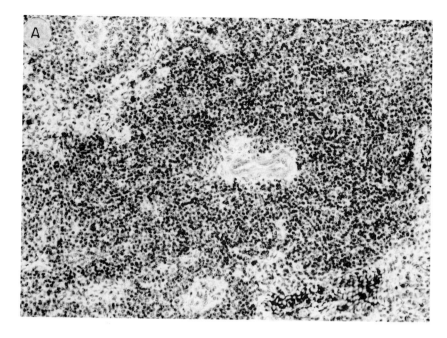

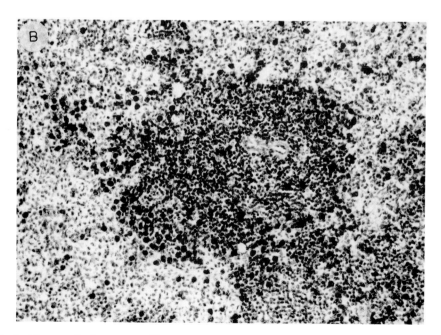

Figure 9.13 Gradual increase in the amount of lymphoid tissue in PALS (a) and PELS (b) of turtles, during autumn. Note that the recovery of the outer part of PELS is not fully complete (b) ($\times$ 110 (a), $\times$ 300 (b)).

Reptilian gut-associated lymphoid tissue (GALT) is the lymphoid mass which is least affected by seasonal variations. Conditions are extremely different among various species. For example, in most lizards, GALT is insensitive to seasonal changes except for slight variations found during summer (Hussein *et al.*, 1978a, b, 1979b). In *Mabuya quinquetaeniata*, rectal nodules decrease in number and size and those of the ileocecal and cloacal accumulations disappear during summer (Hussein *et al.*, 1978b), whereas in *Scincus scincus* they increase (Hussein *et al.*, 1979b). In *Uromastyx aegyptia*, the gut is devoid of lymphoid tissue during winter, except for numerous aggregates which occur in the cecum and appendix (Hussein *et al.*, 1978b). In spring, summer and autumn, numerous lymphoid accumulations appear mostly in the small and large intestines (Hussein *et al.*, 1978b). Finally in the snake *Spalerosophis diadema*, isolated gut-associated lymphoid aggregates are numerous during all seasons, but large patches in the small intestine abound in winter and autumn. They decrease in size and number during spring and summer (Hussein *et al.*, 1979a).

Although available data are restricted to a few species, we assume that season-dependent histological variations observed in the reptilian bone marrow are accompanied by changes in lymphocyte subpopulations. In general, as mentioned above for peripheral blood lymphocytes, seasonal variations in numbers of lymphocytes in central and peripheral lymphoid organs are correlated well with those of thymus-derived lymphocytes, but a small proportion of sIg-bearing lymphocytes survive in peripheral lymphoid compartments. In the lizard *Chalcides ocellatus* thymic cells decrease in viability at the beginning of autumn, which parallels a substantial drop in splenic thymus-derived (TA[+]) lymphocytes. No TA[+] lymphocytes are detected in the spleen during winter but a small proportion of sIg[-] bearing lymphocytes occur in the spleen and peripheral blood.

In spring, TA[+] cells reappear in peripheral lymphoid compartments and their number increases steadily to reach maximal levels by the end of spring (El Ridi and Kandil, 1981; Saad, 1985; Saad *et al.*, 1987; El Ridi *et al.*, 1988). Recent results on seasonal variations in the number of Thy-1-like[+] cells in adult *Chalcides ocellatus*, detected by a rabbit anti-lizard brain antiserum, confirm previous data (Saad *et al.*,

1988). Maximum levels of Thy-1-like[+] cells are observed in late spring through summer. Thereafter from early autumn there is a sharp decline in Thy-1-like[+] cells of the thymus, spleen and peripheral blood. Then, Thy-1-like[+] cells disappear completely as in the thymus and remain at low levels until spring, as in spleen and peripheral blood. Thy-1-like[+] cells in the bone marrow show little change throughout the year.

In the snakes *Spalerosophis diadema* and *Psammophis sibilans*, in spring, when lymphoid tissue peaks in lymphoid organs, TA[+] lymphocytes predominate, constituting 80% and 70% of peripheral blood and splenic lymphocytes, respectively (El Ridi *et al.*, 1988). Before the end of spring, lymphoid organs involute and the percentage of TA[+] cells drops in the periphery. By the beginning of summer, TA[+] lymphocytes are undetectable, but the splenic juxta-arteriolar areas contain a substantial number of sIg[+] lymphocytes. At the end of summer, as thymus and splenic lymphocytes regenerate, the number of TA[+] cells increases gradually in peripheral blood and spleen. Finally, at autumn's end, the thymus begins another cycle of involution, accompanied by loss of TA[+] cells and later of sIg[+] lymphocytes as well (El Ridi *et al.*, 1988).

Birds

Pheasants held in captivity undergo the most rapid body growth from 1½ to 5 months after birth, which correlates with important increases in thymus gland weights (Kirkpatrick, 1944). Thymic weights (higher in males than in females) reached maximum values at about 3½ months in August and September, a time when spermatogenic activity occurs. Wild pheasants caught throughout the year also showed maximum thymus weights in juveniles in the fall. The thymus then regresses through winter until the following June (Anderson, 1970). This period of regression included periods of pre-nesting activity and, for females, laying and incubating eggs. All birds collected during the postnuptial molt period had enlarged thymus glands whose mean weights approached those of juveniles collected in October (Anderson, 1970). Thymi from individual male mallards (*Anas platyrhinchus*) were tenfold larger from July to August than at other times (Hohn, 1947). Likewise, a marked enlargement of the thymus was recorded following the annual breeding

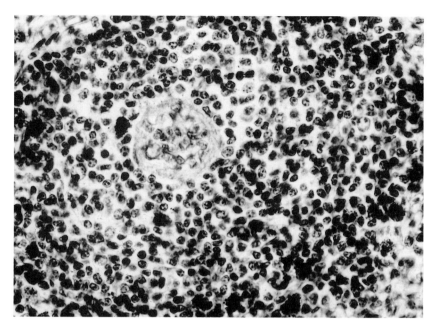

Figure 9.14 Decreased numbers of lymphocytes in the inner zone of the splenic PELS in turtles in early spring (× 200).

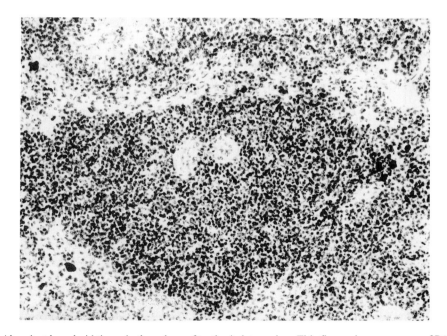

Figure 9.15 Abundant lymphoid tissue in the spleen of turtles in late spring. This figure shows a survey of PALS (× 110).

season in a variety of wild birds, e.g. mallards, robins (*Turdus migratorius*) and house sparrows (*Passer domesticus*) (Hohn, 1956).

Accompanying seasonal fluctuations in thymus weight and histological changes, a remarkable phenomenon, intrathymic erythropoiesis, has been established for a number of different avian species. Relationships between these changes and hormonal levels, mainly sex steroids and thyroxine, have also been claimed (see reviews by Kendall, 1980; Glick, 1984). Season-dependent intrathymic erythropoiesis has been reported in tropical (Kendall and Ward, 1974; Kendall, 1975a, b; Bacchus and Kendall, 1975; Ward and Kendall, 1975) and paleoarctic birds (Kendall and Frazier, 1979 in *Passer domesticus* and *Sturnus vulgaris*; Fonfria *et al.*, 1983 in *Sturnus unicolor*). Likewise, cyclic intrathymic erythropoiesis apparently occurs in rodents (Albert *et al.*, 1965a, b; Kendall, 1980) and humans (Albert *et al.*, 1966; Taylor and Skinner, 1976; Kendall and Singh, 1980) and it can be induced by artificial stimulation of hemorrhage (Kendall, 1978).

Intrathymic erythropoiesis is a cyclic phenomenon which coincides with stages in which blood demand is high, such as during molting and breeding (Kendall, 1980; Fonfria *et al.*, 1983). In the spotless starling, *Sturnus unicolor*, the thymus from hatching to the juvenile period is normal as revealed by active lymphopoiesis. In the post-juvenile molting as well as during mating periods of both sub-adults and adults of successive years, enlarged thymic lobules contain mature and developing erythroid cells in the cortical area. On the contrary, during both the sub-adult periods of the second year and adult molting, the thymus regresses, displaying involuting lobules which contain increased cortical pycnotic cells and epithelial cysts (Fonfria *et al.*, 1983). Furthermore intrathymic erythropoiesis accompanies degeneration in the thymus of *Sturnus unicolor* (Fonfria *et al.*, 1983). These degenerated cells, which are reminiscent of those which have just been described in the thymus of turtles (*Mauremys caspica*) observed in the spring, had abundant tonofilaments and were joined with the neighboring cells by desmosomes, which confirms their epithelial characteristics.

The spleen undergoes substantial variations in size and structure in relationship to the reproductive cycle in the pied flycatcher, *Ficedula hypoleuca*, a small insectivorous passeriform, migratory bird (Silverin, 1981; Fange and Silverin, 1985). In both sexes the spleen has a minimal size in spring, reaching its maximal weight during the egg-laying, incubation and nestling periods. The small spleen of birds examined in spring is quite compact, containing poorly developed red pulp and lymphoid tissue with little or no lymphoid follicles. During the nest-building period, red pulp and splenic lymphoid follicles increase, and at the egg-laying, incubation and nesting periods numerous well-developed lymphoid follicles occur in the parenchyma (Fange and Silverin, 1985). Statistical evaluation shows, additionally, that the number and diameter of follicles per section, and the number of mitoses per follicle in birds examined during the incubation or the nestling periods, are significantly higher than the corresponding data from migrating birds during spring. The red pulp reaches its maximal volume during the incubation period but tends to diminish slightly during the nestling period; individual variations are substantial (Fange and Silverin, 1985). Ultrastructural evidence which supports the observed seasonal changes in histology and cell components, mainly macrophages of the avian splenic lymphoid tissue, probably correlates with the erythropoietic activity, and has also been observed in *Sturnus unicolor* (Fonfria, personal communication).

Mammals

Herein we divert attention away from ectotherms and birds and compare examples of seasonal variations in the immune system of certain mammals, mainly as they relate to hibernation. For during this period in hibernators, their condition mimics in some respects the ectotherm condition. Morphophysiological studies have revealed that the thymus, lymph nodes, spleen and GALT of some mammalian hibernators undergo marked seasonal involution (Alekseeva and Yunker, 1973, 1977; Cirri-Borghi and Arbi-Riccardi, 1961; Fichtelius and Jaroslow, 1969; Shivatcheva *et al.*, 1980; Shivatcheva and Hadjioloff, 1978a, b). Changes in immature European ground squirrels begin in the thymus during early summer and end in the lymph nodes and spleen in autumn (Shivatcheva *et al.*, 1980; Shivatcheva and Hadjioloff, 1978a). Thymic involution persists during the entire hibernating period, whereas involution of other lymphoid organs is limited to the first phase of hibernation (Shivatcheva *et al.*, 1980; Shivatcheva and Hadjioloff, 1987a). GALT also undergoes important seasonal variations whose general features are better expressed in lymphoid tissues of the submucosa where they are concentrated than in the mucosa. In the submucosa, there is a gradual disappearance of cell proliferation in autumn, prior to hibernation, its nearly full arrest during the first half of hibernation and its activation during the second half (Shivatcheva and Hadjioloff, 1987b). Fichtelius and Jaroslow (1969) reported that the very thin intestinal epithelium of hibernating ground squirrels contained many more lymphocytes in winter than that of non-hibernating ones in summer.

Seasonal variations in the thymus of marmots have also been observed (Galletti and Cavallari, 1972). During summer, a richly lymphoid thymus gland is clearly divided into a cortex and a medulla. At the end of September (beginning of autumn) thymic volume decreases, the cortical−medullary demarcation is difficult to discern and numbers of thymocytes are scant. In winter, the thymus in hibernating marmots is reduced to scant rows of epithelial cells and a few Hassall's corpuscles embedded in brown fat. Marmots kept active during hibernation show decreased glands with respect to size but they still have a few lymphocytes which are reminiscent of past activity. The thymus increases again in the spring around the month of May, reaching the histological condition characteristic of summer (Galletti and Cavallari, 1972).

SEASONAL INFLUENCES ON THE IMMUNE REACTIVITIES OF ECTOTHERMIC VERTEBRATES

Introduction

Together with the season-dependent morphological alterations of lymphoid organs, changes occur in immune reactivity of ectothermic vertebrates. Information, however, is scarce and refers exclusively to a few species, mainly reptiles. Actually a systematic study in seasonal cyclicity of humoral and cell-mediated immune reactivity has been observed only in lizards and snakes (Muthukkaruppan *et al.*, 1982; El Ridi *et al.*, 1988).

Fish

With respect to fish and seasons, the summer months are crucial. Russell *et al.* (1976) reported that circulating bacteriophage was more rapidly cleared from nurse sharks in summer than in winter. For an interpretation of these results, the enhancing effect of antibodies elicited at higher temperatures might be important since MacArthur *et al.* (1983) found no significant difference in the rates at which abiotic particles were cleared from plaice acclimated at 5, 12 and 19 °C. Sypek and Burreson (1983) observed contrasting effects, i.e. active phagocytosis of *Trypanoplasma bullocki* in summer flounders, *Paralichthys dentatus*, at 5 °C but without lytic activity in the plasma. Circulating levels of lysozyme (Fletcher and White, 1976), total protein concentration and C-reactive protein (White *et al.*, 1983) in plaice are highest in late summer and also following their active feeding period from March to October (White and Fletcher, 1985).

Even when environmental temperature is held constant, seasonal variations occur in fish humoral immune responses. When antigenic stimulation was performed prior to spring, antibody levels, including bacteriostatic and agglutinating values, tested in *Salmo gairdneri* against formalinized *Aeromonas salmonicida*, were higher than those induced in autumn (Yamaguchi *et al.*, 1981). Prior to winter, however, antibody levels were lower than those from fish immunized prior to spring (Yamaguchi *et al.*, 1981). Agglutinating activity in fish immunized prior to winter appeared first, followed by bacteriostatic activity. Annual variations in the expression of circulating antibodies have also been observed in plaice infected with a digenean parasite (Cottrell, 1977). In this case the antibody concentration peaked in October.

Amphibians

Cyclicity of humoral responses has also been recorded in toads, *Bufo marinus* (Azzolina, 1976) and *Bufo regularis* (Hussein *et al.*, 1984b). The humoral response against a single injection of heterologous erythrocytes is strong during winter but it reaches maximum levels at 49 days post-immunization (Hussein *et al.*, 1984b). In spring, the response is also vigorous and it is accompanied by peak hemagglutinating levels 28 days after injection. In contrast, humoral reactivity is relatively poor during summer and autumn (Hussein *et al.*, 1984b).

Reptiles

Seasonal changes affecting cell viability, antibody titers, numbers of plaque-forming cells (PFCs) and rosette-forming cells (RFCs) have been observed in lizards, snakes (Muthukkaruppan *et al.*, 1982; El Ridi *et al.*, 1988) and turtles (Leceta and Zapata, 1986). In winter, lizards and snakes fail to produce antibodies against T-dependent soluble (human serum albumin (HSA)) or particulate (polyvinylpyrrolidone (PVP)) antigens. Antigen binding and recognition are apparently unaffected but B-lymphocyte proliferation and differentiation are inhibited (Badir and Abdel Khader, 1981). Inhibition did not appear to be due to inherent inability of B-lymphocytes to synthesize or release Ig because a strong anamnestic response could be induced in winter lizards immunized primarily during the optimal season (cited by El Ridi *et al.*, 1988). Splenocytes from winter lizards and snakes cultured *in vitro* with rat erythrocytes (RRBC) under optimal conditions failed to produce antibodies (Saad, 1985; Saad *et al.*, 1987; El Ridi *et al.*, 1988). This failure at antibody production suggests a lack of either T-cells or T-cell-derived lymphokines in winter reptiles. The snake *Psammophis sibilans*, which lacks a summer response to either HSA or RRBC, does produce, however, antibodies against PVP, which supports the view that suppression in summer snakes is not as complete as during winter (El Ridi *et al.*, 1981).

Similar suppression has also been observed in the turtle, *Mauremys caspica*, by Leceta and Zapata (1986), who studied differences in humoral responses against SRBC in summer- and autumn-acclimated lizards. Antibody titers in turtles acclimated during the summer were always below control levels during the primary response, but the secondary response was more vigorous. However, when we consider antibody responses during the summer together with results showing a significant reduction in numbers of PFCs in spleens compared with autumn-conditioned turtles, we suggest an extrasplenic source of antibody-forming cells during secondary responses in summer turtles. Perhaps GALT and bone marrow were important

sources of cells that effected the humoral responses. High titers of agglutinating antibodies are produced, however, during the memory response in summer without regenerating splenic lymphoid tissue, which indicates that splenic involution does not impair a memory response during the summer. Regulation of immune responses during the summer may therefore be attributed to a differential selective effect of seasonal conditions on lymphoid cells and organs and on different phases of the immune response.

With respect to cell-mediated immunity as measured by allograft rejection, the results of various experiments seem equivocal; other factors may be involved. Skin allotransplants in the lizard *Chalcides ocellatus* are tolerated in winter, slowly rejected in mid-June but hardly rejected in summer (Saad and El Ridi, 1984). In another report Worley and Jurd (1979) observed substantial differences in skin allograft survival times in the lizard *Lacerta viridis* maintained in the laboratory when compared to those held in an outdoor environment. Even though the diet, temperature and photoperiod were nearly identical, allograft rejection was quite slow indoors (220−320 days) but much faster (32−64 days) in a more natural, outdoor condition. These variable results support the proposal that adverse environmental and seasonal conditions cause skin allograft rejection to be typically chronic in reptiles, and during extreme conditions allografts are even tolerated (El Ridi *et al.*, 1988).

At the cellular level, which reflects *in vivo* graft rejection patterns, results are also mixed. The proliferative response of lizard (*Chalcides ocellatus*) splenocytes in the one- and two-way mixed leukocyte reaction (MLR) was remarkably vigorous in August through September (Saad and El Ridi, 1984). In contrast, strong reactivity of snake (*Psammophis sibilans*) spleen cells in MLR was observed only in some months of spring and autumn but disappeared in summer and winter (Farag and El Ridi, 1985). Likewise, proliferative responsiveness to Con A is season dependent (Farag and El Ridi, 1986; Saad *et al.*, 1987). In the snake *Spalerosophis diadema*, the response of thymocytes and splenocytes to Con A is highly significant in spring and autumn but impaired during summer and winter (El Ridi *et al.*, 1987).

El Ridi and her colleagues demonstrated that a failure of snake lymphocytes to respond to Con A in winter and in summer may be due to their inability to produce significant amounts of IL-2-like lymphokine (El Ridi *et al.*, 1987). Thus, supernatants from Con A-stimulated cell cultures set up during the spring could restore proliferative responses of either winter or summer Con A-containing splenocytes. This suggests that IL-2-like responsive lymphocytes may persist, while those cells synthesizing this lymphokine or the ability to generate it are absent during adverse seasonal conditions (El Ridi *et al.*, 1987). Taken together, these results seem to indicate that reptiles possess strong cell-mediated immune responses and perhaps an MHC which controls it, but seasonal influences strongly limit their real immune capacities.

CAUSATIVE AGENTS OF SEASONAL MODIFICATIONS OF THE IMMUNE SYSTEM

Introduction

Causative agents which have been proposed to explain season-dependent changes in ectothermic immune systems may be classified into two large groups. First, some workers suggest a direct influence of environmental parameters, basically temperature and photoperiod, on immune reactivity. In contrast, other evidence supports the existence of endogenous rhythms, influenced by environmental variations, which govern the ectothermic immune system. In this last group, attention has been focused primarily on the role played by hormones, mainly sex and non-sexual steroids and thyroxine, on the immune responses. Second, other factors, such as the nutritional stage, healthy conditions of animal housing, stress, pollution, etc., are obviously important parameters affecting seasonal variations in ectothermic immune systems.

Environmental Agents

Light and Temperature

The role of temperature in regulating ectothermic immune responses has been analyzed mostly in fish. In amphibians, immune responses have been compared between hibernating and non-hibernating species (Wright and Cooper, 1980, 1981). Only indirect correlations between changes in immune systems and temperature have been established in reptiles (El Deeb *et al.*, 1980) and we urge the importance of considering those differences obtained from results between *in vivo* and *in vitro* experiments. While it is evident that there is a temperature dependence of *in vitro* assays when using poikilothermic cells, *in vivo* tests emphasize the process of acclimation where endogenous rhythms may be the decisive, controlling factors. Except for information derived from teleosts, mechanisms involved in a presumptive direct influence of temperature on immune responses are little understood. There is a need for more controlled experimental conditions which coordinate light, temperature, season, age and sex when studying immunity.

As early as the 1930s, Nybelin (1935) reported that the immune response is temperature sensitive in ectotherms. At low temperatures, other investigators, some 30 years later, found a reduction in antibody titers (Ambrosius and Shaker, 1964; Cone and Marchalonis, 1972; Paterson and Fryer, 1974; Stolen *et al.*, 1982), still others complete suppression (Barrow, 1955; Fijan and Cvetnic, 1966; Avtalion, 1969; Avtalion *et al.*, 1970), and yet another group only a delay in onset of responses, with or without suppression (Cushing, 1942; Ridgway, 1962; Tait, 1969; Diener and Marchalonis, 1970; Harris, 1973; Rijkers *et al.*, 1980). Adult lampreys, *Petromyzon marinus*, kept at 17 °C, produce detectable anti-O-RBC antibodies earlier and faster than those kept at 9 °C. With time, however, lampreys kept at 9 °C eventually produced peak titers comparable to those observed earlier at 17 °C (Hagen *et al.*, 1985). In general, each species has its own temperature range in which metabolic and physiological processes can normally operate. These thermal tolerance ranges differ considerably from species to species, reflecting individual ecological habitats. Thus, Wright and Cooper (1981) concluded that primary responses of most teleost fish and tropical amphibians and reptiles are temperature dependent, whereas secondary responses are temperature independent within the thermal tolerance range of each species.

There are discrepancies, however, in the immune processes in ectotherms which are sensitive to temperature. Some 40 years ago, Bisset (1948) found that antibody synthesis and its release in ectotherms were affected by temperature. And some 20 years ago,

Avtalion (1969), by contrast, showed that both antibody synthesis and release could occur at low temperature (12 °C) if fish were kept at a high temperature (25 °C) during the latent period of an immune response. To begin with, the processing of antigens by macrophages seems to be affected by temperature. This prompted Avtalion (1981) to suggest that the temperature-sensitive steps in humoral immune responses are probably related to antigen processing by macrophages or to other cell interactions. In contrast, MacArthur et al. (1983) reported that rate of removal of carbon and ^{51}Cr-labeled TRBC (turbot red blood cells) from blood circulation in plaice is not affected significantly within the range of $5-19$ °C. This supports an opposite view that the initial recognition and phagocytosis of antigen is relatively temperature insensitive. Moving a step further in the immune response, by contrast, the anamnestic character of certain fish secondary responses is apparently lost at lower temperatures (Rijkers et al., 1980, 1981b; Stolen et al., 1984). To further support this view, however, Hagen et al. (1985) indicate that lampreys kept at both 9 °C and 17 °C can elaborate a secondary response to antigenic stimulation.

Mechanisms which are responsible for immunosuppressive effects observed at low environmental temperatures in fish are poorly understood. Based upon indirect results from in vivo experiments, the temperature-sensitive step may involve inhibition of carrier-specific helper cells (Avtalion, 1981). Low in vitro temperatures suppress mitogenic responses of T-, but not B-cells in the bluegill, Lepomis macrochirus (Cuchens and Clem, 1977) and in channel catfish (Ictalurus punctatus) leukocytes (Faulmann et al. 1983; Clem et al., 1984), as well as the primary in vitro antibody responses by channel catfish peripheral blood leukocytes to thymus-dependent but not thymus-independent antigens (Miller and Clem, 1984). Apparently low environmental temperatures exert differential inhibitory effects on fish T-cells rather than B-cells (Bly et al., 1986). Two different approaches have been used to better define the precise points where inhibition may originate.

Abbrizzini et al. (1982) found that the in vivo acclimation temperature influences physical properties (i.e. homeoviscosity, fluidity) of lymphocyte plasma membranes in the marine pinfish, Lagadon rhomboides, and of lymphocyte responses to mitogenic stimulation at a given in vitro temperature. It was concluded that the process of homeoviscous adaptation may be an important regulatory factor in immunity. Later, in order to explain this property, Bly et al. (1986) did a comparative analysis of the fatty acid composition of T- and B-cells in channel catfish acclimated to different in vivo temperatures. Channel catfish B- and T-lymphocytes, as well as thrombocytes and erythrocytes, respond to acclimation to lower in vivo temperatures. They will exhibit increases in the levels of unsaturated fatty acids in the phospholipids of these cells with no observed significant differences between T- and B-lymphocytes (Bly et al., 1986).

More recent results indicate that catfish T-cells are more sensitive to the stimulatory effects of exogenous oleic acid but less able to desaturate stearic acid than B-cells (Bly et al., 1988). In any case, actual measurements of the relative fluidities of T- and B-cells are necessary to confirm the suggested differences between both catfish lymphocyte subsets. Recently Bly and her colleagues summarized more extensive results, concluding that low temperature acts to suppress channel catfish primary T-cells but not memory T-cells, B-cells or functions of accessory cells (Bly et al., 1988). Moreover, it appears that the low temperature-sensitive block involves an early step in T-cell activation, although it cannot be attributed to a failure of T-cells to bind or cap ligands or to undergo the plasma membrane modifications necessary for homeoviscous adaptation (Bly et al., 1988). However, to extrapolate these in vitro results to natural conditions it is necessary and important to mention that, in commercial channel catfish ponds, great temperature fluctuations during the spring and autumn months are common (cited by Bly et al., 1987). Such abrupt temperature fluctuations can be expected to result in homeoviscous adaptation and to explain, at least partially, certain seasonally impaired immune responsiveness.

Indirect approaches to the role played by photoperiod in seasonal variations of the ectothermic immune system have been mainly observed in fish, although results are not yet conclusive. Honma and Tamura observed a remarkable coincidence in the cyclic pattern of thymic activity in several teleosts during the annual fluctuation of day length in the Niigata district of Japan (Tamura and Honma, 1974, 1975, 1977; Tamura, 1978). For example, medaka and flat-head goby subjected to complete darkness during June through July show thymic involution which has been observed one month later. In contrast, if fish were confined earlier in April, this caused a gradual increase in thymic volume (Honma and Tamura, 1984). When medaka held under dark conditions were then returned to a normal photoperiod, recovery of thymic volume was found about one month later (Tamura, 1978). A remarkable degeneration of the thymus was also described in the Mexican characin, *Astyanax mexicanus*, kept in dark conditions for one year or more (Rasquin and Rosenbloom, 1954).

Thymic regression followed by its final disappearance can occur in *Plecoglossus altivelis* one or two months earlier in fish if they have been maintained on a short photoperiod (8 L vs 16 D) than in those fish kept on a long photoperiod (16 L vs 8 D) (Honma and Tamura, 1972). The two environmental influences, i.e. temperature and light, do not act alone, thus combined influence of photoperiod and temperature has also been analyzed. Medaka, which display an inactive thymus in winter, undergo a remarkable thymic hyperplasia if they are subjected to a high temperature (25 °C) (Tamura, 1978). In contrast, by combining a high temperature with a long photoperiod one can induce a more effective recovery of the thymus gland (Tamura, 1978). With respect to the immune response, at least one parameter is affected by light. Nakanishi (1986) found a slight elevation in antibody titers in adult rock-fish (*Sebasticus marmuratus*) of both sexes after exposure to a long photoperiod; there was no effect in young adults.

With respect to light and an internal source of regulation, namely the pineal gland, fish and amphibians have been used. Although preliminary, results in frogs (*Rana perezi*) held in complete darkness revealed degenerative areas in the thymus after 7 days; splenic T-dependent areas which surround arterial vessels appear remarkably depleted of lymphocytes at 35 and 42 days (Zapata *et al.*, 1983). Direct effects of light on the immune system are difficult to evaluate and are generally dismissed by most workers who claim, instead, that there is an indirect role of photoperiod on the immune system which is mediated through gonads and/or the pineal gland. A series of experiments using eyeless and pinealectomized medaka, *Oryzias latipes*, supports this hypothesis (Tamura, 1978). In rats, pinealectomy provoked involution of thymic lympho-

cytes but increased epithelial cell numbers and the amount of connective tissue (Csaba and Barath, 1975). At best, these results are preliminary and caution must be taken in interpreting them for the following reasons. Evidence suggests that surgical pinealectomy does not lead to a complete abrogation of levels of melatonin, the principal biologically active mediator together with serotonin of the pineal system. Furthermore, other organs, including the retina and intestine, are also able to produce and release these hormones under similar conditions (discussed by Maestroni and Pierpaoli, 1981). Obviously more controls and extended experimentation are necessary to arrive at more acceptable conclusions.

Endogenous Rhythms

Despite the evident influence of temperature in ectotherm immune responses, data confirm that even at both a constant photoperiod and temperature the immune system undergoes important variations which suggest that endogenous parameters are also playing an influencing role in immune reactions (Yamaguchi *et al.*, 1981; Zapata *et al.*, 1983; Leceta and Zapata, 1986; Nakanishi, 1986). Although a global review of relationships between the neuroendocrine and immune systems escapes the scope of this book, emerging evidence, even in ectotherms, confirms a mutual regulation between both of these homeostatic systems. Thus, we will review existing data on distinct ectothermic classes where regulatory influences of several hormonal systems, including steroids, thyroid hormones and catecholamines have been uncovered. In addition there are other conditions or agents, such as antibiotics, nutrition, pollution or stressors, which probably also modify these immune responses through the neuroendocrine system.

Corticosteroids

Introduction

A role played by corticosteroids in the seasonal modifications of ectotherm immune systems was first claimed by having established correlations between fluctuations in levels of circulating corticosteroids and seasonal immunoreactivity. For immune reactivity, in general, various parameters have been measured which include numbers of peripheral lymphocytes, cellularity of primary and secondary lymphoid organs, humoral and cell-mediated immune responses in fish (Pickering, 1984; Maule *et al.*, 1987), amphibians (Highet and Ruben, 1987) and reptiles (Saad and El Ridi, 1984; Saad *et al.*, 1984, 1987; Saad, 1988; Leceta and Zapata, 1985). These broad categories of changes in immune reactivity will be dealt with in succeeding paragraphs.

Immune Functions and Physiological Variables in Fish

Immune functions and physiological variables in fish that cause alterations in immune functions of salmonids include their inability to generate primary immune responses to *Vibrio anguillarum*. In addition, workers have observed a reduction in relative numbers of splenic lymphocytes and circulating leukocytes during smoltification. These observations seem to be associated with levels of plasma cortisol, but not with changes in gill Na^+, K^+-ATPase activity or plasma T_4 levels, or other physiological variables which measure indices of smoltification (Maule *et al.*, 1987).

Tolerance in Amphibians

In anuran amphibians, the immunotolerant stage observed during metamorphosis has also accounted for increased levels of endogenous corticosteroids during this dramatic transitional period (Highet and Ruben, 1987; Marx *et al.*, 1987). Furthermore, Marx *et al.* (1987) corroborated that this high serum corticosteroid titer is accompanied by a tenfold increase in binding capacity, by metamorphic spleen lymphocytes of radiolabeled dexamethasone, a synthetic corticoid. A fivefold increase in binding occurred in metamorphic larval thymocytes. In contrast cells of pre-metamorphic larvae did not bind this radiolabeled reagent.

Seasonal Variations Correlate with Corticosteroids in Reptiles

Seasonal variations in the immune system of the lizard *Chalcides ocellatus* correlate well with annual variations of circulating glucocorticoids as determined by radioimmunoassay (Saad *et al.*, 1984). Fully developed lymphoid organs and strong immune responses coincide with sustained low levels of serum corticosteroids, which are found in spring through early autumn (Saad *et al.*, 1987). Increase of endogenous corticosteroid levels in October is associated with lysis of most thymocytes, 30–50% of T- and B-lymphocytes in peripheral blood and spleen, impairment of lymphoproliferation to Con A and primary antibody production *in vitro*. High corticosteroid levels persist until January, and coincide with a gradual depletion of the remaining T-lymphocytes and most B-lymphocytes (Saad *et al.*, 1987).

In the turtle *Mauremys caspica*, similar results have been reported (Leceta and Zapata, 1985). The profound involution of thymic and splenic lymphoid tissue during summer thus coincided with high levels of circulating corticosterone, whereas a moderate decrease in lymphoid tissue was difficult to relate with high levels of circulating steroids during the winter (Leceta and Zapata, 1985). Despite this *in vivo* evidence, available information on the effects of corticosteroids on the immune system of ectotherms is sparse and frequently contradictory. The cells directly involved and their underlying mechanisms are also little known.

Deranged Lymphocyte Function After Corticosteriod Treatment in Ectotherms

Marked lymphopenia after corticosteroid treatment has been reported repeatedly in fish (McLeay, 1973b; Johansson-Sjobeck *et al.*, 1978; Anderson *et al.*, 1982; Pickering, 1984; Maule *et al.*, 1987), amphibians (Bennett and Marbottle, 1968; Bennett *et al.*, 1972) and reptiles (Saad *et al.*, 1984; Garrido *et al.*, 1987). Yet Pickering and Pottinger (1985) found no effect of cortisol on numbers of circulating white blood cells in teleosts, and Pickford *et al.* (1971) and Ball and Hawkins (1976) found evidence for corticosteroid-induced leukocytosis. Furthermore, no significant decrease in the number of circulating small lymphocytes was observed in *Rana pipiens* after six weeks of continuous treatment (Rollins and McKinnell, 1980). Slicher (1961) found that in *Fundulus heteroclitus* cortisol caused either lymphopenia or lymphocytosis.

Stress in Fish

Evidence from studies on fish suggests that prolonged

stress or chronic elevation of corticosteroid levels causes lymphocyte depletion from all major lymphoid organs (Rasquin and Rosenbloom, 1954; Robertson *et al.*, 1963; McLeay, 1973a, b; Chilmonczyk, 1982), although differences in magnitude of this response in the various tissues are likely. Although the thymus in general has been claimed as the main lymphoid target for corticosteroids, Chilmonczyk (1982) found earlier modifications in the spleen than in the thymus of *Salmo gairdneri*, and the response observed in thymus of *Astyanax mexicanus* following acute manipulations of the pituitary interrenal system was less severe than in kidneys and spleen (Rasquin, 1951). Similar rapid responses in the kidney and spleen of the perch, *Perca fluviatilis*, were observed after acute stress (Weatherley, 1963), although Tripp *et al.* (1987) demonstrated recently that lymphocytes from the salmonid pronephros possess a different pattern of sensitivity to cortisol from lymphocytes from the spleen.

Lymphopenia After Corticosteroid Treatment in Ectotherms

Corticosteroid administration in *Ambystoma mexicanum* results in a profound lymphopenia of all thymic and splenic lymphocyte populations, with a selectively greater depletion of thymocytes (83%) as compared with splenocytes (50%). This same degree of maximal lymphocytopenia has been observed in young and adult axolotls (Tournefier, 1982). The thymus was the most sensitive organ, although maximum lymphopenia was reached much later than in mammals. This suggests a slow rate of mitosis in axolotls. In *Rana perezi*, dexamethasone treatment induces important morphological changes in lymphoid organs. This consists of thymic involution with abundant lymphocytic pycnosis in the cortex, a reduction in thymic medulla volume, slight lymphopenia in the spleen and possible redistribution of lymphoid elements to bone marrow from peripheral blood and spleen (Garrido *et al.*, 1987). In the lizard, *Chalcides ocellatus*, considerable lymphoid cell destruction has been observed after hydrocortisone administration (Saad *et al.*, 1984). In this instance the majority of thymocytes are killed, whereas bone marrow lymphocytes seem to be resistant by comparison and spleen contains sensitive and resistant populations (Saad *et al.*, 1984).

Injections of cortisol markedly affect cell accumulation in response to glycogen (MacArthur *et al.*, 1984). A threefold increase in circulating cortisol levels was sufficient to cause an anti-inflammatory effect in plaice, *Pleuronectes platessa* (MacArthur *et al.*, 1984). In contrast, hydrocortisone can inhibit the *in vitro* chemoluminescence response which is a measure of respiratory burst and microbicidal activity of striped bass phagocytes (Stave and Roberson, 1985).

In general, humoral immune responses, as measured by numbers of antibody-producing cells and circulating antibody titers, are abrogated by corticosteroid treatment of fish (Anderson *et al.*, 1982; Maule *et al.*, 1987; Tripp *et al.*, 1987), amphibians (Tournefier, 1982) and reptiles (Saad *et al.*, 1984). Only a slight decrease in counts of antigen-binding cells after immunization with SRBC has been reported in urodeles (Ruben and Gwinnell, 1977) and anurans (Ruben and Vaughan, 1974) following hydrocortisone injections. In fish, however, differential effects of cortisol on T-dependent antigens have been observed (Thomas and Lewis, 1987). Cortisol has been shown to induce suppressive effects on hemagglutinating activity to bovine erythrocytes and the development of precipitins against BSA, but no effects were found on the response to *E. coli* OX-174 bacteriophage (Thomas and Lewis, 1987).

The timing of cortisol administration in relation to antigenic challenge is also crucial. In axolotls, for example, hydrocortisone administration did not depress antibody synthesis once it has been initiated. If the injection of hydrocortisone was given eight days before or on the same day as the HRBC injection, the response was remarkably enhanced (Tournefier, 1982). This enhancement may account for the inhibition by hydrocortisone of a suppressive activity usually reported in axolotls or the stimulation of maturation by hydrocortisone of an immature and restricted helper cell population. These hypotheses are obviously not mutually exclusive. In this regard, corticosteroid-dependent inhibition of a T-like suppressor activity has also been reported in *Cyprinus carpio* following cortisol injection (Ruglys, 1985), and an immature population of thymocytes increased markedly after hydrocortisone injections in *Chalcides ocellatus* (Saad *et al.*, 1987). The question of lymphoid cell populations as they relate directly to corticosteroid inhibition will be presented later.

Corticosteroids abrogate the mitogen-stimulated lymphoid proliferation (Grimm, 1985 in *Pleuronectes platessa*; Ellsaesser and Clem, 1987 in *Ictalurus punctatus*; Maule *et al.*, 1987 in *Oncorhynchus kisutch*; Ruben *et al.*, 1985 in metamorphosing *Xenopus laevis*; Highet and Ruben, 1987; Rollins and McKinnell, 1980 in *Rana pipiens*). Likewise, injections of hydrocortisone in the lizard *Chalcides ocellatus* cause a severe impairment of proliferative responses to alloantigens in mixed lymphocyte reactions (MLR) (Saad *et al.*, 1984). A delay in skin allograft rejection also occurred after hydrocortisone injections (Saad *et al.*, 1984) but Tournefier (1982) found no effects of hydrocortisone treatment on allograft rejection in the axolotl; this contrasts with the reported failure of adult thymectomy to impair rejection capacity in urodeles (Fache and Charlemagne, 1975).

Two possible physiological mechanisms, not mutually exclusive, i.e. redistribution of lymphocytes within the lymphoid organs or cytolytic responses, have been offered as explanations for the *in vivo* and *in vitro* effects of corticosteroids on ectothermic vertebrate immune systems. Garrido *et al.* (1987) reported pycnosis of thymic cells but redistribution of lymphocytes from peripheral blood and spleen to bone marrow in dexamethasone-treated frogs. Other workers, in contrast, have suggested that steroids act directly on sensitive cells within various lymphoid organs (Chilmonczyk, 1982). Hydrocortisone-induced depletion of lymphoid elements in *Chalcides ocellatus* has also been explained by direct evidence of cytolytic effects on substantial fractions of both T- and B-cells, without excluding the possibility of lymphocyte redistribution to spleen and bone marrow (Saad *et al.*, 1984).

In any case, the type of corticosteroid doses with respect to duration and season of exposure are essential in defining the response of vertebrate lymphocytes to steroids. Differential sensitivity to distinct corticosteroid has been reported in fish. For example, Ghoneum *et al.* (1986) observed profound alterations in thymic organization of fish treated with deoxycortisone acetate. In contrast, cortisone acetate produced no significant alterations even at higher concentrations and during long periods. Recent results, on the other hand, suggest that the severity of morphological changes induced by dexamethasone treatment of frogs

is seasonally dependent (Garrido *et al.*, 1988). The *in situ* death of cortical thymocytes is quicker and stronger in November than in February. Instances of smaller numbers of pycnotic lymphocytes were observed during later, winter periods.

Two explanations, which are not mutually exclusive, have been proposed in explaining these results: (1) the number of dexamethasone-sensitive resistant lymphocytes differs in lymphoid organs of *Rana perezi* in November and February; and (2) the effects of dexamethasone are modulated differentially by other hormones during both seasons. Moreover, the qualitative effects of dexamethasone treatment on splenic lymphoid populations appear similar in both periods, which may be related mainly to lymphocyte mobilization to other sites. The levels of redistribution, however, seem to be different in February and November, and again sex hormones may be important in understanding the differences (Garrido *et al.*, 1988). In supporting this view, certain earlier observations seem pertinent. Pickford *et al.* (1971) showed that the hematological response to cortisol was dependent on the degree of sexual maturation. Leukocytosis occurred in sexually mature or hypophysectomized fish, whereas leukopenia developed in sexually regressed, intact fish.

Target lymphoid cells for corticosteroids are a matter of discussion. Rollins and McKinnell (1980) suggested that both T-cell and B-cell responses to mitogens can be inhibited by corticosteroids in *Rana pipiens*. In *Rana perezi* both thymic cortex and medulla are corticosensitive. According to one view, immature cortical cells may be more sensitive, being destroyed by dexamethasone, while the mature populations of the thymic medulla are less affected, undergoing no lysis, but they may be redistributed to other sites (Garrido *et al.*, 1987). Ghoneum *et al.* (1986) also described differential sensitivity to corticosteroid treatment in various zones of the teleost thymus. Furthermore, Ellsaesser and Clem (1987) have suggested that resting lymphocytes of fish are more susceptible to the effects of cortisol than stimulated cells.

In contrast, as mentioned above, the proportion of a probable immature population of thymocytes described in *Chalcides ocellatus* increased remarkably after hydrocortisone injection (Saad *et al.*, 1987). These authors also report severe depletion of mature T-lymphocytes of thymus, spleen and peripheral blood after multiple hydrocortisone injections, whereas B-lymphocytes seem to include two distinct subsets: one readily corticosteroid sensitive and the other resistant, even after prolonged exposure to high hydrocortisone levels (Saad et al., 1987). Discrepancies between results on frogs and lizards can be well attributed to differences in the corticosteroid doses, which are higher in lizards.

T-lymphocytes have been claimed as the main, direct, or even indirect target cells for corticosteroids in both fish (Kaatari and Tripp, 1987; Tripp et al., 1987) and amphibians (Highet and Ruben, 1987; Marx et al., 1987). Immunosuppression induced by cortico-steroids during anuran metamorphosis has been attributed to a selective inhibition of T-cell functions (Highet and Ruben, 1987; Marx et al., 1987). Apparently endogenous corticosteroids can induce depression in how antigen presenting cells can function, particularly their capacity to produce IL-1 in response to lectin or antigen activation. This can then lead to a deficiency in IL-2 production and/or expression of its relevant receptors by T-cells in metamorphosing Xenopus. Tripp et al. (1987) also reported that cortisol-dependent inhibition of antibody production may be mediated by inhibiting the expression of a lymphokine-like factor(s) relatively early when these lymphocytes are first induced. The addition of antigen-stimulated culture supernatants demonstrated that cortisol can negatively influence the production of a lymphokine-like factor, released probably by macrophages into the medium of antigen-stimulated lymphocytes. When supernatants from stimulated lymphocytes were added to cortisol suppressed cultures, the cortisol-mediated suppression was completely reversed (Tripp et al., 1987). According to one speculation, the early addition of both antigen and cortisol produces antigen-activated B-cells, which require a second signal (supernatant), the production of which is inhibited by cortisol. Finally, Ellsaesser and Clem have suggested that loss of mitogen responsiveness in fish after stress or intravenously administered cortisol apparently does not result from direct actions. Instead, there could be either a cascade effect which results in the release of a secondary agent (i.e. cAMP) which then directly affects lymphocytes. Or, metabolism of the host fish could result in the release of one or more metabolites which affect lymphocytes (Ellsaesser and Clem, 1987).

Sex Steroids

A role for sex steroids in seasonal changes which affect ectothermic immune systems has been proposed by a few workers; available data are sparse and restricted to a few isolated examples. Information derived from non-salmonid fish indicates that sexual differences in hematology occur in some species (Steuke and Atherton, 1965; Mulcahy, 1970; Ezzat et al., 1974; Fourie and Hattingh, 1976; Burton and Murray, 1979; Murray, 1984) but not in others (van Vuren and Hattingh, 1978). Maturation in both salmonid sexes coincides with prolonged lymphocytopenia (Pickering, 1986). In contrast, no significant variations in frog leukocyte numbers due to sex have been obtained during any season (Harris, 1972).

Differences in thymic organization between male and female rock-fish, Sebasticus marmoratus (Nakanishi, 1986), suggest a regulatory role for sex hormones on the structure of fish lymphoid organs. Substantial regression followed by disappearance of the thymus after sexual maturation have also been reported in other fish (Robertson and Wexler, 1960; Tamura and Honma, 1970; Honma and Tamura, 1972). However, peak thymic activity occurs in many fish in July and it is independent of the breeding season (Tamura and Honma, 1973, 1974, 1975, 1977, 1979; Tamura, 1978; Tamura et al., 1981). Nakanishi (1986) also reported sexual differences with respect to antibody production in rock-fish. Moreover, reactivity of mature females to SRBC was lower than that of males or immature females during the spawning season. Other studies using rock-fish, by contrast, showed no correlation between seasonal changes in immune reactivity and sex hormones such as estradiol-17β, methyltestosterone and progesterone (cited by Nakanishi, 1986). Furthermore, no effects on antibody production were observed after estradiol-17β administration and removal of the ovary during gestation (cited by Nakanishi, 1986).

Remarkable interactions between mothers and fetuses with respect to thymic activities have been reported in several teleosts (Tamura and Honma, 1979 in the guppy; Tamura et al., 1981 in the viviparous surf perch). In the viviparous surf perch, Ditrema termincki, regardless of the period of parturition, the greatest volume of larval thymus occurs one month after hatching. Subsequently there are sexual differences in thymic activity. For example, in males, but never in females, a remarkable involution occurs three months after hatching. It is also of interest that mothers, during the later period of pregnancy, with well-developed embryos, possess a thymus whose volume is larger than during any other stage (Tamura *et al.*, 1981).

In amphibians, Wright and Cooper (1980) described the decreased response of thymic lymphocytes from *Rana pipiens* to mitogens as being coincident with increasing ovarian development. In contrast, orchidectomy in *Rana perezi* during mating, but not later, results in hypertrophy of the thymic cortex (Zapata *et al.*, 1983) and variations in numbers of splenic lymphocytes (Zapata *et al.*, 1983, unpublished). Morphological changes found in the thymus of frogs, *Rana perezi*, in February, which include degeneration of cell microenvironments, have been correlated with high levels of circulating sex hormones (Garrido *et al.*, 1988). Likewise, thymic degeneration in mating turtles, *Mauremys caspica* (Leceta and Zapata, 1985), and the spotless starling, *Sturnus unicolor* (Fonfria *et al.*, 1983), coincides with high levels of testosterone. A third example reports the presence of receptors for gonadal steroids on reticuloepithelial cells rather than on mammalian thymocytes (Pearce *et al.*, 1983; Grossman *et al.*, 1979a, b, 1983). According to one explanation, degeneration of thymic reticulo-epithelial cells, induced by sex hormones, allows changes to occur in thymocyte maturation. Decreased splenic lymphoid tissue without apparent signs of pycnosis and high numbers of lymphocytes in peripheral blood and bone marrow found in *Rana perezi* in February have also been attributed to high levels of circulating sex steroids (Garrido *et al.*, 1988). In mammals, Viklicky *et al.* (1977, 1979) support the view that sex hormones, like glucocorticoids, modify cell distribution in the peripheral blood.

Other evidence supports a contrasting mechanism, i.e. effects of sex steroids on lower vertebrate immune system may be mediated directly by corticosteroids. Pickering and Pottinger (1987) speculated that stimulated interrenal activity during the spawning season increases the susceptibility of salmonid fish to disease; this is mediated by the immunosuppressive effects of cortisol. According to these workers the interrenal tissue was stimulated during the spawning season in both sexually mature male and female brown trout but

not in immature fish kept under identical conditions (Pickering and Pottinger, 1987).

Let us turn now to a brief description of the condition in birds. Finally, a relation between the onset of seasonal regression of avian thymus and increased growth of testes has been claimed (Riddle, 1928; Hohn, 1947; Wolfe *et al.*, 1962). A marked enlargement of the thymus was recorded following the annual breeding season in a variety of wild birds (Hohn, 1956). Thymic regression coincided with the cessation of molting. According to Hohn, increased thyroid activity which is associated with a molt could be responsible for thymic enlargement (see later, thyroid—thymus relationships in birds).

Thyroid

Physiological levels of thyroid hormones are necessary to maintain a responsive immune system in birds. Evidence for a role of thyroid in immune responses of ectothermic vertebrates is less extensive than it is in birds, with the possible exception of anuran amphibians. Du Pasquier and his colleagues have done much to describe immunity in larval *Xenopus laevis* in relation to metamorphosis (Flajnik *et al.*, 1987). Anderson (1970) suggested that thyroid activity is reflected by variations in the lymphoid system. Seasonal variations of thyroid hormone levels associated with molting are correlated well with changes of thymus weight in wild pheasants. Administration of large doses of thyroxine induces both thymic enlargement and molting in the domestic fowl (Anderson, 1970).

There is generally well-documented evidence for positive correlations between thyroid hormone levels and lymphocyte numbers in both peripheral blood and lymphoid organs but the effects on immune responsiveness are less clear. Propylthiouracil (PTU) treatment in birds results in reduced thymus, spleen and bursal weights (Keast and Ayre, 1980; Yam *et al.*, 1981). Hyperthyroid birds have significantly more total leukocytes, specifically lymphocytes, than hypothyroid birds (Bachman and Mashaly, 1987). Moreover, levels of T_3 and T_4 receptors on lymphocytes increase in hypothyroidism but remain unchanged during hyperthyroidism (Lemarchand-Beraud *et al.*, 1977), which suggests that although hormone levels are lower in hypothyroid groups avian lymphocytes may be better able to utilize T_3 and T_4

(Bachman and Mashaly, 1987). In contrast, a low mitogenic response of both spleen and thymus cells following Con A stimulation has been found in PTU-treated chickens (Yam *et al.*, 1981). Nevertheless, no significant correlations occurred between circulating T_3 and T_4 and either PHA or graft-versus-host responses, as markers of cell-mediated immunity (Weetman *et al.*, 1984; Bachman and Mashaly, 1987).

Serum antibody titers and depression of serum T_3 levels appear to be correlated significantly during the primary response to SRBC in budgerigars, *Melopsittacus undulatus*, treated with thiourea (Keast and Ayre, 1980). In contrast, other data show that hypothyroidism induced by either thyroidectomy or antithyroid drugs has no effect on antibody synthesis (Mashaly *et al.*, 1983; Bachman and Mashaly, 1987) or increased immune responsiveness (Scott *et al.*, 1985; Kai *et al.*, 1987). Thyroxine, in addition, has no effects on antibody production in chickens (Marsh, 1983). Recent results explain these discrepancies and amplify our views on relationships between avian thyroid and the immune system. Kai *et al.* (1987) have demonstrated that low doses of propionylthiourea (0.1% and 1%) in the diet stimulate immune responsiveness, whereas a high dose (5%) suppressed it. These results suggest, in addition, that PTU exerts biphasic effects on immune responsiveness in chickens.

Catecholamines

In a few cases, direct innervation of lymphoid organs or possible effects of catecholamines have been mentioned as possible regulatory factors on lymphoid activity in ectotherms, although any possible relationship to seasonal variations is unknown. Hodgson and colleagues have shown that adrenalin stimulates alpha or beta adrenoreceptors of splenic cells from four anuran species, producing an alpha effect (a reduction) in rosette formation in the presence of beta antagonists and a beta effect (an increase) in the presence of alpha antagonists. This same stimulation reduces rosette formation by lymphoid cells from five urodeles (Hodgson *et al.*, 1979). At the organ level, ultrastructural analyses have demonstrated: (1) unmyelinated nerves in thymic trabeculae of the turtle, *Mauremys caspica* (Leceta, 1984); (2) nerve endings, containing norepinephrine-like electron-dense vesicles, close to

free lymphocytes or fixed reticular elements of frog jugular bodies (Zapata *et al.*, 1982). While in mammals changes in local concentrations of neurotransmitters act as regulatory signals capable of modulating immune responses (Besedovsky *et al.*, 1979), their physiological significance in ectotherms remains to be clarified.

Nutrition

Experimental results support the concept that nutrition influences immunity in fish (Durve and Lovell, 1982; Taniguchi, 1983; Fletcher, 1986; Salomoni *et al.*, 1987). In fish, studies have focused on the influence of various diets on immune responsiveness. For example, Durve and Lovell (1982) found that high levels of ascorbic acid mainly at low temperature increased resistance of channel catfish fingerlings to *Edwardsiella tarda*. Moreover, the sera of channel catfish fed with an ascorbic acid-deficient diet have significantly lower levels of complement-mediated hemolytic activity than those of fish fed diets supplemented with ascorbic acid (Li and Lovell, 1985). Ascorbic acid deficiency did not, however, affect intracellular bactericidal activity of phagocytic cells (Li and Lovell, 1985).

In contrast, resident peritoneal macrophages from rainbow trout fed a diet deficient in alpha tocopherol for 16 weeks exhibited significantly decreased phagocytosis of latex beads (Blazer and Wolfe, 1984). Finally differences in protein content of two diets, although their caloric properties were the same, have been recently claimed as responsible for variations found in immune responsiveness of two strains of *Cyprinus carpio* (Salomoni *et al.*, 1987). The importance of either malnutrition or starvation for properly functioning immune systems has been established in reptiles (Salkind, 1915; Borysenko and Lewis, 1979).

Salkind (1915) was among the first workers who observed that starvation caused reversible thymic involution in reptiles. Much later, Borysenko and Lewis (1979) found that nutritional deficiency impaired both humoral and cell-mediated immunity in young snapping turtles (*Chelydra serpentina*). In these animals, the thymus underwent acute involution, whereas splenic lymphocytes were depleted to a lesser extent. To reverse the effects, improved nutrition readily induced recovery of lymphoid organs and immunodeficiency (Borysenko and Lewis, 1979). Stressful conditions, vitamin and mineral deficiencies have also been pointed out as possible direct causative agents of the immunosuppression observed in malnourished turtles (Borysenko and Lewis, 1979).

Antibiotics

In large scale cultures, mainly of fish, antimicrobial drugs often used as food additives are also employed for prophylactic and therapeutic purposes. Unfortunately, based on substantial evidence, antibiotics are known to interfere with the fish immune system (Levy, 1963; Cooper, 1976; Rijkers et al., 1981b; Grondel and Boesten, 1982; Anderson et al., 1984; van Muiswinkel et al., 1985; Grondel and van Muiswinkel, 1985; Grondel et al., 1986). The underlying mechanisms of immunosuppression are poorly understood. Antibiotics and antimetabolites delay fish allograft rejection (Levy, 1963; Cooper, 1976). Oral administration of therapeutic doses of oxytetracycline resulted in normal responses but depressed humoral responses (Rijkers et al., 1981a). Treated fish had, in contrast, increased numbers of granulocytes in the spleen. This prompted the workers to speculate that while specific defense mechanisms may be blocked by antibiotic treatment there may be an increase in the non-specific activity such as that of the phagocytic system.

Stress and Pollution

Under some conditions, seasonal variations which act on ectotherm immune responses may also serve as environmental stressors. A stressor can be any environmental change that affects an organism so that a physiological response is required. In the wild, a stress response may be short term and perhaps advantageous, but prolonged stress can lead to immunosuppression and disease. Effects of stressors on the immune system have been studied mostly in fish (MacArthur et al., 1984; Peters and Schwarzer, 1985). According to one interpretation, the effects might be mediated via the hypothalamus— pituitary — adrenal axis since this axis partially mimics

the immunosuppressive effects of corticosteroids. The mechanisms are complex, so that other biological mediators such as neuropeptides and catecholamines may also be involved.

Regardless of the nature of stress, changes in fish hematological parameters consistently include leuko-cytopenia, lymphopenia and neutrophilia (Finn and Nielson, 1971; Pickford et al., 1971; Bennett and Neville, 1975; Mazeaud et al., 1977; Pickering et al., 1982; Klinger et al., 1983; Tomasso et al., 1983; Angelides et al., 1987). Similar 'symptoms' have been observed in other 'stressed' vertebrates, including wild mammals (Dieterich and Feist, 1980). Evidence concerning the effects of stressors on fish inflammatory processes is scarcely known, but Morgan and Roberts (1976) reported that the Atlantic salmon, Salmo salar, after having been stressed by severe exercise at a high temperature, developed extensive necrotic lesions (at the site where an identification tag was inserted) and a lower chemiluminescence response of head kidney phagocytic cells (Angelidis et al., 1987).

T- and B-lymphocytes, but not IL-1-producing macrophages, seem to be affected by stress (Ellsaesser and Clem, 1986). Only the number of B-cells decreased after stress but those that did remain exhibited much lower levels of sIg (Ellsaesser and Clem, 1986). Results from experiments using T-dependent antigens (TNP-KLH) and those that revealed decreased responses to Con A confirm a stress-induced defect in T cells (Ellsaesser and Clem, 1986). It is, however, remarkable that the effects induced by stress can be mimicked (Ellsaesser, unpublished observations), although a role for interleukins has been suggested in the corticosteroid-dependent immunosuppression (Tripp et al., 1987).

A so-called 'stress pheromone' has been implicated in mediating immune suppression in fish. Pfuderer et al. (1974) found a substance which could be extracted from the flush and the water in which carp had been kept under crowded conditions and which caused depression of heart and growth rates of uncrowded carp. Perlmutter et al. (1973) discovered a similar 'crowding pheromone' in blue gourami, Trichogaster trichopterus. In this species, a reduction in their immune responsiveness to IPN (infectious pancreatic necrosis) virus was found in fish held under crowded conditions. The immune suppression was reversed if the water in which the fish were kept was extracted with methylchloroform.

In relation to fish, pollution, or 'quality' of water could be considered as a form of stress. Thus, agents which pollute, including toxicants, metals, wastes, etc., produce immunosuppression not directly but probably through their stressor properties (Dick and Dixon, 1985; Ellsaesser *et al.*, 1986). Exposure of rainbow trout to copper produces leukopenia, lymphopenia and neutrophilia (Dick and Dixon, 1985), increased susceptibility to enteric red mouth disease (Knittel, 1980) and infectious hematopoietic necrosis (Hetrick *et al.*, 1979). Mechanisms involved in these processes remain unclear.

Distinct evidence supports the view that copper acts similarly to corticosteroid-mediated stressors. However, it has been assumed to be a direct suppressive effect on phagocytic cells (Ellsaesser *et al.*, 1986) which is dependent upon the duration of exposure, a crucial parameter. Thus, immunosuppressive effects have been found after short-term (Knittel, 1980) but not long-term exposure to copper (Hetrick *et al.*, 1979; Viale and Calamari, 1984). In this context, it is interesting that Donaldson and Dye (1975) found that corticosteroid concentrations in *Oncorhynchus nerka* exposed to low concentrations of copper showed a transient elevation during the first 24 hours, with a subsequent return to control values despite the continued presence of the pollutant. The presence of zinc decreased the humoral antibody response of zebrafish, *Brachydanio rerio*, injected with bacterial antigens (Sarot and Perlmutter, 1976). In addition, it seems to markedly decrease the number of circulating thrombocytes in juvenile coho salmon, *Oncorhynchus kisutch* (McLeay, 1975).

Plaice exposed to mercury at 0.3 p.p.m. caused a steady decrease in serum lysozyme over a 7-day exposure and a concomitant lysozymuria (cited by Fletcher, 1986). There is also a significant increase in splenic index by day 6 of exposure which suggests that mercury stimulates proliferation of plaice splenic lymphoid tissue. Mercuric chloride has been reported as mitogenic for human lymphocytes (Caron *et al.*, 1970). Robohm and Nitkawski (1974) reported that cadmium at 12 p.p.m. increased the rate of bacterial uptake in the liver and spleen of the cunner, *Tautogolabrum adspersus*, but it significantly decreased the rates of bacterial killing. However, antibody production against intraperitoneally injected SRBC appeared to be unaffected. In contrast, Robohm (1986) reported reduced antibody responses in cunners after exposure to cadmium.

In contrast, neutrophilia has been observed in rainbow trout after 3 and 9 months of exposure to water heavily contaminated with chlorinated hydrocarbons from the Rhine river (Poels *et al.*, 1980). Likewise, McLeay (1973c) observed neutrophilia in coho salmon, *Oncorhynchus kisutch*, exposed for 25 days to sublethal levels of bleached kraftmill effluent. In this regard, Weeks and Warinner (1984, 1986) found a significant reduction in the phagocytosis of killed bacteria by macrophages from fish taken from polluted areas. Wolke *et al.* (1985) also reported that spleens and livers from winter flounder taken from clean and polluted waters showed significant differences in size, number and pigmentation of macrophage aggregates (melanomacrophage centers). Wolke (1984) was also able to mimic this response under laboratory conditions where fish are exposed to chemical pesticides. Weeks and Warinner (1986) claimed to have found reduced chemotactic activity in macrophages from fish obtained from polluted waters.

Several reports have described the general signs of leukopenia and reduction of splenic weights following exposure to chlorinated hydrocarbon insecticides (Zeeman and Brindley, 1981). Suppression of plaque-forming cells and humoral antibodies induced by DDT was also described by Zeeman (1980). However, no effects on antibody production have been reported in fish taken from water contaminated either with lindane (an organochlorine insecticide), atrazine (a triazine herbicide) (Cossarini-Dunier *et al.*, 1987a, b) or manganese (Cossarini-Dunier, 1987). Furthermore, lindane has no effects on cell-mediated immunity as measured by time of rejection of first- or second-set grafts or phagocytosis, but manganese has an enhancing effect on phagocytosis of bacteria (Cossarini-Dunier, 1987). Remarkably, manganese enhanced phagocytosis of zymosan only at the lowest concentrations (Cossarini-Dunier, 1987). Likewise, halogenated aromatic hydrocarbons affect both humoral (Vos and van Driel Grootenhuis, 1972; Loose *et al.*, 1977; Truelove *et al.*, 1982; Silkworth and Grabstein, 1982) and cellular (Vos and van Driel Grootenhuis, 1972; Chang *et al.*, 1982) but not NK immunity (Cleland and Sonstegard, 1987).

FINAL COMMENT

An integrative hypothesis concerning seasonal mechanisms involved in the regulation of ectothermic vertebrate immune responsiveness is difficult to formulate. From the current available information we conclude that immunity in ectotherms is dramatically influenced by ambient factors. It is necessary to describe immunological responses in ectotherms in the context of defined seasonal and other environmental factors that are properly coordinated with age, sex, light, antigen, dose regimen, etc. Lack of adherence to these variables only complicates the validity of interpretations concerning immune responses in ectothermic vertebrates.

REFERENCES

Abruzzini AF, Ingram LO and Clem LW (1982). Temperature mediated processes in teleost immunity. Homeoviscous adaptation in teleost lymphocytes. *Proc Soc Exp Biol Med* **169**: 12–18.

Albert S, Wolf PL and Pryjma I (1965a). Evidence of erythropoiesis in the thymus of mice. *J Ret Soc* **2**: 30–39.

Albert S, Wolf PL, Pryjma I and Vazquez J (1965b). Variations in morphology of erythroblasts of normal mouse thymus. *J Ret Soc* **2**: 158–171.

Albert S, Wolf PL, Pryjma I and Vazquez J (1966). Erythropoiesis in the human thymus. *Am J Clin Pathol* **45**: 460–464.

Alekseeva GV and Yunker VM (1973). Dynamic of the seasonal morphological changes in the lymph nodes of the red-cheeked suslik. In *Materials of Ecological Morphology*. Nauka. Siberian Dept., Novosibirsk. p 53.

Alekseeva GV and Yunker VM (1977). Seasonal histostructural changes in the thymus of red-cheeked susliks. *Izv Sib Otd Akad Nauk SSSR* **2**: 125–129.

Alvarez F, Razquin B, Villena A, Lopez Fierro P, Herraez PO and Zapata A (1987). Relacion entre los cambios estacionales en los organos linfoides secundarios de la trucha comun *Salmo trutta fario* y la incidencia de infecciones por *Saprolegnia*. *Cuad Marisq Publ Tecn* **8**: 183–192.

Alvarez F, Razquin B, Villena A, Lopez Fierro P and Zapata A (1988). Alterations in the peripheral lymphoid organs and differential leukocyte counts of *Saprolegnia* infected brown trout, *Salmo trutta fario*. *Vet Immunol Immunopathol* **18**: 181–193.

Ambrosius H and Shaker W (1964). Beitrage zur immunobiologie poikilothermer Wirbeltiere I. Immunologische Untersuchungen an Karpfen (*Cyprinus carpio*). *Zool Jb Physiol* **71**: 73 ff.

Anderson DP, Robertson BS and Dixon OW (1982). Immunosuppression induced by a corticosteroid or an alkyating agent in rainbow trout *Salmo gairdneri* administered a *Yersinia ruckeri* bacterin. *Dev Comp Immunol* Suppl **2**: 197–204.

Anderson DP, van Muiswinkel WB and Robertson BS (1984). Effects of chemically induced immune modulation on infectious diseases of fish. In *Chemical Regulation of Immunity in Veterinary Medicine*. Liss: New York. pp 187–211.

Anderson NM (1970). Seasonal changes in thymus weights in ring-necked pheasants. *Condor* **72**: 205–208.

Angelidis P, Baudin-Laurencin F and Youinou P (1987). Stress in rainbow trout *Salmo gairdneri*: effects upon phagocyte chemiluminescence, circulating leucocytes and susceptibility to *Aeromonas salmonicida*. *J Fish Biol* **31** (Suppl A): 113–122.

Avtalion RR (1969). Temperature effect on antibody production and immunological memory in carp (*Cyprinus carpio*) immunized against bovine serum albumin (BSA). *Immunology* **17**: 927–931.

Avtalion RR (1981). Environmental control of the immune response in fish. *CRT Crit Rev Environ Control* **11**: 163–188.

Avtalion RR, Malik Z, Lefler E and Katz E (1970). Temperature effect on immune resistance of fish to pathogens. *Bamidgeh Bull Fish Cul Isr* **22**: 33–38.

Azzolina LS (1976). Cyclicity and memory in the humoral immune response of the marine toad *Bufo marinus*. *Eur J Immunol* **6**: 227–230.

Azzolina LS (1978). Antigen recognition and immune response in goldfish *Carassius auratus* at different temperatures. *Dev Comp Immunol* **2**: 77–86.

Bacchus S and Kendall MD (1975). Histological changes associated with enlargement and regression of the thymus glands of the red-billed *Quelea quelea* L (Plocidae: weaver-birds). *Phil Trans Roy Soc B* **273**: 65–78.

Bachman SE and Mashaly MM (1987). Relationship between circulating thyroid hormones and cell-mediated immunity in immature male chickens. *Dev Comp Immunol* **11**: 203–213.

Badir N and Abdel Khader I (1981). Effect of seasonal changes in humoral immune responses of the lizard *Chalcides ocellatus*. In Solomon JB (Ed), *Aspects of Developmental and Comparative Immunology*. Pergamon Press: Oxford. pp 515–516.

Balduzzi A (1976). Personal communication cited by N Cohen. Phylogenetic emergence of lymphoid tissues and cells. In Marchelonis JJ (Ed), *Lymphocyte Structure and Function*. Part I. Marcel Dekker: New York. pp 149–202.

Ball JN and Hawkins EF (1976). Adrenocortical (interrenal) responses to hypophysectomy and adenohypophysial hormones on the teleost *Poecilia latipinna*. *Gen Comp Endocrinol* **28**: 59–70.

Barrow Jr JH (1955). Social behavior in fresh-water fish and its effect on resistance to trypanosomes. *Proc Natl Acad Sci USA* **41**: 676–679.

Bazan-Kubik I and Skrzypiec Z (1980). Involution saisonniere du thymus de *Rana ridibunda*. *Bull Ann Univ Mariae Curie-Sklodowska, Sect C* **35**: 207 ff.

Bennett MF and Marbottle JA (1968). The effects of hydrocortisone in the blood of tadpoles and frogs, *Rana catesbeiana*. *Biol Bull* **135**: 92−95.

Bennett MF and Neville CB (1975). Effects of cold shock on the distribution of leucocytes in goldfish *Carassius auratus*. *J Comp Physiol* **88**: 213−216.

Bennett MF, Gaudio CA, Johnson AO and Spisso JH (1972). Changes in the blood of newts *Notophthalmus viridescens* following the administration of hydrocortisone. *J Comp Physiol* **80**: 233−237.

Besedovsky HO, del Rey A, Sorkin E, da Prada M and Keller HH (1979). Immunoregulation mediated by the sympathetic nervous system. *Cell Immunol* **48**: 346−355.

Bigaj J and Plytycz B (1981). Ultrastruktura komorek grasiczych zaby. *Przegl Zool* **25**: 489 ff.

Bigaj J and Plytycz B (1984). Endogenous rhythms in the thymus gland of *Rana temporaria* (Morphological study). *Thymus* **6**: 369−373.

Bisset KA (1948). The effect of temperature upon antibody production in cold-blooded vertebrates. *J Path Bact* **60**: 87−92.

Blazer VS and Wolke RE (1984). The effect of tocopherol on the immune response and non-specific resistance factors of rainbow trout (*Salmo gairdneri* Richardson). *Aquaculture* **37**: 1−9.

Bly JE, Buttle TM, Meydrech EF and Clem LW (1986). The effects of *in vivo* acclimation temperature on the fatty acid composition of channel catfish (*Ictalurus punctatus*) peripheral blood cells. *Comp Biochem Physiol* **83B**: 791−795.

Bly JE, Buttke TM, Cuchens MA and Clem LW (1987). Temperature mediated processes in teleost immunity: the effects of temperature on membrane immunoglobulin capping on channel catfish B lymphocytes. *Comp Biochem Physiol* **88A**: 65−70.

Bly JE, Ellaesser CF, Miller NW and Clem LW (1988). Environmental stresses and their influence on channel catfish immune responses. *Proc Fourth ISDCI Congress* Abstract 5.1.

Borysenko M and Lewis S (1979). The effect of malnutrition on immunocompetence and whole body resistance to infection in *Chelydra serpentina*. *Dev Comp Immunol* **3**: 89−100.

Bridges DW, Cech JJ and Pedro DN (1976). Seasonal hematological changes in winter flounder *Pseudopleuronectes americanus*. *Trans Am Fish Soc* **105**: 596−600.

Burton CB and Murray SA (1979). Effects of density on goldfish blood. I. Hematology. *Comp Biochem Physiol* **62A**: 555−558.

Caron GA, Poutala S and Provost TT (1970). Lymphocyte transformation induced by inorganic and organic mercury. *Int Arch Allergy Appl Immunol* **37**: 76−87.

Chang KJ, Hsieh K-H, Tang SY and Tung TC (1982). Immunologic evaluation of patients with polychlorinated

response and its relation to clinical studies. *J Toxicol Environ Health* **19**: 217−223.

Chilmonczyk S (1982). Rainbow trout lymphoid organs: cellular effects of corticosteroids and anti-thymocyte serum. *Dev Comp Immunol* **6**: 271−280.

Cirri-Borghi MB and Arbi-Riccardi R (1976). L'ultrastrutturral del timo del riccio (*Erinaceus europaeus*) durante la veglia nell'ibernazione e nelle varie fasi del risveglio. *Boll Soc It Biol Sper* **52**: 1956−1960.

Cleland GB and Sonstegard RA (1987). Natural killer cell activity in rainbow trout (*Salmo gairdneri*): Effect of dietary exposure to Aroclor 1254 and/or Mirex. *Can J Fish Aquat Sci* **44**: 636−638.

Clem LW, Faulmann E, Miller NW, Ellsaesser CF, Lobb CJ and Cuchens MA (1984). Temperature-mediated processes in teleost immunity: differential effects of *in vitro* and *in vivo* temperatures on mitogenic responses of channel catfish lymphocytes. *Dev Comp Immunol* **8**: 313−322.

Cone RE and Marchalonis JJ (1972). Cellular and humoral aspects of the influence of environmental temperature on the immune response of poikilothermic vertebrates. *J Immunol* **108**: 952−957.

Cooper EL (1976). *Comparative Immunology*. Prentice-Hall: Englewood Cliffs. p. 338.

Cossarini-Dunier M (1987). Effects of the pesticides atrazine and lindane and of manganese ions on cellular immunity of carp (*Cyprinus carpio*). *J Fish Biol* **31** (Suppl A): 67−73.

Cossarini-Dunier M, Monod G, Demael A and Lepot D (1987a). Effects of gamma hexachlorocyclohexane (lindane) on carp (*Cyprinus carpio*). I. Effect of chronic intoxication on humoral immunity in relation with tissue pollutant levels. *Ecotox Environ Safety* **13**: 339−345.

Cossarini-Dunier M, Demael A, Riviere JL and Lepot D (1987b). Investigation on the effects of the herbicide atrazine on carp (*Cyprinus carpio*) Ambro, in press.

Cottrell B (1977). The immune response of plaice (*Pleuronectes platessa* L) to the metacercariae of *Cryptocotyle lingua* and *Rhipidocotyle johnstonei*. *Parasitology* **74**: 93−107.

Csaba G and Barath P (1975). Morphological changes of thymus and the thyroid gland after postnatal extirpation of pineal body. *Endocrin Exp* **9**: 59−67.

Cuchens MA and Clem LW (1977). Phylogeny of lymphocyte heterogeneity. II. Differential effects of temperature on fish T-like and B-like cells. *Cell Immunol* **314**: 219−230.

Cuchens MA, McLean E and Clem LW (1976). Lymphocyte heterogeneity in fish and reptiles. In Wright RK and Cooper EL (Eds), *Phylogeny of Thymus and Bone Marrow—Bursa Cells*. North-Holland: Amsterdam. pp 205−213.

Cushing JE (1942). An effect of temperature upon antibody production in fish. *J Immunol* **45**: 123−126.

Denton JE and Yousef MK (1975). Seasonal changes in haematology of rainbow trout (*Salmo gairdneri*). *Comp*

Biochem Physiol **51A**: 151−153.

Dick PT and Dixon DG (1985). Changes in circulating blood cell levels of rainbow trout *Salmo gairdneri* Richardson, following acute and chronic exposure to copper. *J Fish Biol* **26**: 475−481.

Diener E and Marchalonis JJ (1970). Cellular and humoral aspects of the primary immune response of the toad *Bufo marinus*. *Immunology* **18**: 279−293.

Dieterich RA and Feist DD (1980). Hematology of Alaskan snowshoe hares (*Lepus americanus macfarlani*) during years of population decline. *Comp Biochem Physiol* **66A**: 545−547.

Donaldson EM and Dye HM (1975). Corticosteroid concentrations in sockeye salmon (*Oncorhynchus nerka*) exposed to low concentrations of copper. *J Fish Res Bd Can* **32**: 533−539.

Duguy R (1970). Numbers of blood cells and their variation. In Gans CC and Parsons T (Eds), *Biology of the Reptilia*. Vol 3. *Morphology*. Academic Press: New York.

Durve VS and Lovell RT (1982). Vitamin C and disease resistance in channel catfish (*Ictalurus punctatus*). *Can J Fish Aquat Sci* **41**: 1244−1247.

El Deeb S, El Ridi R and Badir N (1980). Effect of seasonal and temperature changes on humoral response of *Eumeces schneideri* (Reptilia, Sauria, Scincidae). *Dev Comp Immunol* **4**: 753−758.

El Ridi R and Kandil O (1981). Membrane markers of reptilian lymphocytes. *Dev Comp Immunol* Suppl **I**: 143−150.

El Ridi R, Zada S and Kandil O (1980). Lymphocyte structural heterogeneity in the lizard *Chalcides ocellatus*. In Solomon JB (Ed), *Aspects of Developmental and Comparative Immunology I*. Pergamon Press: Oxford. pp 513−514.

El Ridi R, Badir N and El Rouby S (1981). Effect of seasonal variations on the immune system of the snake. *Psammophis schokari*. *J Exp Zool* **216**: 357−365.

El Ridi R, Wahby AF, Saad AH and Soliman MAW (1987). Concanavalin responsiveness and interleukin-2 production in the snake *Spalerosophis diadema*. *Immunobiology* **174**: 177−189.

El Ridi R, Zada S, Afifi A, El Deeb S, El Rouby S, Farag M and Saad AH (1988). Cyclic changes in the differentiation of lymphoid cells in reptiles. *Cell Differentiation* **24**: 1−8.

Ellsaesser CF and Clem LW (1986). Hematological and immunological changes in channel catfish stressed by handling and transport. *J Fish Biol* **28**: 511−521.

Ellsaesser CF and Clem LW (1987). Cortisol induced hematologic and immunologic changes in channel catfish (*Ictalurus punctatus*). *Comp Biochem Physiol* **87A**: 405−408.

Ezzat AA, Shabana MD and Farghally AM (1974). Studies on the blood characteristics of *Tilapia zilli* (Gervias). I. Blood cells. *J Fish Biol* **6**: 1−12.

Fache B and Charlemagne J (1975). Influence on allograft rejection of thymectomy at different stages of larval development in Urodele amphibian *Pleurodeles waltlii* Michah (Salamandridae). *Eur J Immunol* **5**: 155−157.

Fange R and Silverin B (1985). Variation of lymphoid activity in the spleen of a migrating bird, the pied flycatcher (*Ficedula hypoleuca*: Aves, Passeriformes). *J Morphol* **184**: 33−40.

Farag MA and El Ridi R (1985). Mixed leucocyte reaction (MLR) in the snake *Psammophis sibilans*. *Immunology* **55**: 173−181.

Farag MA and El Ridi R (1986). Proliferative responses of snake lymphocytes to concanavalin A. *Dev Comp Immunol* **40**: 561−569.

Faulmann E, Cuchens MA, Lobb CJ, Miller NW and Clem LW (1983). An effective culture system for studying *in vitro* mitogenic responses of channel catfish lymphocytes. *Trans Am Fish Soc* **112**: 673−679.

Fichtelius KE and Jaroslow BN (1969). Changes in the concentration of lymphocytes in the intestinal epithelium of hibernating ground squirrels (*Citellus tridecemlineatus*) *Acta Pathol Microbiol Scand* **77**: 99−102.

Fijan N and Cvetnic S (1966). Immunitetna reactivnost sarana. II. Reaktivnos tokon focline Kod drzanja u ribnjacima. *Vet Arch Zagreb* **3−4**: 100−105.

Finn JP and Nielson NO (1971). The inflammatory response of rainbow trout. *J Fish Biol* **3**: 463−478.

Flajnik MF, Hsu E, Kaufman JF and Du Pasquier L (1987). Changes in the immune system during metamorphosis of *Xenopus*. *Immunol Today* **8**: 58−64.

Fletcher TC (1986). Modulation of non-specific host defenses in fish. *Vet Immunol Immunopathol* **12**: 559−67.

Fletcher TC and White A (1976). The lysozyme of the plaice *Pleuronectes platessa* L. *Comp Biochem Physiol* **55B**: 207−210.

Fonfria J, Barrutia MG, Garrido E, Ardavin MF and Zapata A (1983). Erythropoiesis in the thymus of the spotless starling, *Sturnus unicolor*. *Cell Tissue Res* **232**: 445−455.

Fourie Fle R and Hattingh J (1976). A seasonal study of the haematology of carp (*Cyprinus carpio*) from a locality in the Transvaal, South Africa. *Zool Afr* **11**: 75−80.

Galletti G and Cavallari A (1972). The thymus of marmots: spontaneous, natural seasonal thymectomy? *Acta Anat* **83**: 593−605.

Gardner GR and Yevich PP (1969). Studies on the blood morphology of three estuarine cyprinodontiform fishes. *J Fish Res Bd Can* **26**: 433−447.

Garrido E, Gomariz RP, Leceta J and Zapata A (1987). Effects of dexamethasone on the lymphoid organs of *Rana perezi*. *Dev Comp Immunol* **11**: 375−384.

Garrido E, Gomariz RP, Leceta J and Zapata A (1988). Different sensitivity to the dexamethasone treatment of the lymphoid organs of *Rana perezi* in two different seasons. *Dev Comp Immunol* **13**: 57−64.

Ghoneum MH, Egami N, Ijiri K and Cooper EL (1986). Effect of corticosteroids on the thymus of the fish *Oryzias latipes*. *Dev Comp Immunol* **10**: 35−44.

Glick B (1984). Interrelation of the avian immune and neuro-endocrine systems. *J Exp Zool* **232**: 671−682.

Grimm AS (1985). Suppression by control of the nitrogen-induced proliferation of peripheral blood leucocytes from plaice (*Pleurodeles platessa* L.). In Manning MJ and Tatner MF (Eds), *Fish Immunology*. Academic Press: London. pp 253−272.

Grondel JL and Boesten HJAM (1982). The influence of antibiotics on the immune system. I. Inhibition of the mitogenic leukocyte response *in vitro* by oxytetracycline. *Dev Comp Immunol* Suppl 2: 211−216.

Grondel JL and van Muiswinkel WB (1985). Immunological defence mechanisms as a target for antibiotics. In *Comparative Veterinary Pharmacology, Toxicology and Therapy*. 3rd EAVPT Congress, Ghent (Abstract). p 145.

Grondel JL, Nouws JFM and Haenen OLM (1986). Fish and antibiotics: Pharmacokinetics of sulphadimidine on carp (*Cyrinus carpio*). *Vet Immunol Immunopathol* 12: 281−286.

Grossman CJ, Sholiton LJ and Nathan P (1979a). Rat thymic estrogen receptor. I. Preparation, location and physiochemical properties. *J Steroid Biochem* 11: 1233−1240.

Grossman CJ, Sholiton LJ, Blaha GC and Nathan P (1979b). Rat thymic estrogen receptor. II. Physiological properties. *J Steroid Biochem* 11: 1241−1246.

Grossman CJ, Sholiton LJ and Roselle GA (1983). Dihydrotestosterone regulation of thymocyte function in the rat mediastinum by serum factors. *J Steroid Biochem* 19: 1459−1467.

Hagen M, Filosa MF and Youson JH (1985). The immune response in adult sea lamprey (*Petromyzon marinus*). The effect of temperature. *Comp Biochem Physiol* 82A: 207−210.

Harris JA (1972). Seasonal variations on some hematological characteristics of *Rana pipiens*. *Comp Biochem Physiol* 431: 975−989.

Harris JE (1973). The immune response of dace *Leuciscus leuciscus* (L) to injected antigenic materials. *J Fish Biol* 5: 261−276.

Hetrick FM, Knittel MD and Fryer JL (1979). Increased susceptibility of rainbow trout to infectious hematopoietic necrosis virus after exposure to copper. *Appl Environ Microbiol* 37: 198−201.

Highet AB and Ruben LN (1987). Corticosteroid regulation of IL-1 production may be responsible for deficient immune suppressor function during the metamorphosis of *Xenopus laevis*, the South African clawed toad. *Immunopharmacology* 13: 149−155.

Hodgson RM, Clothier RH and Balls M (1979). Adrenoreceptors, cyclic nucleotides, and the regulation of spleen cell antigen binding in urodele and anuran amphibians. *Eur J Immunol* 9: 289−293.

Hohn EO (1947). Seasonal cyclical changes in the thymus of the mallard. *Exp Biol* 24: 184−191.

Hohn EO (1956). Seasonal recrudescence of the thymus in adult birds. *Can J Biochem Physiol* 34: 90−101.

Holzapfel RA (1937). The cyclic character of hibernation in frogs. *Quart Rev Biol* 12: 65−87.

Honma Y and Tamura E (1972). Studies on the endocrine glands of a salmonid fish, the Ayu, *Plecoglossus altivelis* Temminck et Schlegel. VIII. Degenerative changes in the thymus of Koayu exposed to artificial photoperiods. *Bull Jap Soc Scient Fish* 38: 995−1005.

Honma Y and Tamura E (1984). Histological changes in the lymphoid system of fish with respect to age, seasonal and endocrine changes. *Dev Comp Immunol* Suppl 3: 239−244.

Hussein MF, Badir N, El Ridi R and Akef M (1978a). Differential effects of seasonal variation on lymphoid tissue of the lizard *Chalcides ocellatus*. *Dev Comp Immunol* 2: 297−311.

Hussein MF, Badir N, El Ridi R and Akef M (1978b). Effects of seasonal variation on lymphoid tissues of the lizards, *Mabuya quinquetaeniata* Licht. and *Uromastyx aegyptia*. *Dev Comp Immunol* 2: 469−479.

Hussein MF, Badir N, El Ridi R and Akef M (1979a). Lymphoid tissues of the snake *Spalerosophis diadema* in the different seasons. *Dev Comp Immunol* 3: 77−89.

Hussein MF, Badir N, El Ridi R and El Deeb S (1979b). Effect of seasonal variations on immune system of the lizard *Scincus scincus*. *J Exp Zool* 209: 91−96.

Hussein MF, Badir N, El Ridi R and Afifi A (1984a). Immune system of the gecko, *Tarentola annularis* in the different seasons. *Bull Fac Sci Cairo Univ* 52: 17−29.

Hussein MF, Badir N, Zada S, El Ridi R and Zahran W (1984b). Effect of seasonal changes on immune system of the toad *Bufo regularis*. *Bull Fac Sci Cairo Univ* 52: 181−192.

Jakubow K, Gromadzka-Ostrowska J and Zalewska B (1984). Seasonal changes in the haematological indices in peripheral blood of chinchilla (*Chinchilla laniger* L). *Comp Biochem Physiol* 78A: 845−853.

Johansson-Sjobeck ML, Larsson A, Lewander K and Lidman U (1978). Hematological effects of cortisol in the European eel *Anguilla anguilla* L. *Comp Biochem Physiol* 60A: 165−168.

Kaatari SL and Tripp RA (1987). Cellular mechanisms of glucocorticoid immunosuppression in salmon. *J Fish Biol* 31 Suppl A: 129−132.

Kai O, Imada M, Imada Y and Sato K (1987). Effects of the thyroid status on the immune system of the chicken. *Jap Poultry Sci* 24: 150−159.

Kapa E, Olah I and Toro I (1968). Electron-microscopic investigation of the thymus of adult frog (*Rana esculenta*). *Acta Biol Acad Sci Hung* 19: 203−213.

Keast D and Ayre DJ (1980). Antibody regulation in birds by thyroid hormones. *Dev Comp Immunol* 4: 323−330.

Kendall MD (1975a). Sizes and numbers of nuclei in the cortex of thymus glands of the red-billed weavers *Quelea quelea*. *Cell Tissue Res* 164: 233−249.

Kendall MD (1975b). EMMA-4 analysis of iron in the cells of the thymic cortex of weaver bird (*Quelea quelea*). *Phil Trans Roy Soc B* 273: 79−82.

Kendall MD (1978). The effect of haemorrhage on the cell populations of the thymus and bone marrow in wild starlings (*Sturnus vulgaris*). *Cell Tissue Res* 190: 459−479.

Kendall MD (1980). Avian thymus glands: a review. *Dev Comp Immunol* 4: 191−210.

Kendall MD and Frazier JA (1979). Ultrastructural studies on erythropoiesis in the avian thymus. I. Description of all cell types. *Cell Tissue Res* **199**: 37−61.

Kendall MD and Singh J (1980). The presence of erythroid cells in the thymus gland of man. *J Anat* **130**: 183−199.

Kendall MD and Ward P (1974). Erythropoiesis in an avian thymus. *Nature (London)* **249**: 366−367.

Kirkpatrick CM (1944). Body weights and organ measurements in relation to age and season in ring-necked pheasants. *Anat Rec* **89**: 175−194.

Klinger H, Delventhal H and Hilge V (1983). Water quality and stocking density as stressors in fish: some new data with a general review. *Trans Am Fish Soc* **106**: 201−212.

Knittel MD (1980). Heavy metal stress and increased susceptibility of steelhead trout (*Salmo gairdneri*) to *Yersinia ruckeri* infection. In Eaton JG, Parrish PR and Hendricks AC (Eds), *Aquatic Toxicology*. ASTM STP 707, American Society for Testing and Materials: Philadelphia. pp 321−327.

Leceta J (1984). Cambios estacionales en el sistema inmune de *Mauremys caspica*. Papel regulador del sistema neuroendocrino. Doctoral thesis, Complutense University, Madrid.

Leceta J and Zapata A (1985). Seasonal changes in the thymus and spleen of the turtle *Mauremys caspica*. A morphometrical light and microscopical study. *Dev Comp Immunol* **9**: 653−668.

Leceta J and Zapata A (1986). Seasonal variations in the immune response of the tortoise *Mauremys caspica*. *Immunology* **57**: 483−487.

Leceta J, Villena A, Rasquin B, Fonfria J and Zapata A (1984). Interdigitating cells in the thymus of the turtle *Mauremys caspica*. Possible relationships to macrophages. *Cell Tissue Res* **238**: 381−385.

Leceta J, Garrido E, Torroba M and Zapata A (1988). Seasonal modifications affecting the thymic cell microenvironments in the turtle *Mauremys caspica*. An ultrastructural study. *Cell Tissue Res* **256**: 213−219.

Lemarchand-Beraud T, Holm AC and Scazziga BR (1977). Triiodothyroxine nuclear receptors in lymphocytes from normal hyper-and hypothyroid subjects. *Acta Endocrinol* **85**: 44−54.

Levy L (1963). Effects of drugs on goldfish scale homograft survival. *Proc Soc Exp Biol Med* **114**: 47−50.

Li Y and Lovell RT (1985). Elevated levels of dietary ascorbic acid increase immune responses in channel catfish. *J Nutr* **115**: 123−131.

Loose LD, Pittman KA, Benitz KF and Silkworth JB (1977). Polychlorinated biphenyl and hexachlorobenzene induced humoral immunosuppression. *J Ret Soc* **22**: 253−271.

MacArthur JI, Fletcher TC and Thomson AW (1983). Distribution of radiolabeled erythrocytes and the effect of temperature on clearance in the plaice (*Pleuronectes platessa* L.). *J Ret Soc* **34**: 13−21.

MacArthur JI, Fletcher TC, Pirie BJS, Davidson RJL and Thomson AW (1984). Peritoneal inflammatory cells in plaice *Pleuronectes platessa* L.: effects of stress and endotoxin. *J Fish Biol* **35**: 69−81.

Maestroni GJM and Pierpaoli W (1981). Pharmacologic control of the hormonally mediated immune response. In Ader R (Ed), *Psychoneuroimmunology*. Academic Press: New York. pp 405−428.

Mahajan CL and Dheer JS (1979). Seasonal variations in the blood constituents of an air-breathing fish, *Channa punctatus* Bloch. *J Fish Biol* **14**: 413−417.

Marsh JA (1983). Assessment of antibody production in sex-linked and autosomal dwarf chickens. *Dev Comp Immunol* **7**: 535−544.

Marx M, Ruben LN, Nobis C and Duffy D (1987). Compromised T-cell functions during anuran metamorphosis: the role of corticosteroids. In Cooper EL, Langlet C and Bierne J (Eds), *Developmental and Comparative Immunology*. Progress in Clinical and Biological Research, Vol 233. Alan R Liss: New York. pp 129−140.

Mashaly MM, Youtz SL and Wideman RF (1983). Hypothyroidism and antibody production in immature male chickens. *Immunol Comm* **22**: 551−563.

Maule AG, Schreck CB and Kaatari SL (1987). Changes in the immune system of coho salmon (*Oncorhynchus kisutch*) during the parr-to-smolt transformation and after implantation of cortisol. *Can J Fish Aquat Sci* **44**: 161−166.

Mazeaud MM, Mazeaud F and Donaldson EM (1977). Primary and secondary effects of stress in fish: some new data with a general review. *Trans Am Fish Soc* **106**: 201−212.

McKnight IM (1966). A hematological study on the mountain whitefish *Prosopium williamsoni*. *J Fish Res Bd Can* **23**: 45−64.

McLeay DJ (1973a). Effects of ACTH on the pituitary−interrenal axis and abundance of white blood cell types in juvenile coho salmon *Oncorhynchus kisutch*. *Gen Comp Endocrinol* **21**: 431−440.

McLeay DJ (1973b). Effects of cortisol and dexamethasone on the pituitary−interrenal axis and abundance of white blood cell types in juvenile coho salmon *Oncorhynchus kisutch*. *Gen Comp Endocrinol* **21**: 441−450.

McLeay DJ (1973c). Effects of a 120h and 25 day exposure to kraft pulp mill effluent on the blood and tissues on juvenile coho salmon (*Oncorhynchus kisutch*). *J Fish Res Bd Can* **32**: 2357−2364.

McLeay DJ (1975). Variations in the pituitary−interrenal axis and the abundance of circulating blood-cell types in juvenile coho salmon *Oncorhynchus kisutch* during stream residence. *Can J Zool* **53**: 1882−1891.

Miller NW and Clem LW (1984). Temperature-mediated processes in teleost immunity: differential effects of temperature on catfish *in vitro* antibody responses to thymus-dependent and thymus-independent antigens. *J Immunol* **133**: 2356−2359.

Morgan RIG and Roberts RJ (1976). The histopathology of salmon tagging. IV. The effect of severe exercise on the induced tagging lesion in salmon parr at two temperatures. *J Fish Biol* **8**: 289−292.

Mulcahy MF (1970). Blood values in the pike *Esox lucius* L. *J Fish Biol* **2**: 203−209.

Murachi S (1959). Hemoglobin content, erythrocyte sedimentation rate and hematocrit of the blood in young carp (*Cyprinus carpio*). *J Fac Fish Anim Husb Hiroshima Univ* **2**: 241–247.

Murray SA (1984). Hematological study on the bluegill *Lepomis macrochirus* Raf. *Comp Biochem Physiol* **78A**: 181–191.

Muthukkaruppan VR, Borysenko M and El Ridi R (1982). Reticuloendothelial system. Structure and function in reptiles. In Cohen N and Sigel MM (Eds), *The Reticuloendothelial System. A Comprehensive Treatise.* Vol. 3. *Phylogeny and Ontogeny.* Plenum Press: New York.

Nakanishi T (1986). Seasonal changes in the hormonal immune response and the lymphoid tissues of the marine teleost *Sebasticus marmoratus*. *Vet Immunol Immunopathol* **12**: 213–223.

Nybelin GC (1935). Uber Agglutininbildung bei Fischen. *Z Immun Forsch* **84**: 74–79.

Paterson WP and Fryer JL (1974). Effect of temperature and antigen dose on the antibody response of juvenile coho salmon (*Oncorhynchus kisutch*) to *Aeromonas salmonicida* endotoxin. *J Fish Res Bd Can* **31**: 1743–1749.

Pearce PT, Khalid BA and Funder JW (1983). Progesterone receptors in rat thymus. *Endocrinology* **113**: 1287–1291.

Perlmutter A, Sarot DA, Uy M, Fillozola RJ and Seeley RJ (1973). The effect of crowding on the immune response of the blue gourami (*Trichegaster trichopterus*) to infectious pancreatic necrosis (IPN) virus. *Life Sci* **13**: 363–375.

Peters G and Schwarzer R (1985). Changes in hemopoietic tissues of rainbow trout under influence of stress. *Dis Aquat Org* **1**: 1–10.

Pfuderer P, Williams P and Francis AA (1974). Partial purification of the crowding factor from *Carassius auratus* and *Cyprinus carpio*. *J Exp Zool* **187**: 375–382.

Plisalix C (1885). Recherches sur l'anatomie et la physiologie de la tete chez les ichthyopsides. *Arch Zool Exp Gen* **13**(2): 369–464.

Pickering AD (1984). Cortisol induced lymphocytopenia in brown trout, *Salmo trutta* L. *Gen Comp Endocrinol* **53**: 252–259.

Pickering AD (1986). Changes in blood cell composition of the brown trout *Salmo trutta* L. during the spawning season. *J Fish Biol* **29**: 335–347.

Pickering AD and Pottinger TG (1985). Cortisol can increase the susceptibility of brown trout *Salmo trutta* L. to disease without reducing the white blood cell count. *J Fish Biol* **27**: 611–619.

Pickering AD and Pottinger TG (1987). Lymphocytopenia and interrenal activity during sexual maturation in the brown trout *Salmo trutta* L. *J Fish Biol* **30**: 41–50.

Pickering AD, Pottinger TG and Christie P (1982). Recovery of the brown trout *Salmo trutta* L. from acute handling stress: a time-course study. *J Fish Biol* **20**: 229–244.

Pickford GE, Srivastava AK, Slicher AM and Pang PKT (1971). The stress response in the abundance of circulating leucocytes in the killifish, *Fundulus heteroclitus*. III.

The role of the adrenal cortex and a discussion of the leucocyte-stress syndrome. *J Exp Zool* **117**: 109–118.

Plytycz B and Bigaj J (1983). Seasonal cyclic changes in the thymus of the adult frog *Rana temporaria*. *Thymus* **5**: 327–344.

Poels CLM, van der Graag MA and van der Kerkhoff JFJ (1980). An investigation into the long term effects of Rhine water on rainbow trout. *Water Res* **14**: 1029–1035.

Rasquin P (1951). Effects of carp pituitary and mammalian ACTH on the endocrine and lymphoid system of the teleost *Astyanax mexicanus*. *J Exp Zool* **117**: 317–334.

Rasquin P and Rosenbloom L (1954). Endocrine imbalance and tissue hyperplasia in teleosts maintained in darkness. *Bull Am Mus Nat Hist* **104**: 359–426.

Riddle O (1928). Studies on the physiology of reproduction in birds. XXII. Growth of the gonads and bursii Fabricii in doves and pigeons, with data for body growth and age at maturity. *Am J Physiol* **86**: 248: 265.

Ridgway GJ (1962). The application of some special immunological methods to marine population problems. *Am Nat* **96**: 219–224.

Rijkers GT, Frederix-Wolders EM and van Muiswinkel WB (1980). The immune system of cyprinid fish. Kinetics and temperature dependence of antibody-producing cells in carp (*Cyprinus carpio*). *Immunology* **41**: 91–97.

Rijkers GT, van Oosterom R and van Muiswinkel WB (1981a). The immune system of cyprinid fish. Oxytetracycline and the regulation of humoral immunity in carp. *Vet Immunol Immunopathol* **2**: 281–290.

Rijkers GT, Wiegerick JAM, van Oosterom R and van Muiswinkel WB (1981b). Temperature dependence of humoral immunity on carp (*Cyprinus carpio*). In Solomon JB (Ed), *Aspects of Developmental and Comparative Immunology I.* Pergamon Press: Oxford. pp 233–240.

Robertson OH and Wexler BC (1960). Histological changes in the organs and tissues of migrating and spawning Pacific salmon (genus *Oncorhynchus*). *Endocrinology* **66**: 222–239.

Robertson OH, Hane S, Wexler BC and Rinfret AP (1963). The effect of hydrocortisone on immature rainbow trout (*Salmo gairdneri*). *Gen Comp Endocrinol* **3**: 422–436.

Robohm RA (1986). Paradoxical effects of cadmium exposure on anti-bacterial antibody responses in two fish species: inhibition in cunners (*Tautogolabrus adspersus*) and enhancement in striped bass (*Morone saxatilis*). *Vet Immunol Immunopathol* **12**: 251–262.

Robohm RA and Nitkowski MF (1974). Physiological response of the cunner *Tautogolabrus adspersus* to cadmium. IV. Effects on the immune system. *NOAA Tech. Rep NMFS SSRF-681*: 15–20.

Rollins LA and McKinnell RG (1980). The influence of glucocorticoids on survival and growth of allografted tumors in the anterior eye chamber of leopard frogs. *Dev Comp Immunol* **4**: 283–294.

Ruben LN and Gwinnell EM (1977). The effects of hydrocortisone and bacterial lipopolysaccharide on the anti-erythrocyte response in the spleens of adult *Triturus viridescens*. *J Exp Zool* **200**: 137–142.

Ruben LN and Vaughan MR (1974). The effect of hydro-cortisone on the sheep red cell response in adult *Xenopus laevis*, the South African clawed toad. *J Exp Zool* **190**: 229–236.

Ruben LN, Buenafe A, Oliver S, Malley A, Barr K and Lukas D (1985). Suppression in *Xenopus laevis*: thymus inducer, spleen effector cells. *Immunology* **54**: 65–70.

Ruglys MP (1985). The secondary immune response of young carp *Cyprinus carpio* L. following injection of cortisol. *J Fish Biol* **26**: 429–434.

Russell WJ, Taylor SA and Sigel MM (1976). Clearance of bacteriophage in poikilothermic vertebrates and the effect of temperature. *J Ret Soc* **19**: 91–96.

Saad AH (1985). Corticosteroids and immune system of the lizard *Chalcides ocellatus*. PhD thesis, Faculty of Science, Cairo University.

Saad AH (1988). Corticosteroids and immune systems of non-mammalian vertebrates: A review. *Dev Comp Immunol* **12**: 481–494.

Saad AH and El Ridi R (1984). Mixed leukocyte reaction, graft-versus-host-reaction and skin allograft rejection in the lizard *Chalcides ocellatus*. *Immunobiology* **166**: 484–493.

Saad AH, El Ridi R, Zada S and Badir N (1984). Effects of hydrocortisone on immune system of the lizard *Chalcides ocellatus*. II. Differential action on T and B lymphocytes. *Dev Comp Immunol* **8**: 835–844.

Saad AH, El Ridi R, El Deeb S and Soliman MAW (1987). Corticosteroids and immune system in the lizard *Chalcides ocellatus*. In Cooper EL, Langlet C and Bierne J (Eds), *Developmental and Comparative Immunology*. Alan R Liss: New York. pp 129–140.

Saad AH, El Deeb S and Zapata A (1988). Seasonal variations and corticosteroid sensitivity in the Thy-1[+] lymphoid population of the lizard *Chalcides ocellatus*. *Thymus* **12**: 3–9.

Salkind J (1915). Contributions à histologiques à la biologie comparée du thyme. *Arch Zool Exp Gen* **2**: 81–332.

Salomoni C, Fiorentino M and Palenzona DL (1987). Effects of diet, sham immunization and bleeding on the immune response kinetics for two strains of *Cyprinus carpio*. *J Fish Biol* **31** (Suppl A): 93–99.

Sarot DA and Perlmutter A (1976). The toxicity of zinc to the immune response of the zebrafish *Brachydanio rerio* injected with viral and bacterial antigens. *Trans Am Fish Soc* **105**: 456–459.

Scott T, van der Zijpp A and Glick B (1985). Effect of thiouracil-induced hypothyroidism on the humoral immunity of New Hampshire chickens. *Poultry Sci* **64**: 2211–2217.

Shivatcheva TM and Hadjioloff AI (1987a). Adaptive seasonal involution of the ground squirrel thymus. *Thymus* **10**: 251–255.

Shivatcheva TM and Hadjioloff AI (1987b). Seasonal involution of gut-associated lymphoid tissue of the European ground squirrel. *Dev Comp Immunol* **11**: 791–799.

Shivatcheva TM, Goranov IT and Hadjioloff AI (1980). Seasonal involution of the thymus of the European ground squirrel (*Citellus citellus* L.). *CR Acad Bulg Sci* **33**: 1685 ff.

Silkworth JB and Grabstein EM (1982). Polychlorinated biphenyl immunotoxicity: dependence on isomer planarity and the Ah gene complex. *Toxicol Appl Pharmacol* **65**: 109–115.

Silverin B (1981). Reproductive effort as expressed in body and organ weights, in the pied fly catcher. *Ornis Scand* **12**: 133–139.

Slicher AM (1961). Endocrinological and haematological studies in *Fundulus heteroclitus* (Linn). *Bull Bingham Oceanogr Collect* **17**: 3–55.

Srivastava AK and Agrawal V (1981). Seasonal and diurnal variations of blood cell types on a freshwater teleost *Colisa fasciatus*. *Comp Physiol Ecol* **6**: 19–24.

Stave JW and Roberson BS (1985). Hydrocortisone suppresses the chemiluminescent response of striped bass phagocytes. *Dev Comp Immunol* **9**: 77–84.

Steuke EW and Atherton CR (1965). Use of microhematocrit values to sex largemouth bass. *Prog Fish Cult* **27**: 87–89.

Stolen JS, Gahn T and Nagle J (1982). The humoral antibody formation to erythrocyte antigens in three species of flatfish. *Dev Comp Immunol Suppl* **2**: 101–106.

Stolen JS, Gahn T, Kasper V and Nagle JJ (1984). The effect of environmental temperature on the immune response of a marine teleost (*Paralichthys dentatus*). *Dev Comp Immunol* **8**: 89–98.

Sypek JP and Burreson EM (1983). Influence of temperature on the immune response of juvenile summer flounder, *Paralichthys dentatus*, and its role in the elimination of *Trypanoplasma bullocki* infections. *Dev Comp Immunol* **7**: 277–286.

Tait NN (1969). The effect of temperature on the immune response in cold-blooded vertebrates. *Physiol Zool* **42**: 29–35.

Tamura E (1978). Studies on the morphology of the thymus in some Japanese fishes. *Spec Publ Sado Marine Biological Station*, Niigata University. pp 1–75.

Tamura E and Honma Y (1970). Histological changes in the organs and tissues of the gobiid fishes throughout their life span. III. Hemopoietic organs in the ice-goby *Leucopsarion petersi* Hilgendorf. *Bull Jap Soc Sci Fish* **36**: 661–669.

Tamura E and Honma Y (1973). Histological changes in the organs and tissues of the gobiid fishes throughout their life-span. V. Seasonal changes in the branchial organs of the flat-head goby in relation to sexual maturity. *Bull Jap Soc Sci Fish* **39**: 1003–1011.

Tamura E and Honma Y (1974). Histological changes in the organs and tissues of the gobiid fish throughout their life-span. VI. Seasonal changes in the lymphopoietic organs of the flat head goby. *Bull Jap Soc Sci Fish* **40**: 447–455.

Tamura E and Honma Y (1975). Histological changes in the organs and tissues of the gobiid fishes throughout their life-span. VII. Seasonal changes in the hemopoietic organs of the fork tongue goby. *Bull Jap Soc Sci Fish* **41**: 413−422.

Tamura E and Honma Y (1977). Histological changes in the organs and tissues of the gobiid fish throughout their life span. VIII. Seasonal changes in the thymus of four species of gobies. *Bull Jap Soc Sci Fish* **43**: 963−974.

Tamura E and Honma Y (1979). Seasonal changes in the thymus of young guppy (Abstract). *Ann Meet Jap Soc Sci Fish* p 101.

Tamura E, Honma Y and Kitamura Y (1981). Seasonal changes in the thymus of the viviparous surfperch, *Ditrema temmincki*, with special reference to its maturity and gestation. *Jap J Ichthyol* **28**: 295−303.

Taniguchi M (1983). Effects of the food quality on the appearance of yellowtail streptococcicosis. *Bull Jap Soc Sci Fish* **49**: 363−366.

Taylor CR and Skinner JM (1976). Evidence for significant hematopoiesis in the human thymus. *Blood* **47**: 305−313.

Thomas P and Lewis DH (1987). Effects of cortisol on immunity in red drum *Sciaenops ocellatus*. *J Fish Biol* **31** (Suppl A): 123−128.

Tomasso JR, Simco BA and Davis KB (1983). Circulating corticosteroid and leukocyte dynamics in channel catfish (*Ictalurus punctatus*) during net confinement. *Tex J Sci* **35**: 83−88.

Toro I, Olah I, Rohlich P and Viragh SZ (1969). Electron microscopic observations on myoid cells of the frog's thymus. *Anat Rec* **165**: 329−341.

Tournefier A (1982). Corticosteroid action on lymphocyte subpopulations and humoral immune response of axolotl (urodele amphibian). *Immunology* **46**: 155−162.

Tripp RA, Maule AG, Schreck CB and Kaatari SL (1987). Cortisol mediated suppression of salmonid lymphocyte responses *in vitro*. *Dev Comp Immunol* **11**: 565−576.

Truelove J, Grant D, Mes J, Tryphanos H, Tryphanos L and Sawidzka Z (1982). Polychlorinated biphenyl toxicity in the pregnant *Cynomolgus* monkey: a pilot study. *Arch Environ Contam Toxicol* **11**: 583−588.

van Muiswinkel WB, Anderson DP, Lamers CHJ, Egberts E, Loon van JJA and Ijssel JP (1985). Fish immunology and fish health. In Manning MJ and Tatner MF (Eds), *Fish Immunology*. Academic Press: London. pp 1−8.

van Vuren JHJ and Hattingh J (1978). A seasonal study of the haematology of wild freshwater fish. *J Fish Biol* **13**: 305−313.

Viale G and Calamari D (1984). Immune response in rainbow trout *Salmo gairdneri*, after long-term treatment with low levels of Cr, Cd, and Cu. *Environ Pollut (Ser A)* **35**: 247−257.

Viklicky V, Polackova M, Vojtiskova M, Draber P and Khoda ME (1977). Immunosuppressive effect of an antiandrogenic steroid (cyproterone acetate) in mice. *Folia Biol Praha* **23**: 145−157.

Viklicky V, Pokorna Z, Draker P, Polackova M and Vojtiskova M (1979). Mechanism of immune suppressive action of the anti-androgenic steroid cyproterone acetate (CA). *Proc 4 Symp Immunology of Reproduction*, p 806.

von Braunmulh A (1926). Uber einige myelolymphoide und lymphoepitheliae organe der anuren. *Letsch Mikrosk Anat Forch* **4**: 635−688.

Vos JE, van Driel and Grootenhuis L (1972). PCB-induced suppression of the humoral and cell-mediated immunity in guinea pigs. *Sci Total Environ* **1**: 289−302.

Ward P and Kendall MD (1975). Morphological changes in the thymus of young and adult red-billed queleas (*Quelea quelea*) (Aves). *Phil Trans R Soc B* **273**: 55−64.

Weatherley AH (1963). Thermal stress and interrenal tissue in the perch *Perca fluviatilis* (Linnaeus). *Proc Zool Soc Lond* **141**: 527−555.

Weeks BA and Warinner JE (1984). Effects of toxic chemicals on macrophage phagocytosis in two estuarine fishes. *Mar Environ Res* **14**: 327−335.

Weeks BA and Warinner JE (1986). Functional evaluation of macrophages in fish from a polluted estuary. *Vet Immunol Immunopathol* **12**: 313−320.

Weetman AP, McGregor AM, Ludgate M and Hall R (1984). Effect of triiodothyroxine on normal human lymphocyte function. *J Endocrinol* **101**: 81−86.

White A and Fletcher TC (1985). Seasonal changes in serum glucose and condition of the plaice *Pleuronectes platessa* L. *J Fish Biol* **26**: 755−764.

White A, Fletcher TC and Pepys MB (1983). Serum concentrations of C-reactive protein and serum amyloid P component in place (*Pleuronectes platessa* L) in relation to season and injected lipopolysaccharide. *Comp Biochem Physiol* **74B**: 453−458.

Wolfe HS, Sheridan SA, Bilstad NM and Johnson MA (1962). The growth of lymphoidal organs and the testes of chickens. *Anat Rec* **142**: 485−494.

Wolke RE (1984). Using fish as pollution monitors. *University of Rhode Island Marine Resources Information*, p 136.

Wolke RE, Murchelano RE, Dickstein CD and George CJ (1985). Preliminary evaluation of the use of macrophage aggregates (MA) as fish health monitors. *Bull Environ Contam Toxicol* **35**: 222−227.

Worley RTS and Jurd RD (1979). The effect of a laboratory environment on graft rejection in *Lacerta viridis*, the European green lizard. *Dev Comp Immunol* **3**: 653−665.

Wright RK and Cooper EL (1980). Temperature and immunological memory in anuran amphibians. In Manning MJ (Ed), *Phylogeny of Immunological Memory*. Elsevier/North-Holland Biomedical Press: New York. pp 155−166.

Wright, RK and Cooper EL (1981). Temperature effects on ectotherm immune responses. *Dev Comp Immunol* **5** (Suppl 1): 117−122.

Yam D, Heller D and Snapir DJ (1981). The effect of the thyroidal state on the immunological state of the chicken. *Dev Comp Immunol* **5**: 483−490.

Yamaguchi N, Teshima C, Kurashige S, Saito T and Mitsuhashi S (1981). Seasonal modulation of antibody formation in rainbow trout (*Salmo gairdneri*). In Solomon JB (Ed), *Aspects of Developmental and Comparative*

Immunology. Pergamon Press: Oxford. pp 483—484.

Zapata A, Villena A and Cooper EL (1982). Direct contacts between nerve endings and lymphoid cells in the jugular body of *Rana pipiens*. *Experientia* **38**: 623—624.

Zapata A, Garrido E, Leceta J and Gomariz RP (1983). Relationships between neuroendocrine and immune system in amphibians and reptiles. *Dev Comp Immunol* **7**: 771—774.

Zeeman MG (1980). Effects of DDT upon the hematology and immunology of the goldfish (*Carassius auratus*). PhD dissertation. Logan: Utah State University. p 133.

Zeeman MG and Brindley WA (1981). Effects of toxic agents upon fish immune systems: A review. In Sharma RP (Ed), *Immunological Considerations in Toxicology*. Vol II. CRC Press: Boca Raton, Florida. pp 1—60.

10

Recapitulations and Directions

INTRODUCTION

In the other chapters, we have reviewed the main histophysiological aspects of cells, tissues and organs involved in vertebrate immune responses and herein we will present some general conclusions. Especially striking is the abundance of distinct lymphohemopoietic organs, functionally equivalent to bone marrow, occurring in lower vertebrates, particularly in fish. There is little understanding of their immune significance though their basic histological organization and even ultrastructural features are relatively well known. Furthermore, the classification as central or primary lymphoid organs (thymus, bone marrow/bursa of Fabricius) and peripheral or secondary lymphoid organs (spleen, lymph nodes, GALT) assumed for homothermic vertebrates, mainly birds, cannot be applied so strictly yet to ectotherms, where many lymphoid tissues are truly a mixture of lymphohemopoietic organs, actually a chimeric condition.

THE GENESIS OF VERTEBRATE IMMUNITY— SITES OF HEMOPOIESIS, LYMPHOID PRECURSOR STEM CELLS, BONE MARROW AND BURSA OF FABRICIUS

The immunological condition of Agnatha deserves special attention where typical T- and B-like cell reactivities have repeatedly been documented but morphologically identifiable thymus, bone marrow and spleen

are lacking. In myxinoids, hemopoietic aggregates of the intestinal lamina propria and the central mass of the pronephros are the main lymphohemopoietic organs. Both organs resemble both structurally and functionally bone marrow of homothermic vertebrates, which exhibits a capacity for hemopoiesis, but in the intestine granulopoiesis predominates. The pronephros houses, in addition, mature and developing erythrocytes, lymphocytes and plasma cells. Despite the possession of these several cell types, the immunological significance of both organs is unknown.

In lampreys, the lymphohemopoietic system, like other physiological systems, undergoes profound modifications during their complex life-cycle. These changes indicate the importance of cell microenvironments in determining the lymphohemopoietic capacity of distinct organs. In larval ammocoetes, both typhlosole and opisthonephros are the principal lymphohemopoietic organs. The transformation of the intestine during metamorphosis, which includes changes in the epithelium, development of villi and improved circulatory patterns, supports an increased connective tissue of the lamina propria and disappearance of sinusoids. Consequently, the organ loses its lymphohemopoietic capacity. A similar condition will occur in the opisthonephros. The nephric fold in ammocoetes houses developing blood cells in a connective tissue stroma which surrounds tubules or even adipocytes. At the beginning of metamorphosis, the larval opisthonephros regresses, thus revealing greatly reduced blood sinuses, degenerated renal tubules and increasing stromal connective tissue. At the end of metamorphosis, the recently formed mature opistho-nephros has no lymphohemopoietic capacity, although in old specimens the organ becomes again a hemopoietic locus. In contrast, the supraneural body represents the most important hemopoietic locus in adult lampreys. The evolution of this organ is in obvious contrast to that exhibited by the typhlosole and opisthonephros. Until premetamorphosis the supraneural body is not lymphohemopoietic, but in young lampreys numerous lymphohemopoietic aggregates begin to appear in it. Despite these differences in the time when they acquire hemopoietic functioning, the typhlosole, opisthonephros and supraneural body show a similar histological organization. This similarity is established on the basis of stroma, reticular cells and sinusoidal blood vessels, which resemble the cell microenvironments of bone marrow which are known to be inductive.

In any case, the most striking condition of Agnatha is the lack of a thymus or thymic equivalents. Meticulous structural studies have confirmed the absence of a thymus gland in these primitive vertebrates despite pioneer reports signaling (1) lymphoid infiltrates into the velar muscle complex of Pacific hagfish or (2) lymphoid accumulations in the lamprey's pharynx which may act as thymus equivalents. The obvious question is: when these organisms without an apparently functional thymus do mount typical T-dependent immune responses or its corollary, is a thymus really necessary for normal development and function of vertebrate T-lymphocytes? Some data derived from higher vertebrates which are thymusless push us to question also the central immunological function of the thymus gland.

Table 3.1 enumerates a range of lymphohemopoietic organs in fish and amphibians that assume the functional role of mammalian bone marrow, which houses and serves as a site for differentiating hemopoietic stem cells. The list may be extended by adding recent reports which have demonstrated a meningeal lymphohemopoietic tissue in the sting-ray *Dasyatis akajei* (Chiba *et al.*, 1988). As in the case of lymphohemopoietic organs of Agnatha, the histological organization of all these organs resembles the cell microenvironments of bone marrow. Consequently, probably all vertebrates, including those without bone marrow, possess loci where blood stem cells are able to find adequate cell conditions for their safe keeping and nutrition that will, in turn, promote differentiating

blood cell lineages, some of which will surely include immunocompetent cells.

Unfortunately, except for the teleost kidney, the immunological role of all these organs (with microenvironments) is scarcely understood. Improved histophysiological and immunological studies which will focus on the immune system of these primitive fish will provide invaluable information on the phylogenetic origins of vertebrate immune responses. Obviously, a first unresolved problem is the source of lymphoid cell precursors in ectothermic vertebrates. Despite some reports which claim that the teleost pronephros, urodelean liver and anuran embryonic mesoderm are sources of lymphocyte precursors, little confirmed information is available. In the next few years, new data may be obtained which may have been derived from these and other experimental models that are relatively easy to keep under laboratory conditions (e.g. lampreys, dogfish, teleosts, urodeles and reptiles) and whose precursor cells may be amenable to cultivation *in vitro*.

The special condition of the avian immune system is characterized by the existence of the bursa of Fabricius, a lymphoid organ unique to birds. The structure and function of the bursa of Fabricius have been extensively studied in *Gallus domesticus*; however, some pioneer studies in other species have demonstrated important anatomical and histological variations on the common pattern found in chickens. Currently unknown, the immunological significance in a wider range of avian species deserves further investigations. The bursa of Fabricius, as the thymus, undergoes an involution during aging, a process that is characterized by decreased weight, mucoid involution and replacement of lymphoid cells by fibrotic tissue. Little is known about the regulatory mechanisms, although hormones, mainly sex steroids, have been implicated. However, the aged bursa of Struthioniformes, remarkably, undergoes metaplasia rather than involution.

Three histological stages are recognized chronologically during the embryonic development of the bursa of Fabricius: the formation of the anlage, the follicular appearance and the maturation of the follicles. Mesenchyme—epithelium interactions seem to be crucial for the appearance of lymphoid follicle, although the true inductive mechanisms are poorly established. Besides, although the bursa of Fabricius is clearly a lymphoid organ, the surrounding mesenchyme houses transitional, active granulopoiesis as well as discrete erythropoiesis which disappear at hatching. Whether common or specific committed hemopoietic precursors are involved in these distinct functions is still controversial.

As in the thymus—the other central lymphoid organ of vertebrates—epithelial–lymphoid interactions are essential for normal development and function of the bursa of Fabricius. Thus, in the three principal areas of the bursa of Fabricius—the follicle-associated epithelium (FAE), the follicular cortex and medulla— intimate interactions occur between the epithelia and the lymphoid elements. The follicle-associated epithelium is formed by long cells exhibiting an endocytic capacity. They make contact basically with the reticuloepithelial cells which form the supporting network of the follicular medulla. A mesenchymatous or epithelial nature has been postulated for the bursal follicle-associated epithelium, where there is evidence to support both views. The functional significance of FAE is also a matter of discussion. Some workers point out the need for antigenic transport through the FAE in order to induce bursal lymphopoiesis and B-cell differentiation. Instead, true antigenic stimulation could accelerate the development of lineages of antibody-forming cells.

Although the ultrastructural organization of the bursal follicles is well known, recent reports have described the presence of non-lymphoid cells within it, the immunological significance of which requires further clarification. Dendritic-like cells may be the first cells which colonize the bursal epithelium and they may represent either antigen-presenting cells or monocyte–macrophage precursors. Secretory-like cells observed in the chicken's bursal medulla by Glick and Olah (1987) related to the ellipsoid-associated reticulum cells which are involved in antigen trapping and processing in chicken spleen. However, recent immunohistochemical data do not support this relationship.

During the last few years, analyses using monoclonal antibodies reactive for bursal stroma, B-lymphocytes and their precursors have enhanced our knowledge of the ontogenetic development and immune function of the bursa of Fabricius. Recent immunohistochemical studies using monoclonal antibodies against bursal stroma have revealed developmental relationships between adult medulla and embryonic surface epithelium, while monoclonal anti-bodies directed against adult cortex have also been shown to stain the embryonic lamina propria.

Lymphoid differentiation in the bursal follicle depends on migration of blood-derived precursors from extrabursal mesenchyme. Chemotacting and immobilizing humoral factors have been involved in the bursal colonization by lymphoid stem cells. These precursors, already committed to the B-cell lineage, express Ia-antigen and other non-Ig, non-BL, B-lymphocyte determinants similar to L-22 or Bu-1a, contain unrearranged Ig genes and appear first in the lamina propria of 10-day embryos and on day 12 in developing epithelial buds. The CB-1 homodimer, as well as the CB-2 and HNK-1 antigens, are expressed exclusively on intrabursal B-cells but are lost when B-lymphocytes migrate to peripheral lymphoid organs. Other markers, including BU-1, CB-3, CB-5 and sIg, are, however, expressed on B-cells throughout the body and some of them, such as CB-5, on plasma cells. The number of lymphoid stem cells which colonize a bursal follicle is small, and although B-cell proliferation is rapid only 15% of the cells produced in it will migrate to the periphery, with most new cells dying in situ. On the other hand, intrabursal B-cell maturation occurs independently in each follicle, deriving additional cortical and medullary cells in the same follicle from the same precursors.

The avian bursa of Fabricius seems to function as both a central lymphoid organ during ontogeny and an antibody-producing, peripheral lymphoid organ after hatching, especially in the per-anum antigen stimulation. The peripheral function of the bursa has been proposed as serving to create an antibody repertoire necessary for host survival in a given environment. As a central lymphoid organ, the specific function of the bursa is to generate clonal and isotypic diversity and not initiation of B-cell development. This consequently implies that Ig gene rearrangements during development occur exclusively within the bursa. Moreover, since the mechanisms of generating Ig variability in birds seem to be different from those in mammals, a likely conclusion is that the functions of the bursa are to provide an environment where rapid cell divisions will allow the generation of diversity from a limited germ-line repertoire by the accumulation of somatic modifications.

A striking, non-follicular region which probably plays an important role in immune responses via cloacal antigenic stimulation occurs after hatching, in the bursal duct. This area, sometimes called the diffusely infiltrated lymphoid area, shows typical characteristics, which include presence of postcapillary venules and interdigitating cells, a highly developed reticular fiber stroma and immuno-identification of T-lymphocytes, in T-dependent areas of peripheral lymphoid organs. Nevertheless, despite their strategic location, which ensures intimate contact with environmental antigens, their role in the repeatedly demonstrated antibody production by the bursa is unclear.

ANOTHER PRIMARY ORGAN—WAS THE THYMUS NECESSARY?

The thymus gland is present in all vertebrates except perhaps for the Agnatha; thus it appears for the first time in Chondrichthyes. There are minimal structural differences between the distinct vertebrate classes—the most relevant are: the absence of a clear cortex—medulla demarcation in teleosts, Apoda and Urodela and the lack of typical Hassall's bodies in all ectotherms. Special attention should be given to the thymus of teleostean fish, which retains its embryological connection with the pharyngeal cavity during adult life and where attempts to establish histological correlations with higher vertebrate thymus, particularly mammals, is almost impossible. Nevertheless recent histochemical and ultrastructural studies on the thymus of *Salmo gairdneri* have demonstrated the existence of non-lymphoid cell microenvironments in various zones which are histophysiologically equivalent to those described in the thymic cortex and medulla of higher vertebrates (Castillo *et al.*, 1989a, b; Rasquin *et al.*, 1989). The possible arrival of antigenic material into the thymic parenchyma through the pharyngeal epithelium, due to anatomical proximity, is an important functional aspect of the teleost thymus which remains, however, still unresolved.

In contrast, minimal anatomical differences related to thymic location, number of thymic lobes and number of pharyngeal pouches involved in the embryonic development have been reported between different vertebrate species. Especially notable is the condition of some primitive mammals which show two thymus glands—one thoracic and another cervical. Moreover, the immunological importance of the vertebrate thymus is emphasized by the fact that in most vertebrates it is the first organ to become lymphoid during ontogeny. Despite these morphological variations, functional evidence from teleosts, amphibians and reptiles supports the view that the thymus of ectothermic vertebrates plays, in general, the same immunological role as it does in mammals.

Information on the origin of lymphoid stem cells, ways of migration to T-cell precursors to the thymus and those factors involved in its colonization, are limited and are mainly restricted to some anuran species (see review by Katagiri and Tochinai, 1987). Stem cells enter the larval *Xenopus* thymus at 3–4 days of age (Tochinai, 1978; Kurihara and Kato, 1986) and monoclonal antibodies produced against T-cell specific antigens detect the first positive T-cells at stage 48 (7 days old) with a sharp increase until stage 49 (10 days old) (Nagata, 1986).

By using chimeras produced between diploid and triploid tailbud embryos, dorsal lateral plate and ventral blood island mesoderms have been identified as two different loci which supply hemopoietic precursors (Maeno *et al.*, 1985a, b). The dorsolateral plate mesoderm contributes to the major hemopoietic population of advanced larvae and adults, while the ventral blood islands supply the major hemopoietic cells in early larvae and a minor population in advanced larvae and adults. Thus, at the neural fold stage, precursor cells of larval thymocytes are localized in both of these hemopoietic compartments, whereas those for erythrocytes occur only in the ventral blood island region (Kau and Turpen, 1983). Ventral blood island-derived cells enter the circulation around stage 35/36 when just the circulatory system is established. Some of these cells leave the blood vessels around the jugular vein and/or internal carotid artery to migrate through the mesenchyme to the thymic anlage. It is unknown if chemotactic factors, as those recently reported in birds and mammals, contribute to this migration. Ventral blood island-derived cells migrate also to the liver, where B-lymphocyte precursors are housed, and differentiate in anurans (Hadji-Azimi *et al.*, 1982). On the other hand, Turpen and Smith (1986) have recently provided circumstantial evidence indicating that thymocytes and thymic accessory cells could arise from a bipotential precursor that diverges into these separate lineages after colonization of the epithelial thymic rudiment.

The thymus in all vertebrates is an encapsulated

organ, the parenchyma of which contains a non-lymphoid stroma and abundant maturing thymocytes. There are three major components of the thymic stroma: (1) fibroblasts which form the connective tissue capsule and the thymic trabeculae; (2) epithelial cells which constitute the main support elements in both cortex and medulla, and an additional heterogeneous population of medullary cells whose true function still remains to be resolved; (3) blood-borne cells which include monocytes/macrophages, interdigitating cells and dendritic-like cells. Moreover, myoid cells, plasma cells, mast cells and granulocytes occur in the vertebrate thymus.

Apart from the above-mentioned mechanical supporting function, thymic epithelial cells have been implicated in mammals in the phenomenon of intrathymic positive and negative selection which triggers the differentiation of thymocytes. The process has been structurally related to the *in vitro* and *in vivo* identification of lymphostromal complexes, which contain developing thymocytes and nurse-epithelial cells. In *Xenopus laevis*, Holtfreter and Cohen (1987) identified thymic nurse cell-like structures in mechanically dissociated tadpole thymuses as an intact thymocyte-filled multistromal cell rather than a single cell compartment. On the other hand, Flajnik *et al.* (1985) demonstrated that chimeric *Xenopus*, produced by joining the anterior portion of one 24-hour embryo which contains the thymic epithelial anlage to the posterior region of an MHC-incompatible embryo source of hemopoietic stem cells, exhibited thymus glands composed of epithelium of one MHC and thymocytes of the other one. Recently, Horton *et al.* (1987) pointed out that, in addition to epithelial cells, a whole range of stromal cell types remain after introducing a foreign thymus into a thymectomized larva which probably influences one of the differentiating thymic structures.

Further research must therefore be focused on a more reliable, structural, phenotypical and functional characterization of stromal cells which constitute the thymic cell microenvironments in ectothermic vertebrates. In any case, the condition is extremely striking in anuran amphibians, i.e. *Xenopus*, since it has been demonstrated that class II molecules are present throughout ontogeny, while class I antigens appear at metamorphosis (Flajnik *et al.*, 1987). The obvious question is, as the allogeneic recognition and sub-sequent responses are expressed by larvae, how can they discriminate the MHC antigens to self and non-self without their own MHC? Flajnik and colleagues have speculated that this condition may be advantageous for tadpoles in order to protect themselves against autoimmunity. If tadpoles expressed class I molecules and therefore generated MHC-restricted cytotoxic T-cells directed against viral antigens, these might cross-react on the newly arising minor H antigens, which might induce autoimmune reactions. We could add, though, that autoimmune phenomena have not been demonstrated in anuran amphibians, unless we assume that the metamorphic event, although triggered by hormonal changes, is at the same time an autoimmune event. Therefore, it is becoming increasingly important to determine conclusively whether or not anuran tadpoles possess class I restricted cytotoxic T-lymphocytes.

Available data on the function of intrathymic macrophages, dendritic-like cells and interdigitating cells are almost non-existent in non-mammalian vertebrates. In chickens, there are apparently two populations of thymic accessory cells: one with typical characteristics of macrophages, which does not express Ia molecules, and the other which shows surface class II MHC determinants but is devoid of phagocytic capacity. As mentioned earlier, in *Xenopus* precursors of these accessory cells seem to predominate within the thymic rudiment together with the first wave of lymphocytes. The presence of thymic interdigitating cells has been reported in a few species of birds, reptiles and anuran amphibians. They resemble, morphologically, those found in central and peripheral lymphoid organs of mammals, although no Birbeck's granules have been observed in ectotherms. Nevertheless, the origin of interdigitating cells, their immunological functions and relationships to other blood-borne cells, such as macrophages and dendritic-like cells, remains unknown, even in mammals.

One of the most exciting features of the vertebrate thymus is the existence of a myriad of medullary epithelial cell types whose function is scarcely understood. Some of these cells exhibit an apparently secretory-like capacity as mucus cells or thymic hormone-producing elements. Immunohistochemical or functional evidence of hormonal factors in non-mammalian thymus has been reported in a few species of teleosts and urodelan amphibians and in chickens.

Most workers have considered Hassall's corpuscles to be absent in the thymus of ectothermic vertebrates, although frequently found groups of medullary epithelial cells or degenerative epithelial cysts have repeatedly been claimed as their precursors or equivalents. Even in the avian thymus, the occurrence of true Hassall bodies is controversial. Additionally, their immunological significance is obscure.

Uni- and multicellular epithelial cysts are, on the contrary, constant components of the thymic medulla of all vertebrates. Especially remarkable is the finding in the thymus of *Xenopus laevis*, later confirmed in *Bufo calamita* and *Rana pipiens* (Barrutia *et al.*, 1989), of epithelial cysts containing thyrotropin-releasing hormone and 5-hydroxytryptamine which resemble skin glands morphologically. Likewise, multinucleated giant cells, found in the thymus of the natterjack, *Bufo calamita*, may be related to presumptive antigen-presenting cells in the spleen of this same toad and they may play a role in the above-mentioned MHC-restricted education of thymocytes. From the demonstration of endocrine-like cells in the thymus of some non-mammalian vertebrates arises the subject of the phylogeny of the neuroendocrine — immune relationships which are now known to exist in mammals. A role for endocrine-like cells in the regulation of immunological functions of the thymus in ectothermic vertebrates could be confirmed by further experiments.

Immature, mature and degenerative myoid cells are frequent in the thymus of all vertebrates, although the assumption of a greater number in ectothermic vertebrates than in endotherms has not been confirmed. Nevertheless, they are especially abundant in some amphibians and reptiles. The results of pioneer work on the origin of thymic myoid cells disagree, but recent experiments using quail — chick chimeras have determined that myoid cells originate from neural crest. In addition, the functional significance of thymic myoid cells is unclear. They have been claimed as an intrathymic source of muscle-specific self-antigens, although their reported role, if any, in the autoimmune disease myasthenia gravis is still not clear.

Although the presence of intrathymic plasma cells has repeatedly been reported in numerous vertebrates, little attention has been paid to their immunological significance. Some workers, however, have emphasized that although low, the number of thymic plasma cells is not functionally irrelevant, which suggests that they may represent a subset of B-lymphocytes which rest in or pass through the thymus as a necessary mechanism for the regulation of immune responses.

Erythroid cells usually occur in the thymus (most probably in association with circulatory channels) but a strict thymic erythropoietic capacity has been only occasionally reported, especially in birds and more recently in some teleost species. Remarkably, this thymic erythropoiesis seems to be a cyclic event and it may be related to seasonal variations which are mediated through the sex steroid hormones. As one explanation, the process implicates drastic changes in the thymic cell microenvironment, which includes degeneration of cortical reticuloendothelial cells, thus favoring erythropoiesis versus lymphopoiesis.

Finally, a morphological description of the hemato-thymic barrier has been provided in some ectothermic vertebrates, but experimental evidence of such a barrier is lacking in ectotherms. Besides, recent reports in mammals (Nieuwenhuis *et al.*, 1988) question the physiological significance of the arrival of antigens into the thymic parenchyma and further research must clarify this claim.

MOVING TO THE SECONDARY ORGANS— THE SPLEEN AND BLOOD FLOW AS AN IMPORTANT COMPONENT FOR INITIATING IMMUNE RESPONSES

The spleen is a large organ present in all gnathostomes and its immunological role increases progressively throughout vertebrate phylogeny. It assumes, nevertheless, other hemopoietic functions, especially in ectothermic vertebrates, including erythropoiesis, granulopoiesis and thrombopoiesis. Thus, the vertebrate spleen undergoes histophysiological changes in order to assure an increasing diversity and specialization of its functions.

The spleen is found in all vertebrates, even in primitive holocephalans where it is free in the peritoneal cavity, associated frequently with the pancreas. Except in Dipnoi, it is located within the wall of the stomach and in the anterior region of the intestine. Apparently, this primitive condition may be related to blood vascular dynamics of the foregut and yolk. Furthermore, the histological organization of lungfish spleen is also strikingly primitive.

The spleen in elasmobranchs is a large organ with a well-developed lymphoid component which develops important immunological functions. Ultrastructural and immunohistochemical studies confirm that the spleen is the main site for antibody production in elasmobranchs. On the contrary, the splenic lymphoid tissue is not highly developed in teleosts, and its immunological importance has been questioned. Although the teleost spleen shows histological changes after primary and secondary immunization, and antigen-binding cells and antibody-producing cells have been detected, at least in some teleost species, splenectomy has no effect on immune responses.

In contrast to more immediate immunological functions, special attention should be directed to the structure and biological significance of melanomacrophage centers (MMCs), aggregations of closely packed macrophages which contain heterogeneous inclusions, the most frequent being melanin, hemosiderin and lipofucsin that have been reported in lymphoid organs of fish, mainly teleosts. Apart from trophic functions and a relation with iron – hemoglobin catabolism, MMCs have been correlated with fish immunological reactivity. They are closely associated with lymphocyte aggregates in teleostean lymphoid organs, and ultrastructural and immunohistochemical studies demonstrate that they participate in trapping and processing of antigenic and non-antigenic materials. Nevertheless, though a phylogenetic relationship of the MMCs to germinal centers of endothermic vertebrates is claimed by some comparative immunologists, it is not assumed by others, who consider them instead as domains where numerous physiological products are non-specifically processed and stored.

Splenic morphology in amphibians shows important differences not only between the three main groups but even among various families of the same group. A primitive condition, resembling that of teleosts, is evident in Apoda and Urodela. It consists of small lymphoid aggregates, poorly demarcated, that, however, increase considerably in size and number after immunization. In this regard, typical T- and B-like mediated reactions may be elicited *in vitro* by urodelan splenocytes, but absence of the spleen in these amphibians apparently does not affect allograft rejection.

With some exceptions, the amount of lymphoid tissue is also scarce in anuran amphibians, which prompted Cooper and Wright (1976) to suggest that a trend from primitive to a more advanced white pulp condition developed from a diffuse to a concentrated arrangement of lymphoid elements. A clear distinction between red and white pulp is lacking in primitive anurans but a highly elaborated white pulp, exhibiting a primitive marginal zone formed by flat reticular cell processes, occurs in *Xenopus laevis* and *Bufo calamita*. Moreover, antigen-trapping dendritic-like cells are evident in both species, although some workers have located them in *Xenopus laevis* inside the lymphoid follicles, whereas in *Bufo calamita* they occur in the red pulp immediately surrounding the white pulp. Interdigitating cells have also been found in the splenic lymphoid follicles of *Bufo calamita*.

Thus two histological and probably functional patterns of splenic organization may be proposed in anurans. In *Xenopus*, a member of the primitive family Pipidae, lymphoid tissue surrounding splenic arteries seems to be T-independent. T-like lymphocytes occur near the marginal zone, inside lymphoid follicles, or they form a perifollicular layer. Giant, dendritic, XL-cells located inside the follicles collect and retain antigen – antibody complexes, which have been previously processed by free macrophages of red pulp, where they collaborate with T- and B-lymphocytes. In *Bufo calamita* and probably in *Bufo bufo*, the white pulp consists of an inner T-independent zone and an outer zone where T-lymphocytes predominate. Toward the T-dependent area, giant cells of the red pulp send out cell processes in order to present previously phagocytosed and processed antigens to T-like lymphocytes. This histological regionalization which has been observed in anuran amphibians, though requiring further, functional confirmation, represents an important step in the phylogenetic evolution of the vertebrate spleen.

Histological and ultrastructural changes, including pyroninophilia, increased appearance of lymphoblasts, developing and mature plasma cells, occur in the anuran amphibian spleen after immunization. The morphology can vary, nevertheless, depending upon the antigen. As a result, production of antibodies can be detected by immunofluorescence and enumerated by the PFC assay, a rather common assay when analyzing the anuran spleen. Furthermore, splenocytes may be stimulated by various mitogens, which attests to a difference in cell types required for PHA and Con A responses; these cells can show mixed leukocyte reactivity and express delayed hypersensitivity reactions. Alloreactive cells, on the other hand, occur in the anuran spleen and both the spleen and thymus of *Xenopus laevis* contain apparently suppressor cells which regulate the timing and intensity of allograft rejection. Despite these immunological capacities, it has been claimed that splenectomy in anurans, as in urodeles, has no marked effects on anuran immunological responses. Recently a T-cell growth-like factor has been obtained from cultures of PHA-stimulated adult *Xenopus* splenocytes. Furthermore, splenocyte subpopulations have been characterized using their capacity to bind an anti-human IL-2 receptor antibody. Coupling these findings with recombinant DNA-produced IL-2 will enable additional molecular analysis of ectothermic vertebrate immune reactions.

The incipient compartmentalization reported in some anuran species increases in the reptilian spleen. In some reptiles, mainly turtles, the spleen is composed primarily of white pulp, whereas in others both the red and white pulp are well developed. In addition, the chelonian spleen shows a clear demarcation between red and white pulp, and white pulp shows a morphofunctional regionalization characterized by the presence of both periarteriolar (PALS) and periellipsoidal lymphoid sheaths (PELS), which have been identified in several species.

This regionalization is also evident at the cellular level. For example, in PALS, small lymphocytes, lymphoblasts and interdigitating cells predominate. In PELS, two areas can even be distinguished. In its inner zone, small and medium lymphocytes occur, where they are associated with large dendritic cells, whereas the outer zone contains less lymphoid elements but reticular cells and macrophages abound. Both zones of PELS are demarcated by a discontinuous layer of flat reticular cells, similar to those which occur within the limits between the red and white pulp. Various functional approaches have demonstrated that this histological zonation in reptilian spleen reflects the distribution of lymphocyte subpopulations. Thus, PALS of reptiles consists predominantly of T-cells whereas in PELS B-lymphocytes occur.

Furthermore, trapping and retention of immune complexes by splenic dendritic cells of *Chrysemys scripta elegans* and *Phyton reticulatus* confirm that they resemble mammalian follicular cells. Thus, although involving different non-lymphoid cells in the process, all ectothermic vertebrates, including fish, amphibians and reptiles in which germinal centers are absent, possess the antigen-trapping and processing capacity.

The role played by various lymphoid organs, mainly the spleen, in the reptilian immune responses is unclear. A wide range of variability, perhaps due to species-specific differences, has been observed in the kinetics of humoral responses, and the classical experiments of splenectomy have produced certain contradictory results. Thus, a direct correlation between an increasing histological complexity of the spleen and the immune capacity of reptiles has not been satisfactorily established. In contrast, splenocytes are involved in mixed lymphocyte and graft-versus-host reactions, and undergo strong proliferative responses after mitogenic stimulation. Furthermore, as in anurans, a soluble lymphokine has been isolated from the Con A conditioned medium of cultured spleen cells.

The histological organization of splenic lymphoid tissue in birds, probably governed by a complex pattern of vascularization in which the so-called Schweigger—Seidel sheaths of ellipsoids detach, resembles that described in reptiles rather than that of mammals, although the avian condition is even more elaborate; it even contains germinal centers for the first time. Thus, in the chicken spleen, three compartments can be recognized: (1) PALS occupies areas around central arteries up to the middle portion of the penicilliform capillaries and incorporates germinal centers in association with tertiary arteries; (2) perivenous lymphoid tissue, apparently an extension of the PALS, which occurs along the course of large veins in red pulp; and (3) periellipsoidal lymphoid tissue which is arranged in a less defined region around connective tissue walls of ellipsoids. In this area, non-lymphoid elements referred to as ellipsoid-associated cells (EACs) may be related to antigen trapping.

As reported in other vertebrates, histological regionalization of the avian spleen has a specific distribution of T- and B-lymphoid subpopulations. Thus, numerous studies have pointed out PELS as bursa dependent whereas PALS and perivenous lymphoid tissue are thymus dependent. As in mammals, T- and B-cell cooperation occurs during germinal center formation. In birds, however, mechanisms governing antigen distribution from ellipsoids where it may be trapped from blood circulation and into germinal centers are a matter of discussion. Specifically striking and different from mammals is the fact that birds are apparently unable to discriminate between antigenic and non-antigenic material which is processed by similar mechanisms.

In summary, the spleen, together with the thymus—the most primitive lymphoid organ which is found in vertebrate phylogeny— is involved in the trapping and processing of antigens in close association with blood vascular channels, but a gradual morphofunctional compartmentalization leads to increasing levels of efficiency in its immunological functions.

WHAT ABOUT FLOW OF LYMPH AND CONNECTIONS TO OTHER SECONDARY CENTERS SUCH AS LYMPH NODES?

Contrary to the spleen, present in all gnathostomatous vertebrates, lymph nodes are peripheral lymphoid organs, exclusive to endothermic vertebrates, which reach their full development in eutherian mammals. Although it is difficult to establish phylogenetic equivalents in ectothermic vertebrates, lymph- or vein-associated lymphoid accumulations may be found in anurans and reptiles. In addition, certain primitive lymphoid organs, the so-called lymphomyeloid (LM) organs, of advanced anurans (i.e. *Rana* and *Bufo* sp.) trap and process antigens, eliciting strong immune responses in a functional condition which resembles that of mammalian lymph nodes.

In larval anurans, the lymph gland and ventral cavity bodies, the main LM organs, occupy branchial regions, while in adults the jugular, procoracoid and prepericardial bodies occur in the throat and axillary regions. Apart from these anatomical differences, the histological organization of all anuran LM organs shows a similar pattern composed of cell cords which contain numerous lymphocytes, lymphoblasts, plasma cells, macrophages and antigen-presenting cells, arranged between enlarged sinusoids; occasionally thin-walled lymph vessels have been observed.

Various experimental results suggest that lymph glands are a source of T- and B-stem cells and that they serve as both a blood- and lymph-filtering organ. Immune functions of ventral cavity bodies are unknown. They occur as small lymphoid aggregates in variable number in the branchial region of several anuran species, diminishing rapidly and disappearing at the end of metamorphosis. Jugular bodies change following immunization. Their dendritic cells retain antigens extracellularly, and PFCs which form against both soluble and particulate antigens have been observed. Thus, although morphologically different from mammalian lymph nodes, the jugular bodies provide a locus where lymphoid cells can accumulate and respond to stimulation by antigens. Additional information supports the view that jugular bodies are also sites for long-term antigen retention.

Reptiles represent a more advanced situation in the phylogenetic origin of lymph nodes. In the gecko, *Gehyra variegata*, lymphoid tissue is closely associated with the lymphatic and blood systems in the axillae. Moreover, lymphoid tissue which is found in the wall of the cardinal lymphatic of the snake *Elaphe quadrivirgata* resembles lymphoid nodes of the domestic fowl. The immune function of these aggregates is, nevertheless, completely unknown. In any case, this condition represents a fundamental difference to that of LM organs in amphibians, which are known to filter blood primarily rather than lymph.

In birds, lymph-filtering lymphoid accumulations have been categorized into three histological types which might reflect distinct developmental stages. The smallest lymphoid aggregates appear as lymphoid infiltrates in fat without lymphatic sinuses. A second type has a similar histological condition but it contains germinal centers, which probably result from antigenic stimulation. The most complex lymphoid accumulations represent well-developed discrete organs containing lymph sinuses, in which lymph filtration, antigen trapping and germinal centers occur.

In this progression, the last step is the evolution of lymph nodes, which occurs in primitive mammals, the monotremes (i.e. echidna). While in eutherian mammals (e.g. mice) a single lymph node contains many nodules and lies in the path of a lymphatic vessel, in the echidna several nodules occur within the lumen of a lymphatic vessel, where they are suspended by a vascular bundle. Furthermore, echidna nodules are composed mainly of small lymphocytes, without primary lymphoid follicles in their periphery, and an inner medulla is also lacking. This histological condition of monotreme lymph nodes reflects a primitive efficiency in the trapping and processing of antigens from lymph.

IMMUNE COMPONENTS ASSOCIATED WITH THE EPITHELIUM

All vertebrates, including Agnatha, contain isolated lymphoid cells scattered in the lamina propria and epithelium of the gut, but more or less organized lymphoid aggregates appear for the first time in the Chondrichthyes. Even during ontogeny, scattered lymphocytes and macrophages accumulate in the dogfish spiral valve, increasing gradually until they reach the category of true lymphoid accumulations in both primitive and bony fish. Is the nature of their non-encapsulated infiltrates, a condition that practically occurs in GALT of all ectotherms, although in some classes, mainly reptiles, it reaches maximal development? A striking condition has, however, been reported in *Agama stellio*, a lizard without GALT, the immunological condition of which has been compared to that of early, bursectomized chickens. The immune function of reptilian GALT is controversial and may be species specific. Whereas certain evidence suggests a more important role for GALT than for spleen, other authors report scarce PFCs in both the cloacal complex and intestine of reptiles.

In birds, the GALT is extensive, including, apart from the bursa of Fabricius, the cecal tonsil, Peyer's patches and other lymphoid aggregates in the urodeum, proctodeum and elsewhere in the gut. The histological organization of avian GALT resembles profoundly that found in mammals, although its immunological function remains obscure. In both avian Peyer's patches and cecal tonsils, occurrence of a lymphoepithelium which contains M-cells—an important step in the evolution of vertebrate GALT—has been reported. Although in some ectotherms, mainly teleosts and turtles, epithelial cells associated with intestinal lymphoid aggregates resemble morphologically mammalian M-cells, functional evidence for the existence of lymphoepithelial and T-independent areas demonstrates the advanced condition of avian GALT.

Information on the phylogeny of mucosal associated lymphoid system, consisting in mammals of lymphoid tissue of the gut, respiratory, urinary and genital tracts, mammary and salivary glands, is almost reduced to the above summarized structure of gut-associated lymphoid tissue (GALT), but functional evidence is currently emerging. In this regard, two questions must be emphasized in the future. Is there a common mucosal immune system in ectothermic vertebrates, specifically in fish where numerous reports have demonstrated natural and induced specific Ig in gut, bile and skin? If so, can this system be traced throughout vertebrate phylogeny as a specific Ig for mucosae which resembles the secretory IgA of mammals?

Several results claim the existence of a local immune system in fish. Antigens administered into the gut lead to an increase in the numbers of intraepithelial leukocytes (Davina *et al.*, 1982) and induce the production of specific antibodies in the mucosae and bile (Fletcher and White, 1973; Schachte, 1978; Kawai *et al.*, 1981; Rombout *et al.*, 1986; Hart *et al.*, 1987). In contrast, administration of antigens via the gut produces either low or undetectable serum antibody titers (Fletcher and White, 1973; Pyle and Dawe, 1985; Rombout *et al.*, 1986) or it can induce a protective immune response in skin mucus (Amend and Johnson, 1981; Johnson and Amend, 1983). Also bath immunization of catfish (*Ictalurus punctatus*) with the soluble antigen DNP−HoSA (horse serum albumin) enhances secretory immunity but is not effective for stimulating the systemic immune system (Lobb, 1987). Furthermore, the titer of mucosal antibodies increases independently of the systemic humoral antibody response (Lobb, 1987). In this regard, works determining the specific activities of the Ig in mucus, bile and serum of the sheepshead, *Archosargus probatocephalus*, following the intravenous administration of radiolabeled Ig indicated that the Ig found in the secretions was predominantly the result of local synthesis (Lobb and Clem, 1981c).

Lebacq-Verheyclen *et al.* (1972, 1974) reported a special secretory Ig in chickens, occurring in bile, saliva, seminal plasma, lacrimal fluids and intestinal contents. It was produced by most of the plasma cells from intestinal lamina propria and seemed to be homologous mammalian IgA. Further studies claimed, however, that the Ig of chicken bile did not possess antigenic properties common to the IgA of mammals (Hadge and Ambrosius, 1983). Moreover, an analysis of the degree of antigenic relationship between the Ig of IgA class and the 7S IgY of birds, reptiles and anuran amphibians determined the existence of close evolutionary connections of these IgY-type Ig to the mammalian IgA class (Hadge and Ambrosius, 1984).

Nevertheless, IgM or IgM-like molecules appear to mediate gut immunity of most non-mammalian vertebrates. An Ig of IgM class has been reported in the bile of various fish (Underdown and Socken, 1978; Lobb and Clem, 1981b; Hadge, 1985), amphibians (Jurd, 1977; Hadge and Ambrosius, 1988) and reptiles (Vaerman et al., 1975; Hadge, 1985). In chicks, Ng and Higgins (1986) isolated an Ig fraction which resembled serum IgM but carried additional epitopes of unknown nature. The intestinal Ig of the Australian catfish (DiConza and Halliday, 1971) and the biliary Ig of the dogfish (Hart et al., 1987) and sheepshead (Lobb and Clem, 1981c) are antigenically similar to serum Ig. In contrast, the biliary Ig of the sheepshead occurs as a dimer and the molecular weights of the heavy chain of biliary and serum Ig differ.

On the other hand, in most non-mammalian species, a secretory component (SC) has not been isolated. A preliminary study reported a similar protein in the intestinal contents of chickens (Watanabe et al., 1975), but its absence was noted in the Ig of bile (Watanabe et al., 1975; Kobayastri and Hirai, 1980). Recently an 80-kD protein described in some biliary Ig molecules has been considered as the SC of chicken secretions (Peppard et al., 1986). An SC has not been detected in the intestine and biliary system of either elasmobranchs (Hart et al., 1987) or teleosts (Lobb and Clem, 1981c). In contrast, it has been described in the mucus of the sheepshead (Lobb and Clem, 1981a), and the serum of the nurse shark, *Ginglyomostroma cirratum*, has a high affinity for mammalian SC (Underdown and Socken, 1978). More information is necessary in order to confirm the occurrence of a mucosal immune system in non-mammalian vertebrates as well as to know the true nature of its molecular and cellular components, but the above reported evidence firmly suggests it.

WHAT DOES THE MILIEU DO TO THE IMMUNE SYSTEM? THE CASE FOR HORMONES, TEMPERATURE AND LIGHT

We have considered it necessary to dedicate one chapter of this book to seasonal changes that affect the histophysiology of vertebrate immune systems as well as to the analysis of their presumptive causative agents, i.e. photoperiod, temperature, endogenous neuroendocrine rhythms. In that chapter we pointed out that, in general, the structural and functional information available on immune responses of ectothermic vertebrates is oversimplified and does not reflect the physiological condition which occurs in nature. Unfortunately, the data are scarce and restricted to a few species from various vertebrate classes, making it difficult to support general speculations. In any case, histological and functional changes in the immune system of ectothermic vertebrates are currently well defined, although in many cases the evidence is indirect and the results controversial, reflecting probably distinct methodological approaches and/or species-specific differences.

Causative agents are also a matter of discussion, but our opinion supports strongly an indirect influence of environmental factors, mainly photoperiod and temperature through the neuroendocrine system, on vertebrate immune reactivity. In this regard, the demonstrated role of steroids, mainly corticosteroids, in modulating seasonal variations and stress responses of the ectotherm immune system is especially valuable, as well as possible mediation by processes of IL-2-like and IL-2-receptor molecules which has been recently reported in some ectotherms. Nevertheless, the effects of temperature on teleost immune responses mediated by modifications in the homeoviscosity of lymphocyte surface membranes deserve further attention. Additional information on the lymphocyte subpopulations directly involved in seasonal variations of immune systems will permit a better knowledge of the basic mechanisms. In conclusion, we would like to emphasize strongly that further results on the structure and/or function of ectothermic immune systems must be defined in the context of seasonal and other environmental factors.

REFERENCES

Amend DF and Johnson KA (1981). Current status and future needs of *Vibrio anguilarium* bacterium. *Dev Biol Standard* **49**: 403–417.

Barrutia MG, Torroba M, Fernandez MJ, Vicente A and Zapata A (1989). Macrophages and epithelial cells of the thymus gland. An ultrastructural study in the natterjack *Bufo calamita*. *Tissue and Cell* **21**: 65–81.

Castillo A, Lopez-Fierro P, Zapata A, Villena A and Razquin BE (1989a). Post-hatch development of the thymic microenvironments in the rainbow trout *Salmo gairdneri*: An ultrastructural study. *Am J Anat* in press.

Castillo A, Razquin BE, Lopez-Fierro P, Alvarez F, Zapata A and Villena AJ (1989b). Enzyme- and immuno-histochemical study of the thymic stroma in the rainbow trout, *Salmo gairdneri* Rich. *Thymus* in press.

Chiba A, Torroba M, Honma Y and Zapata A (1988). Occurrence of lympho-hemopoietic tissue in the meninges of the stingray *Dasyatis akajei* (Elasmobranchii, Chondrichthyes). *Am J Anat* **183**: 268–276.

Cooper EL and Wright RK (1976). The anuran amphibian spleen. An evolutionary model for terrestrial vertebrates. In Battisto JW and Streilein (Eds), *Immuno Aspects of the Spleen*. Elsevier/North-Holland Biomedical Press: Amsterdam. pp 47–60.

Davina JHM, Parmentier HK and Timmermans LPM (1982). Effect of oral administration of *Vibrio* bacteria on the intestine of cyprinid fish. *Dev Comp Immunol* Suppl **2**: 157–166.

DiConza JJ and Halliday WJ (1971). Relationship of catfish serum antibodies to immunoglobulin on mucus secretions. *Aust J Exp Med Biol Sci* **49**: 517–519.

Flajnik MF, Du Pasquier L and Cohen N (1985). Immune responses of thymus lymphocyte embryonic chimeras: studies on tolerance and major histocompatibility complex restriction in *Xenopus*. *Eur J Immunol* **15**: 540–547.

Flajnik MF, Hsu E, Kaufman JF and Du Pasquier L (1987). Changes in the immune system during metamorphosis of *Xenopus*. *Immunol Today* **8**: 58–64.

Fletcher TC and White A (1973). Antibody production in the plaice *Pleuronectes platessa* after oral and parenteral immunization with *Vibrio anguillarum* antigens. *Aquaculture* **1**: 417–428.

Glick B and Olah I (1987). Contribution of a specialized dendritic cell, the secretory cell, to the microenvironment of the bursa of Fabricius. In Weber WT and Ewert DL (Eds), *Avian Immunology*. Alan R Liss Inc: New York, pp 53–66.

Hadge D (1985). Zur Evolution der Immunglobuline. *Allerg Immunol* **31**: 231–243.

Hadge D and Ambrosius H (1983). Evolution of low molecular weight immunoglobulins. III. The immunoglobulin of chicken bile—not an IgA. *Mol Immunol* **20**: 597–606.

Hadge D and Ambrosius H (1984). Evolution of low molecular weight immunoglobulins. IV. IgY-like immunoglobulins of birds, reptiles and amphibians, precursors of mammalian IgA. *Mol Immunol* **21**: 699–707.

Hadge D and Ambrosius H (1988). Comparative studies of the structure of biliary immunoglobulins of some avian species. II. Antigenic properties of the biliary immunoglobulins of chicken, turkey, duck and goose. *Dev Comp Immunol* **12**: 319–329.

Hadji-Azimi I, Schwager J and Thiebaud C (1982). B lymphocyte differentiation in *Xenopus laevis* larvae. *Dev Biol* **90**: 253–258.

Hart S, Wrathmell AB, Doggett TA and Harris JE (1987). An investigation of the biliary and intestinal immunoglobulin and the plasma cell distribution in the gall bladder and liver of the common dogfish *Scyliorhinus canicula* L. *Aquaculture* **67**: 147–155.

Holtfreter HB and Cohen N (1987). *In vitro* behavior of thymic nurse cell-like complexes from mechanically and enzymatically dissociated frog tadpole thymuses. *Am J Anat* **179**: 342–355.

Horton JD, Russ JH, Aitchison P and Horton TL (1987). Thymocyte stromal cell chimaerism in allothymus-grafted *Xenopus*: developmental studies using the *Xenopus borealis* fluorescence marker. *Development* **100**: 107–117.

Johnson KA and Amend DF (1983). Efficacy of *Vibrio anguillarum* and *Yersinia ruckeri* bacterins applied by oral and anal intubation of salmonids. *J Fish Dis* **6**: 473–476.

Jurd RD (1977). Secretory immunoglobulins and gut-associated lymphoid tissue in *Xenopus laevis*. In Solomon JB and Horton JD (Eds), *Developmental Immunobiology*. Elsevier/North-Holland Biomedical Press: Amsterdam, pp 307–319.

Katagiri CH and Tochinai S (1987). Ontogeny of thymus-dependent immune responses and lymphoid cell differentiation in *Xenopus laevis*. *Dev Growth Differ* **29**: 297–305.

Kau CL and Turpen JB (1983). Dual contribution of embryonic ventral blood island and dorsal lateral plate mesoderm during ontogeny of hemopoietic cells in *Xenopus laevis*. *J Immunol* **131**: 2262–2266.

Kawai L, Kusuda R and Itami T (1981). Mechanisms of protection in ayu orally vaccinated for vibriosis. *Fish Pathol* **15**: 257 ff.

Kobayashi K and Hirai H (1980). Studies on subunit components of chicken polymeric immunoglobulins. *J Immunol* **124**: 1695–1704.

Kurihara K and Kato S (1986). Immigration of lymphoid precursor cells into the thymic rudiment in *Xenopus*. *Experientia* **42**: 179–181.

Lebacq-Verheyden A-M, Vaerman J-P and Heremans JP (1972). A possible homologue of mammalian IgA in chicken serum and secretions. *Immunology* **22**: 165–175.

Lebacq-Verheyden A-M, Vaerman J-P and Heremans JP (1974). Quantification and distribution of chicken immunoglobulins IgA, IgM and IgG in serum and secretions. *Immunology* **27**: 683–692.

Lobb CJ (1987). Secretory immunity induced in catfish *Ictalurus punctatus*, following bath immunization. *Dev Comp Immunol* **11**: 727–738.

Lobb CJ and Clem LW (1981a). Phylogeny of immunoglobulin structure and function. XI. Secretory immunoglobulins in the cutaneous mucus of the sheepshead *Archosargus probatocephalus*. *Dev Comp Immunol* **5**: 587–596.

Lobb CJ and Clem LW (1981b). Phylogeny of immunoglobulin structure and function. XII. Secretory immunoglobulins in the bile of the marine teleost *Archosargus probatocephalus. Mol Immunol* **18**: 615−619.

Lobb CJ and Clem LW (1981c). The metabolic relationships of the immunoglobulins in fish serum, cutaneous mucus and bile. *J Immunol* **127**: 1525−1529.

Maeno M, Todate A and Katagiri CH (1985a). The localization of precursor cells for larval and adult hemopoietic cells in *Xenopus laevis* in two regions of embryos. *Dev Growth Differ* **27**: 137−148.

Maeno M, Tochinai S and Katagiri CH (1985b). Differential participation of ventral and dorsal lateral mesoderms in the hemopoiesis of *Xenopus*, as revealed in diploid−triploid or interspecific chimeras. *Dev Biol* **110**: 503−508.

Nagata S (1986). Development of T lymphocytes in *Xenopus laevis*. Appearance of the antigen recognized by an anti-thymocyte mouse monoclonal antibody. *Dev Biol* **114**: 389−395.

Ng PL and Higgins DA (1986). Bile immunoglobulin of the duck (*Anas platyrhynchos*). I. Preliminary characterization and ontogeny. *Immunology* **58**: 323−327.

Nieuwenhuis P, Stot RJM, Wagenaar JPA, Wubbena AS, Kampinga J and Karrenbeld A (1988). The transcapsular route: a new way for (self) antigens to by-pass the blood thymus barrier? *Immunol Today* **9**: 372−375.

Peppard JV, Hobbs SM, Jackson LE, Rose ME and Mockett AP (1986). Biochemical characterization of chicken secretory component. *Eur J Immunol* **16**: 225−229.

Pyle SW and Dawe DL (1985). Immune response of channel catfish *Ictalurus punctatus* to bacterial and protozoan antigens administered by three routes. *Aquaculture* **46**: 1−10.

Rasquin BE, Castillo A, Lopez-Fierro P, Alvarez F, Zapata A and Villena AJ (1989). Ontogeny of IgM-producing cells in the lymphoid organs of *Salmo gairderni*: an immuno- and enzyme-histochemical study. *J Fish Biol* submitted.

Rombout JH, Blok LJ, Lamers CH and Egberts E (1986). Immunization of carp (*Cyprinus carpio*) with a *Vibrio anguillarium* bacterin: indications for a common mucosal immune system. *Dev Comp Immunol* **10**: 341−351.

Schahte JH (1978). Immunization of channel catfish *Ictalurus punctatus* against two bacterial diseases. *Mar Fish Rev* **40**: 18.

Tochinai S (1978). Thymocyte stem cell inflow in *Xenopus laevis* after grafting diploid thymic rudiments into triploid tadpoles. *Dev Comp Immunol* **2**: 627−635.

Turpen JB and Smith PB (1986). Analysis of hemopoietic lineage of accessory cells in the developing thymus of *Xenopus laevis*. *J Immunol* **136**: 412−421.

Underdown BJ and Socken DJ (1978). A comparison of secretory component−immunoglobulin interactions amongst different species. *Adv Exp Med Biol* **107**: 503−511.

Vaerman J-P, Picard J and Heremans JF (1975). Structural data on chicken IgA and failure to identify the IgA of the tortoise. *Adv Exp Med Biol* **54**: 185−195.

Watanabe H, Kobayashi K and Isayama Y (1975). Peculiar secretory IgA system identified in chickens. II. Identification and distribution of free secretory component and immunoglobulins of IgA, IgM and IgG in chicken external secretions. *J Immunol* **115**: 998−1001.

Index